EXPLOSIVE CALISTHENICS

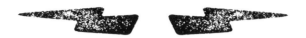

SUPERHUMAN POWER, MAXIMUM SPEED AND AGILITY, PLUS COMBAT-READY REFLEXES– USING BODYWEIGHT-ONLY METHODS

THE THIRD VOLUME IN THE *CONVICT CONDITIONING* SERIES

⟱ PAUL "COACH" WADE ⟱

PRAISE FOR EXPLOSIVE CALISTHENICS

"The first physical attribute we lose as we age is our ability to generate power. Close behind is the loss of skilled, coordinated movement. Both of these losses lead to frailty and devastating falls in old age. The fix is never to lose these abilities in the first place! Paul Wade's *Explosive Calisthenics* is the best program for developing power and skilled movement I have seen. Just as with his previous two books, the progressions are masterful with no fancy equipment needed.

You don't have to achieve a full back flip or kip up to get HUGE benefit from mastering the early progressions. It doesn't matter if you are a 20-year old looking to push your power and agility to new heights or approaching middle age, trying to slow the hands of time. Do yourself a favor and get this amazing work. This book will be the gold standard for developing bodyweight power, skill, and agility."
—**CHRIS HARDY**, D.O. MPH, CSCS, author, *Strong Medicine*

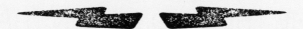

"Martial arts supremacy is all about explosive power and speed, and you will possess both once you've mastered the hardcore exercises in *Explosive Calisthenics*. Take your solo training to a level you never even imagined with these teeth-gritting, heart-palpating exercises—from a master of the genre."
—**LOREN W. CHRISTENSEN**, author of over 50 books, including *Fighting Power: How to Develop Explosive Punches, Kicks, Blocks,* and *Grappling and Speed Training: How to Develop Your Maximum Speed for Martial Arts*

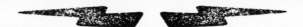

"*Explosive Calisthenics* by Paul 'Coach' Wade is a masterfully constructed roadmap for the attainment of power, functional speed, and agility. The book is extreme in that only a small percentage of the population would be able or willing to fully take the challenge, but at the same time, brilliant in that the path proceeds methodically and progressively from relatively simple to extremely advanced, allowing a discretionary endpoint for each individual.

The book is also refreshingly raw. The exercises are all done using only bodyweight and little in the way of equipment. There are only five moves to master and yet each is a proverbial double-edge sword—at the same time dangerous yet potentially transformative.

Take this on and I doubt you will ever again be satisfied with the mundane bench press or the other exercise machines found in the typical gym."
—**PATRICK ROTH**, M.D., author of *The End of Back Pain: Access Your Hidden Core to Heal Your Body,* Chairman of Neurosurgery at Hackensack University Medical Center and the director of its neurosurgical residency training program.

"Once again, Paul 'Coach' Wade, inspires with a life-changing approach to fitness that relies only on the weight of one's body. In his comprehensive new book, *Explosive Calisthenics*, he presents how calisthenics can and should be taken to the next level. Starting as he always does, with history of the early practitioners of bodyweight training, *Explosive Calisthenics* explains the widely misunderstood difference between 'strength' and 'power' as perhaps the key theme. This crucial distinction is what defines truly functional exercise as a life-long endeavor that has been a fountain of youth since ancient times.

To that, Wade ties his dynamic calisthenics to popular disciplines including my own, martial arts—drawing on exercises specific to the combative arts, but applicable to any physical activity. Wade also includes basic jumps, rolls, and somersaults as key parts of the regimen. Correctly, Wade prefers not to define these as 'gymnastics' but as whole-body explosive power and speed training. While this may not be for everyone at first, I would encourage the calisthenics-advanced non-gymnast, to give these 'explosive' movements a try.

Of particular note to me as a long-time proponent of time-tested, more functional fitness training, I very much appreciated Wade's discussion of developing the senses as a fundamental part of *Explosive Calisthenics*. As a professional, more traditional martial artist and Chen Taijiquan practitioner, development of the senses through exercises that utilize whole-body movement and stringent eye-hand-foot coordination practices, Wade's presentation of total senses development as part of advanced calisthenics training is fantastic to see.

And lastly, Wade's emphasis on solo training, which he explains so well, is something not to be over-looked. The importance of solo training not only builds true functional fitness, but as Wade describes, provides an inner strength and focus that spoke directly to me as a traditional martial artist. In my teachings I've always maintained that relying on no one else or any apparatus other than your own body for core training is what truly separates the master from the student and from those who can't let go of psychological and physical baggage that holds them back, from those whom depend on nothing other their own strength. Wade's discussion of this ageless wisdom is magnificent to see and is to me the heart and soul of *Explosive Calisthenics*."
—STEPHAN BERWICK, author *True Strength Yang*

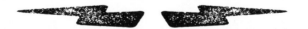

"*Explosive Calisthenics* is an absolute Treasure Map for anybody looking to tear down their body's athletic limitations. Who doesn't want to be able to kip to their feet from their back like a Bruce Lee? Or make a backflip look easy? Paul makes you want to put down the barbells, learn and practice these step-by-step progressions to mastering the most explosive and impressive bodyweight movements. The best part is? You can become an absolute Beast in under an hour of practice a week. Way to go, Paul! AROO!"
—JOE DISTEFANO, **Spartan Race,** Director of Training & Creator of the **Spartan SGX Certification**

"*Explosive Calisthenics* continues the epic saga of the Convict Conditioning opus, which has become a staple for any bodyweight training library. If you've applied all the incredible techniques taught in the first two books, you'll be able to maximize your training with even more impressive moves. Coach Wade offers up a blueprint for pushing your workouts to a whole new level. Lots of books say they are taking things to a whole new level—this one really does.

Where books one and two laid a strong foundation with exercises like muscle-ups and human flags, *Explosive Calisthenics* literally brings in the explosiveness by introducing flips and other power-based moves. With his usual step-by-step guides and clear instructions, Wade covers an extensive list of exercises with progressions and regressions that makes this book perfect for both beginners and advanced calisthenics enthusiasts. Holding true to the Dragon Door style, the pics are bold and easy to follow. I'm inspired to go do some flips right now!"

—**MIKE FITCH,** creator, *Global Bodyweight Training*

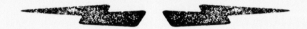

"Your body is the ultimate 'training tool'. Paul Wade shows you how to transform your own body and turn it into a weapon! I've taken these methods and applied them to the training of my athletes as well as my own training and the bottom line is that they work. The workouts and exercises deliver. They are powerful and results driven.

If you are done wasting your time on fads and gimmicks and simply want a training program that works BIG time. This is it."

—**ZACH EVEN-ESH,** author *The Encyclopedia of Underground Strength and Conditioning*

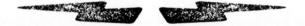

"Coach Wade saved the best for last! *Explosive Calisthenics* is the book all diehard Convict Conditioning fans have been waiting for. There has never been anything like it until now!

With his trademark blend of old-school philosophy, hard-earned wisdom and in-your-face humor, Coach expands his infamous system of progressive bodyweight programming to break down the most coveted explosive moves, including the back flip, kip-up and muscle-up. If you want to know how far you can go training with just your own bodyweight, you owe it to yourself to get this book!"

—**AL KAVADLO,** author, *Stretching Your Boundaries*

"*Explosive Calisthenics* is aptly-named. This book is a power-boosting 'smart-bomb' that delivers a payload of immensely practical info. The content is not only interesting and unique, it practically screams at you to try it out. You will love the skills and their associated progressions. For multi-sport athletes, prospective parkour-enthusiasts, budding badasses and aspiring ninja warriors everywhere, here is your textbook!"
—MIKE GILLETTE, author, *Rings of Power*

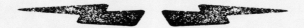

"Paul Wade's series Convict Conditioning continues with the newest addition, *Explosive Calisthenics*. I applaud the loss of the convict/prison shtick and we get to explore what Wade does best: he progresses a movement from the basic and simple to, in this case, it's most complex (and awesome). The chapter on programming, the sets and reps of things, has a series of rules that you will instantly claim as your own.

"I can't believe we abandoned traditional calisthenics in our schools and training programs, but this book is the best argument I know for carrying signs in front of schools proclaiming 'No More Dodgeball' and 'Calisthenics Progressions for All!'"
—DAN JOHN, author, *Never Let Go*

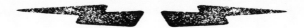

"I have found in my work with world-class athletes that they have a common skill; the ability to generate explosive power. Paul Wade's new book shows you not only how to generate explosive power, but how to direct and control it as well. If you have ever wanted to join the rank of super-human, this book gives you the road map of how to get there. The progressions allow anyone to master the skills of the athletic elite. Plus you'll also learn Speed Hacks that will give you lightning quick reflexes and Animal Drills for agility. Get this book and become amazing!"
—JON BRUNEY, author, *Neuro-Mass*

EXPLOSIVE CALISTHENICS

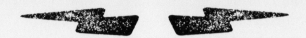

SUPERHUMAN POWER, MAXIMUM SPEED AND AGILITY, PLUS COMBAT-READY REFLEXES– USING BODYWEIGHT-ONLY METHODS

© Copyright 2015, Paul "Coach" Wade
A Dragon Door Publications, Inc. production
All rights under International and Pan-American Copyright conventions.
Published in the United States by: Dragon Door Publications, Inc.
5 East County Rd B, #3 • Little Canada, MN 55117
Tel: (651) 487-2180 • Fax: (651) 487-3954
Credit card orders: 1-800-899-5111 • Email: support@dragondoor.com • Website: www.dragondoor.com

ISBN 10: 0-938045-83-0   ISBN 13: 978-0-938045-83-0
This edition first published in February, 2015
Printed in China

Book design and cover by Derek Brigham • www.dbrigham.com • bigd@dbrigham.com

DISCLAIMER: The author and publisher of this material are not responsible in any manner whatsoever for any injury that may occur through following the instructions contained in this material. The activities, physical and otherwise, described herein for informational purposes only, may be too strenuous or dangerous for some people and the reader(s) should consult a physician before engaging in them.

— Contents —

Foreword by John Du Cane

Dedicated to John Du Cane,

The world's greatest innovator in fitness.

FOREWORD

By John Du Cane

The greatest fitness writers grab you by the wrist—and yank you into a new vision of what it means to excel as a human being. These writers inspire you to transcend your self-imposed physical limitations and to fly high in your athletic aspirations. These writers open up whole new vistas of potentiality for you—and dare you to dream big.

These rare writers challenge you to separate yourself from the herd of also-ran followers—to become leaders, survivors and winners in the physical game of life. But they don't just challenge and inspire you. They give you the means, the secrets, the science, the wisdom, the blueprints, the proven methods and the progressions—that make success inevitable, when you supply YOUR end in consistent, diligent, skillful application.

These writers each possess their own potent, soulful, visceral voice. They are artists in their expression. They resonate profoundly with their own distinct vibe. You can feel the implicit truth of their message in every sentence they write.

Now—sad to say—I don't need all of my ten digits to count out the fitness writers who have rocked my world in this manner. And I'll bet you don't either… Such writers are as rare as the most iconic of athletes, the Michael Jordans of their domain…

And if God chopped off all of my digits, except for my right forefinger—and asked me to point at the greatest modern writer in fitness? Without a nanosecond's of hesitation I would point at **Paul Wade.**

I pride myself at recognizing true excellence in the world of fitness writing—but I almost jumped out of my skin with excitement when I first laid eyes on Paul's *Convict Conditioning* in September, 2008. CC had greatness stamped all over it. Here was a work that could change the fitness landscape big time—and most assuredly it did. Now a legendary international bestseller, Convict can lay claim to be the Great Instigator when it comes to the resurgence of interest in bodyweight exercise mastery.

And—while *Convict Conditioning 2* cemented Paul's position as the preeminent authority on bodyweight exercise—there is no doubt in my mind that his magisterial new accomplishment, *Explosive Calisthenics* is going to blow the doors off, all over again.

What makes *Explosive Calisthenics* so exciting—and so profound in its implications?

See, it goes back to the laws of brute survival. It's not "Only the strongest shall survive". No, it's more like: "Only the strongest, quickest, most agile, most powerful and most explosive shall survive." To be a leader and dominator and survivor in the pack, you need to be the complete package.

Traditional martial arts have always understood this necessity of training the complete package—with explosive power at an absolute premium. And resilience is revered: the joints, tendons, muscles, organs and nervous system are ALL conditioned for maximum challenge.

Really great athletes are invariably that way too: agile as all get-go, blinding speed, ungodly bursts of power, superhuman displays of strength, seemingly at will...

How do you excel as a martial artist, as an athlete—or really at almost anything? You excel by relentlessly building your foundation and fundamentals. You excel by relentlessly practicing the **skills** it takes to master the moves. No one gets great by half-hearted, inconsistent application or by employing some special "hack" that's going to magically transform you into a monster. Get real.

Note the word "skill." The foundation and fundamentals center first around the building of power and speed. But *Explosive Calisthenics* does a masterful job of elucidating the skill-practices needed to safely prepare for and master the more ambitious moves.

So, *Explosive Calisthenics* is for those who want to be winners and survivors in the game of life. Explosive Calisthenics is for those who want to be the Complete Package: Powerful, Explosive, Strong, Agile, Quick and Resilient.

But—the hallmark of greatness—*Explosive Calisthenics* doesn't just inspire you with the Dream of being the Complete Package. It gives you the complete blueprint, every detail and every progression you could possibly want and need to NAIL YOUR DREAM and make it a reality. YOU, the Complete Package—it's all laid out for you step by step.

Frankly, I shake my head at Paul Wade's brilliance...the wisdom and sheer practicality...the compelling authoritativeness... the clarity. There's been an enduring conspiracy theory that I am actually Paul Wade. That I secretly wrote *Convict Conditioning* and concocted a whole trumped-up marketing shtick to sell it with. Too funny! But, God, if only I could be that brilliant myself!

I am aware of how many hundreds of thousands of people around the world are now stronger and healthier as a result of Paul Wade's first two volumes in the Convict Conditioning series. That's wonderful to know and to contemplate. I am proud to have helped get the message out.

Now—for those who have the balls and the will and the fortitude to take it on—comes the next stage: *Explosive Calisthenics*. The chance not only to be strong and healthy but to ascend to the Complete Package. If you want it, then here it is...

John Du Cane

John Du Cane, owner and CEO, Dragon Door Publications

DISCLAIMER!

Fitness and strength are meaningless qualities without *health*. With correct training, these three benefits should naturally proceed hand-in-hand. In this book, every effort has been made to convey the importance of safe training technique, but despite this all individual trainees are different and needs will vary. Proceed with caution, and at your own risk. **This warning applies *even more* where power training is involved, and high velocity exercises are undertaken.** Your body is your own responsibility—look after it. All medical experts agree that you should consult your physician before initiating a training program. Be safe!

This book is intended for entertainment purposes only. This book is not biography. The names, histories and circumstances of the individuals featured in this book have accordingly been changed either partially or completely. Despite this, the author maintains that all the exercise principles within this volume—techniques, methods and ideology—are valid. Use them, and become the best.

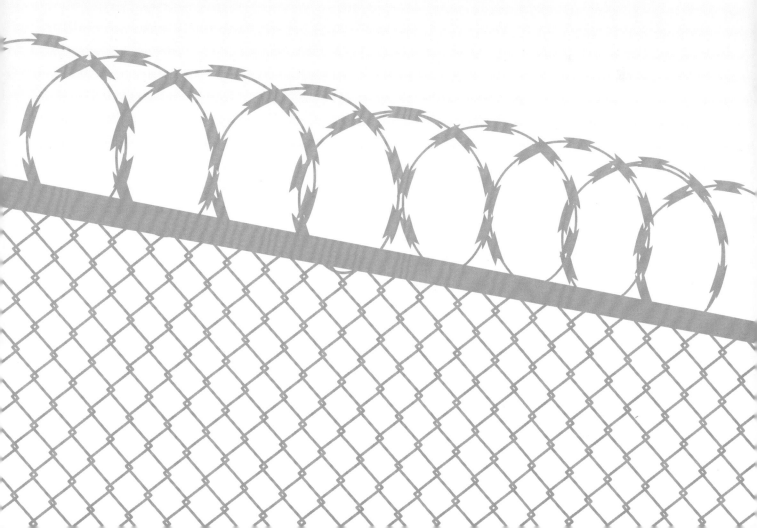

PART 1

POWER, SPEED, AGILITY

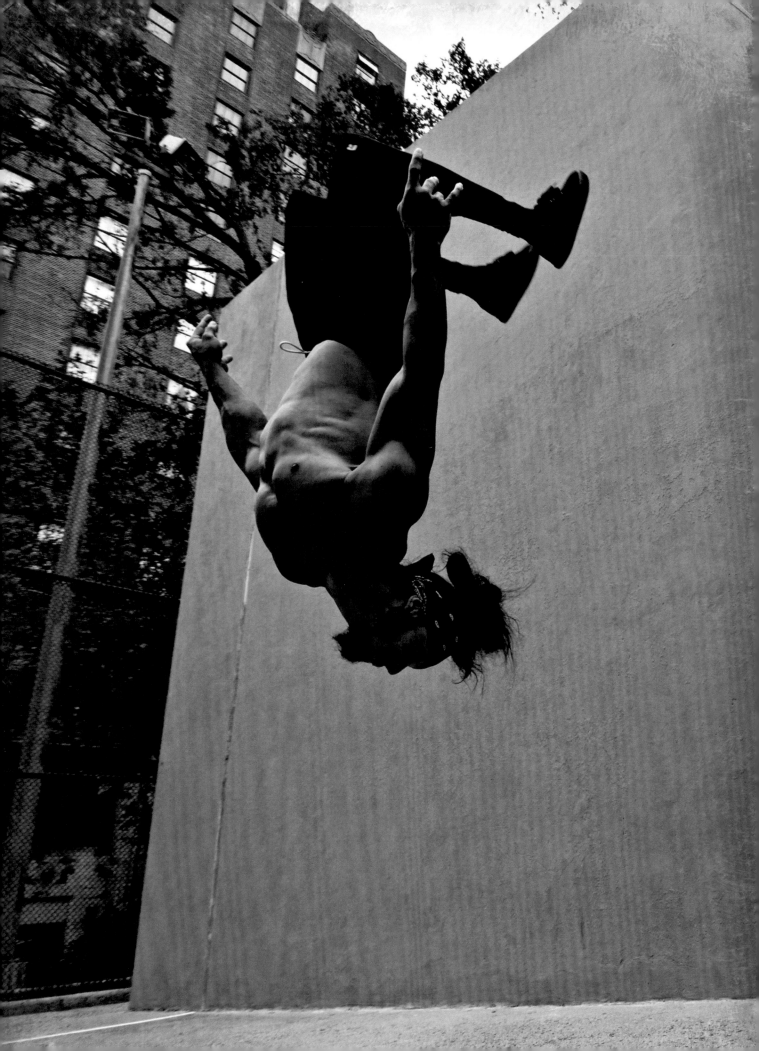

1
POWER UP!
THE NEED FOR SPEED

First things first: *Who the hell am I to be teaching you how to build incredible bodyweight power and speed?*

Fair question. My name is Paul Wade, and it's probably more helpful to tell you what I'm not— I'm *not* a certified personal trainer; I'm *not* a famous champion athlete; and I'm sure as damn *not* some scientist with a million PhDs who wrote a doctorate on *nerve transmissions and their relationship to plyometric overload*. (Woah! I impressed myself there. A little.)

I'm not disrespecting any of these folks I mentioned. They all have their own types of knowledge, in many ways superior to mine. If you want to buy books by men and women like that, there are plenty. But my education was very different. I learned what I learned about bodyweight training from close to twenty years of obsessive workouts spread out in American institutions like San Quentin, LSP ("the Alcatraz of the South"), and USP Marion. (If you understand jails, that probably sounds like a weird spread. It might make more sense if you understand that I was initially incarcerated for possession plus intent to manufacture, and later trafficking across state lines, which is a federal offense.)

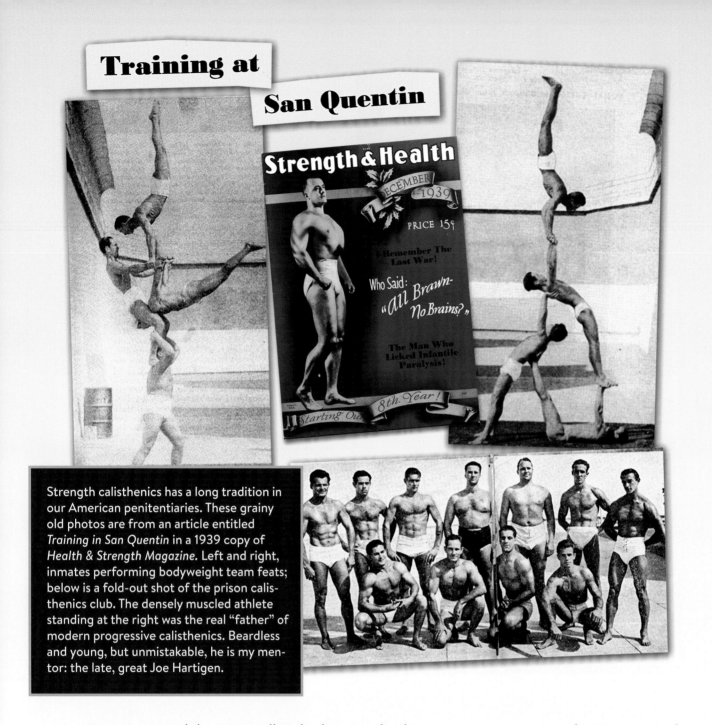

Training at
San Quentin

Strength & Health
DECEMBER 1939
PRICE 15¢

I Remember The Last War!

Who Said: "All Brawn—No Brains?"

The Man Who Licked Infantile Paralysis!

Starting Our 8th Year!

Strength calisthenics has a long tradition in our American penitentiaries. These grainy old photos are from an article entitled *Training in San Quentin* in a 1939 copy of *Health & Strength Magazine*. Left and right, inmates performing bodyweight team feats; below is a fold-out shot of the prison calisthenics club. The densely muscled athlete standing at the right was the real "father" of modern progressive calisthenics. Beardless and young, but unmistakable, he is my mentor: the late, great Joe Hartigen.

I'm going to end the prison talk right there. My books are *not* an attempt to make prisons sound like kick-ass gladiator schools. They really aren't. There's nothing *gangsta* about me, kid. In some circles, however, American prisons are still sources of great knowledge in bodyweight training, because the cell athletes within them have very little else to work with. (This was particularly true of older generations of inmates.)

My mission in life over the past ten years has been to spread as much of this useful knowledge as I can, to any athletes around the world who might be interested. Aside from my writings, I choose to remain fairly anonymous, for reasons intelligent people can probably guess at. I cannot go back in time and correct my own messed up, hurtful, destructive actions. But to bring something good from those dark years—this I can try to do.

The bottom line: if you are expecting instruction from an officially certified expert who can tell you every type of amino acid, and who reads (and understands!) every new scientific study on training that comes out, you picked up the wrong book. But I hope you'll stick with me for a few pages anyways—I'd like to get to know ya, kid.

Besides, who knows? With luck, I might even be able to teach you a thing or two the certified guys missed.

WHAT ARE "EXPLOSIVE CALISTHENICS"?

This manual focuses on three major athletic qualities:

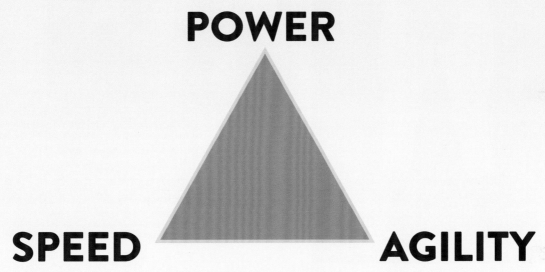

In the remainder of this chapter, I'll explain these three qualities by giving you some working definitions. There are, of course, alternative potential definitions for these qualities. These are just the ones I choose to use with my athletes. They are direct, easy to understand, and pretty simple. (Like me!)

POWER IS THE ABILITY TO MOVE WITH STRENGTH X SPEED.

The term *power* often confuses athletes, because it is so often used (incorrectly) as a synonym for *strength*. In fact, many hugely strong men—ironically termed "powerhouses"—are lacking in power compared to smaller athletes. Power is strength *and* speed, blended.

It may sound crazy to say that strength doesn't require power, but it's true. At its purest level, strength requires zero speed. Imagine a man holding up a crashed vehicle, so that his child can safely crawl out from underneath—this would require massive *strength*, but no *power*, since there was no movement and therefore no *speed* involved.

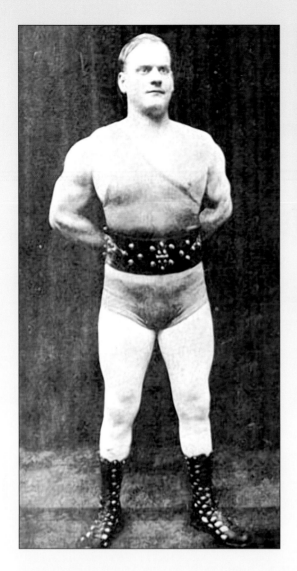

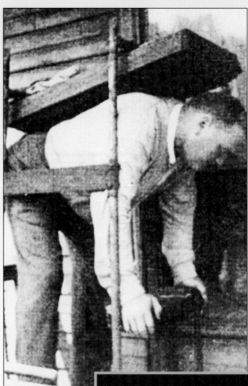

Strongman Warren Lincoln Travis built a machine that allowed him to hold huge weights on his back—the "back lift". He worked up to 4240 lbs! Incredible *strength*, but no *power*—he wasn't moving.

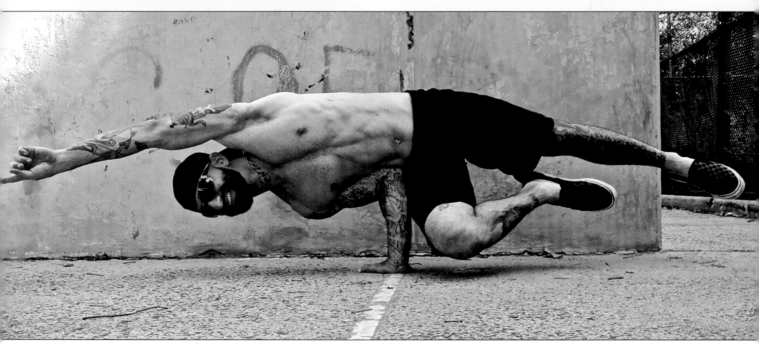

EXPLOSIVE CALISTHENICS

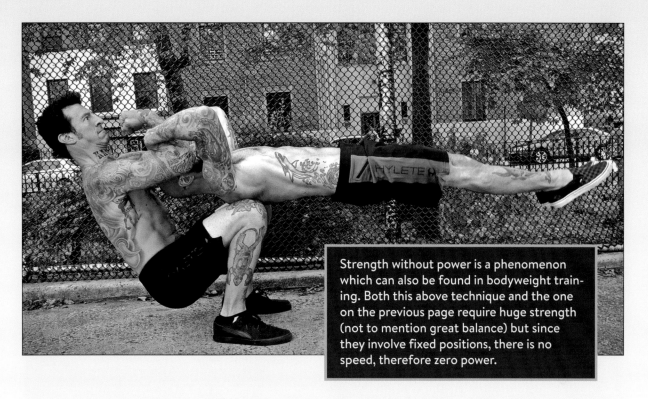

Strength without power is a phenomenon which can also be found in bodyweight training. Both this above technique and the one on the previous page require huge strength (not to mention great balance) but since they involve fixed positions, there is no speed, therefore zero power.

Next, imagine a kung fu master whipping out a backfist with such rapidity that he can "punch out" a candle flame, several feet away. Such a feat would require great *speed*, but since the moving arm is under very little load—just the inertia of its own mass—there's not much *strength*, and therefore not much *power*.

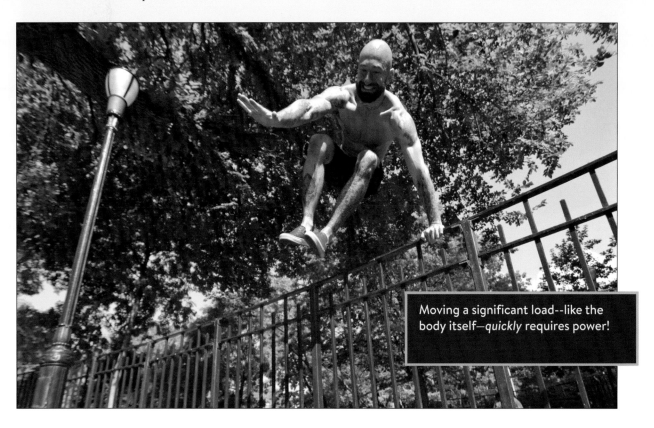

Moving a significant load--like the body itself—*quickly* requires power!

Genuine power lies somewhere in the middle. It is the sum of speed *and* strength. The greater the load, the more strength and less speed. The lower the load, the more speed and less strength. This "middle road" of true power is best achieved not by performing light, load-less drills (like punching or kicking) nor by trying to snap up gigantic barbells. The best *golden mean* is the one given to us by Mother Nature: moving your body's own weight quickly, the way an acrobat or parkour master does. This is the true meaning of *power* in athletics.

FUNCTIONAL <u>SPEED</u> IS THE ABILITY TO MOVE THE BODY QUICKLY OVER A SHORT DISTANCE.

Let me say something that might sound strange, at first: I'm not really interested in *pure* speed. What do I mean by "pure" speed? Here's legendary Olympic coach Al Murray to give us the answer:

> *One talks of speed, and of an athlete being the fastest in the world, but this can often be incorrect. To say that a man is fast because he covers many miles in a record time is extremely misleading as this is principally endurance. But when a man is fast over a very short distance, or in performing a single action like punching, kicking, leaping, springing or turning, then this to me is speed.*
>
> — Al Murray M.S.R.G., *Modern Weight-Training* (1963)

Some training manuals take this idea too far—they focus heavily on pure speed "tricks" like flipping coins and catching them, or catching a slide rule dropped by another athlete. Unfortunately, this kind of *pure speed* is useless, because it's only in exceptional circumstances that we need to move just one limb, or one part of the body. *The body evolved to move as a whole.* That's why I'm much more interested in *functional speed*, which is about moving the *entire body* as quickly as the limits of your frame will allow.

This book will teach you how to move your *entire body* with lightning speed. In the real world—in sports or a survival situation—displacing *part* of your body isn't good enough, no matter how quick you can do it. Imagine:

- A soldier diving to avoid a line of fire
- Jumping over an obstacle
- A fighter dodging an oncoming opponent
- Getting over a wall quickly to escape danger
- Twisting in mid-air to land safely

These are examples of "real world" speed. The entire body is moved. That's why, in this manual the drills will focus on moving your *entire body* as fast as possible. (You can see that speed and power overlap here: moving the entire body quickly requires *power*, due to the body's mass.)

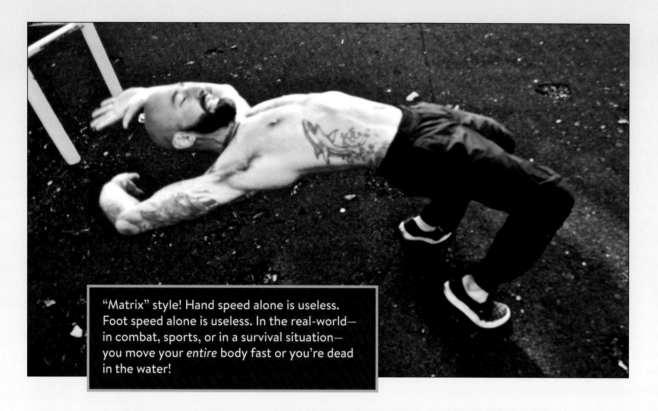

"Matrix" style! Hand speed alone is useless. Foot speed alone is useless. In the real-world—in combat, sports, or in a survival situation—you move your *entire* body fast or you're dead in the water!

<u>AGILITY</u> IS THE ABILITY TO ALTER THE BODY'S DIRECTION IN A RAPID, COORDINATED MANNER.

One problem with the modern "plyometrics" trend is that the drills develop *power*, but not *agility*. An athlete can have great power but still lack agility. Powerful athletes can quickly explode their body in *one* direction, but lack the ability to *alter their movement at high velocity* with other muscles. Whenever multiple-directions or velocities are required in rapid succession, agility is involved. (In this sense, agility can be seen as *complex power*, as opposed to *simple power*, which expresses in a single basic direction.)

Take for example a back flip. An athlete can have a *huge* vertical leap (*power*), and yet be completely incapable of a back flip (*power + agility*). Why? Because their nervous system lacks the ability to switch direction and bring in alternate muscle groups with the balance, speed and precision required to pull off the skill. The same is true for kip-ups, front flips, and—to some extent—muscle-ups.

This book contains drills which will lead you to a *very* high level of agility. Whereas power can be trained very simply—in a similar way to peak strength—agility should be trained like a *skill*. Part III of this book will explain the difference and teach you the distinct training methods you'll need for optimal power AND agility.

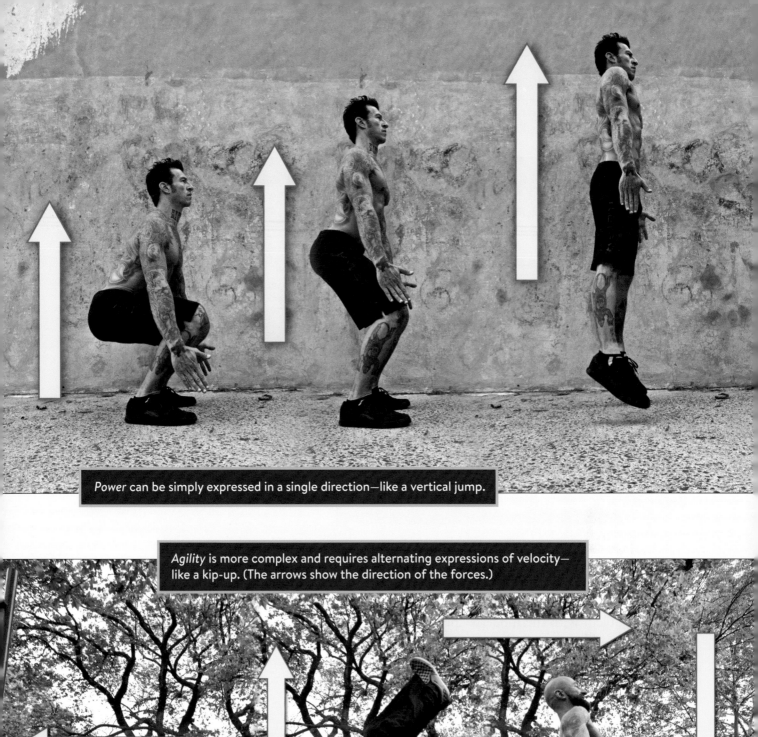

Power can be simply expressed in a single direction—like a vertical jump.

Agility is more complex and requires alternating expressions of velocity—like a kip-up. (The arrows show the direction of the forces.)

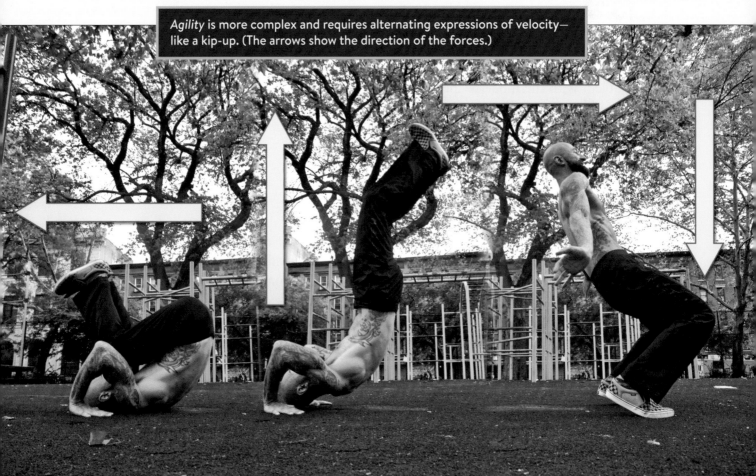

IT'S ALL IN THE REFLEXES

In this manual I occasionally refer to a fourth quality: *reflexes*. Often, laypeople and athletes misuse the term *reflexes*. The common use relates to the ability to respond defensively to an external situation like an *oncoming object*—such as dodging a punch or catching an arrow in mid-flight. This is not quite right; in reality, reflexes perform a more basic, less theatrical task. *They are our body's automatic movements in response to any stimuli.*

Imagine walking down the stairs, and accidentally missing a step. Whether you fall on your face, or your leg automatically stabilizes itself depends on the quality of your reflexes. The reflexes move faster than the mind, because they bypass the mind; they come directly from the nervous system. When something happens so fast that the mind can't react to it, the reflexes take over, and the nervous system makes thousands of instantaneous calculations and readjustments to keep the body safe.

If all this happens when you make a misstep, how hard do the reflexes have to work to make sure your arms fire at exactly the right time during a handspring? Or to ensure you land safely after a front flip?

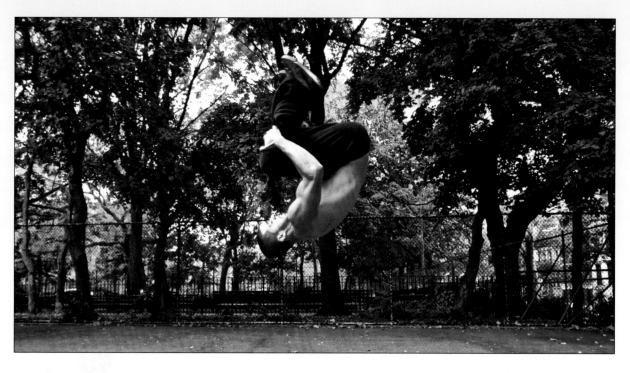

To keep a long story short, if you want to generate high levels of power, speed and agility, your reflexes need to level up to the same degree. They will do this automatically as you practice. After you initiate ballistic power movements *voluntarily*, there is a host of *involuntary* stuff that needs to happen—stuff that happens quicker than the conscious mind can process. When you perform an explosive pushup, flip or kip-up, you need to readjust and land—and this happens in a fraction of a second. You are essentially training your reflexes to do this job for you. Although many of our reflexes are innate—also called *natural*, or *unconditioned reflexes*—we can also train our nervous system to react more efficiently to different situations—these are called *conditioned reflexes*.

The take-home? If you train right using the drills in this book, your movement reflexes will automatically ramp up to black belt level—and you don't need to catch a single arrow, ninja-boy.

LIGHTS OUT!

Most gym-trained athletes build strength, but *true* athleticism—and youthful movement—will always be out of reach for them because they don't truly understand how to build the three major explosive qualities: *power*, *functional speed*, and *agility*. (Your *reflexes* are also crucial, and can be seen as the sum of your development of these three.)

If you follow the teachings in this book, you *can* build all these qualities: faster *and* more efficiently than you can build strength! Anybody who can move can rapidly learn to build awesome levels of power—the kind of explosive power normally most people only see in wild animals or superhero comics. But modern methods won't cut it. You need to ditch the kind of un-functional strength movements trainers get paid to teach at the gym. You have to go back to the hardcore basics and do it the *right* way. What's the "right" way?

That's up next.

2

EXPLOSIVE TRAINING
FIVE KEY PRINCIPLES

When I last left jail, I took a look around to see how athletes were training to build explosive power and strength. What I found was—to be honest—a *real mess*. Many of the traditional calisthenics methods which have been used for centuries to build power and total-body agility—the kind of methods drawn from classical martial arts, for example—had fallen by the wayside. Instead, folks were using modern gimmicks like cones, elastic bands and other devices.

What makes matters worse is that only a tiny, tiny percentage of folks who work out train for explosiveness anyway; and those athletes who *do* train for speed, power and agility tend to do it as an afterthought—because they need these qualities for football, combat, or another sport that requires them. Sadly, most folks who hit the gym don't even train for speed/power at all! They have been taught to build their training around *bodybuilding movements*, performed with external weights and machines. Because these techniques are performed with a slow, smooth speed, and by isolating muscles (or groups of muscles) they actually de-condition the muscles and nervous system from moving quickly, or in an integrated manner. Yeah, you heard me—most modern, in-gym training is making people *slower*! If you think about it, you'll know what I'm saying is true.

Combined with the epidemic of obesity, there's no doubt about it—modern Americans are the slowest, least agile members of our species in history.

It doesn't have to be this way. You *can* teach your body to be the lightning-fast, explosive, acrobatic, super-hunter your DNA is coded to make you. In this book, I'm going to teach you a *system* for developing speed, power and agility. Because of my background, this system is based on a handful of unbeatable principles:

- Use **bodyweight**
- Go **Spartan**
- Apply **total-body** training
- Focus on a **small group of exercises**
- Be **progressive**

Let's look at each of these five principles, briefly.

USE BODYWEIGHT

Why are pure, traditional, bodyweight methods so important? Despite what you may think, I do *not* emphasize traditional bodyweight arts because I spent most of my career training in a cell, devoid of equipment. I emphasize them because they are the *superior* method of physical development—*in all cases*.

Take explosiveness. An athlete cannot be classed as an explosive athlete unless he (or she) possesses the three qualities I mentioned in the first chapter—power, functional speed, and agility—to a very high degree. Yet very few methods used today are capable of generating these qualities *together*.

Let's look at three major modern methods, and compare them to calisthenics explosives (like flips, muscle-ups and kip-ups). The three methods most commonly seen today are:

- Box work (i.e., plyometric box jumps or box pushups)
- Cone training (i.e., zig-zagging around cones in a sports field or hall)
- Olympic lifting (i.e., the so-called "fast" lifts like snatches, cleans, jerks)

To see if these methods build the three qualities needed for our definition of an explosive athlete, we need to ask three questions, based on the definitions I laid out in the previous chapter:

— POWER: Does the athlete need to move with strength *and* speed?
— FUNCTIONAL SPEED: Is the *entire body* moved, quickly?
— AGILITY: Does the body have to *change direction* at high velocity?

METHOD	POWER	FUNCTIONAL SPEED	AGILITY
Box Work	✔	✔	✘
Cone Training	✘	✔	✔
Olympic Lifting	✔	✘	✘

Check out the table above. These questions should make it pretty clear that *none* of the three methods builds complete explosiveness:

- *Box work* (plyometrics) builds **power** because a load is moved quickly; it also builds functional **speed** because the entire body is moved. But box work does little for **agility**, since the majority of techniques are just variations on the athlete going up and down—there is no change of the body's angle, which is essential for real agility.

- *Cone training* builds **agility** because the body is forced to radically alter its direction at high velocity; it also builds functional **speed**, because the entire body is moving rapidly. But since the load demands are fairly low—not much different from running—it cannot build **power.** (One of the reasons why cone drills are popular in schools is because of the low load demands—these exercises are pretty safe, and anybody can participate, no matter how weak they are.)

- *Olympic lifting* builds **power**, because it requires high strength used as quickly as possible. But there is no true **agility** required, because the body doesn't appreciably change its direction—the weight just goes up and down. Also, the feet remain on the floor—or very close to it—during Olympic lifts, therefore the criteria of functional **speed** (rapid total-body movement) is not fulfilled. The body doesn't move very far at all.

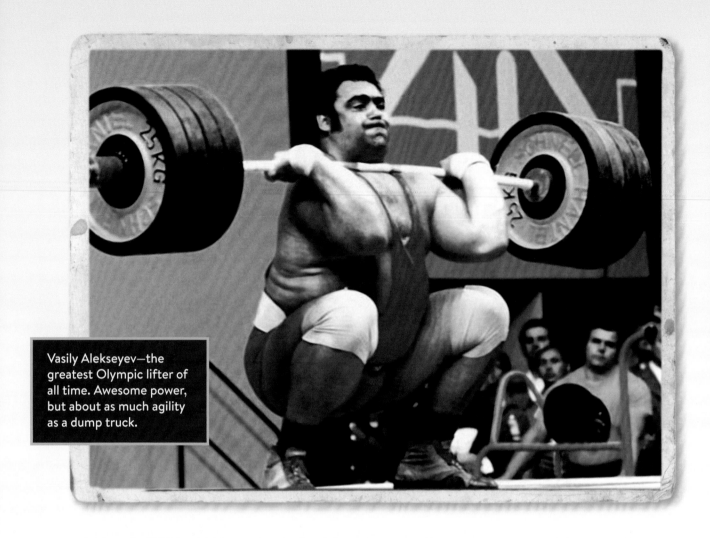

Vasily Alekseyev—the greatest Olympic lifter of all time. Awesome power, but about as much agility as a dump truck.

If you understood what I meant in the first chapter, it will be clear to you now that none of these three methods build complete explosiveness.

Now, compare these three with calisthenics explosive methods: *kip-ups, front flips, back flips* and *muscle-ups*—the four skill-based movement-types in this manual.*

METHOD	POWER	FUNCTIONAL SPEED	AGILITY
Explosive Calisthenics	✔	✔	✔

*The first two movement-types—power jumps and power pushups—should be seen as a form of basic training/conditioning, to be approached *before* the four movement-types which follow them. I discuss this training hierarchy more on page 272.

These exercises win hands-down, since they all require a *load* (the body's mass) to be moved *quickly*—**power**. They also require the *entire body* to be moved *rapidly*—functional **speed**. Finally, the **agility** criterion is also met perfectly because the body must *change its direction at high velocity*. This is very obviously true for flips and kip-ups, where the body must fire in different directions to lift off, rotate and land; but it is also true for the muscle-up—the initial "kipping" movement requires the body to quickly alter directions. (See page 212 for more information on kipping.)

Remember that these definitions are my own—*power*, *functional speed* and *agility* are fairly standard criteria for what comprises "explosiveness" in an athlete, but you can develop your own approach if you wish. I'm just showing you the way *I* think, and how I train my athletes.

Also, please understand that I'm not putting any of these other methods—weight-lifting, etc.—down. Each may be valuable in its own field—for example, box jumps teach basic power, strength athletes can certainly benefit from the Olympic work, and the cone stuff is useful in specialist sports like soccer. But if an athlete wants to become as *explosive as possible*—and possess the three qualities of explosiveness—each of these methods is lacking. The traditional calisthenics approach is not. I'm also not saying that these methods are negative or counter-productive.

GO SPARTAN

As well as being the most *efficient* means of explosive training, traditional bodyweight-only methods are also the most *convenient*. They are low or zero-tech—meaning they require no unusual equipment. At most, the "Explosive Six" drills in this book require you to have access to a floor, a wall, and a horizontal bar for hanging.

If they expect to learn explosive flips, for example, in a modern club, beginners are given rubber bands to help them with muscle-ups; gymnasts use foam rubber mats and blocks, and wedges and supports and cables and all kinds of similar devices. I understand *why* modern coaches lean on this stuff—for insurance purposes. It projects a powerful illusion of safety. (And it *is* an illusion. You can break your neck training on a foam mat, just the same as you can on grass, if you are not training with discipline.)

If you're new to bodyweight training, and are worried that you'll need a gymnastics club or a ton of commercial equipment to able to safely learn power feats like flips, kip-ups and muscle-ups, I would remind you of a truth: *a thousand generations of our ancestors mastered these techniques—and perfectly—a thousand years before Christ*. Certainly, well before any of this junk was even thought of. In my opinion, they're worse than useless. These toys only get in the way. Avoid them.

Training Spartan also means training *solo*. This is something that is very important to me. I've had some incredible instructors throughout my training career, but I've more or less *trained* alone. For me, the effort and discipline in solitude is a spiritual aspect of my training. That's why none of the drills in this book demand a spotter, or partner for assistance. *Not one*. That's not the way gymnastics is typically taught, today. But this book is not about gymnastics—it's about progressive calisthenics. The two are different.

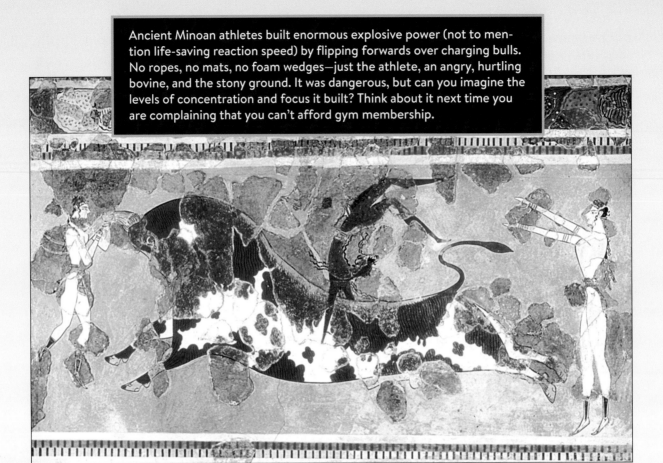

Ancient Minoan athletes built enormous explosive power (not to mention life-saving reaction speed) by flipping forwards over charging bulls. No ropes, no mats, no foam wedges—just the athlete, an angry, hurtling bovine, and the stony ground. It was dangerous, but can you imagine the levels of concentration and focus it built? Think about it next time you are complaining that you can't afford gym membership.

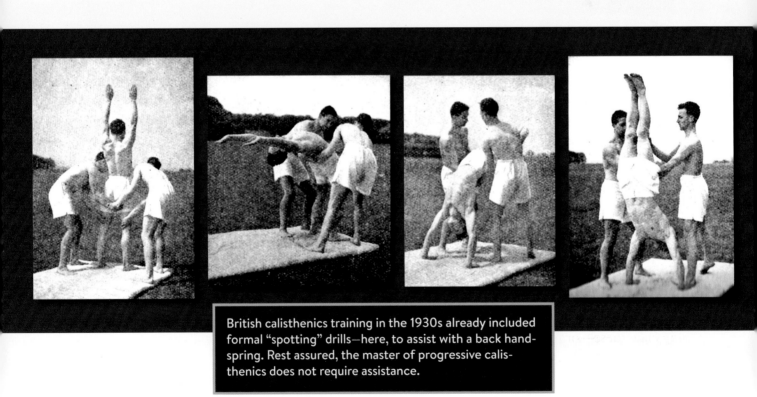

British calisthenics training in the 1930s already included formal "spotting" drills—here, to assist with a back handspring. Rest assured, the master of progressive calisthenics does not require assistance.

EXPLOSIVE CALISTHENICS

I don't care if you live in your parents' basement, or if you are in a small military encampment in Afghanistan. Find something to hang from, and you have everything you need to become a master of explosive calisthenics.

APPLY TOTAL-BODY TRAINING

In the real world, you never need just a quick arm, or a quick foot. Some folks talk about boxers having "fast hands" but this is a misnomer; in reality, a boxing punch involves the entire body, the legs, waist, torso, shoulders and arms. Everything needs to be fast, or there is no speed. The same is true for kicking—ask any martial artist with "fast feet" and they'll tell you the waist and upper-body are just as important in generating speed.

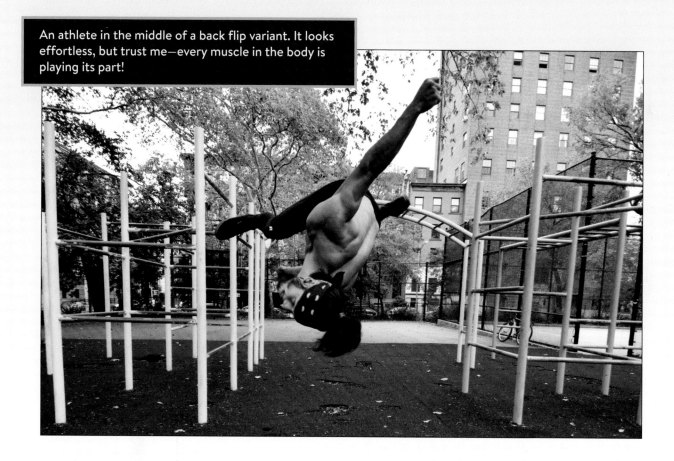

An athlete in the middle of a back flip variant. It looks effortless, but trust me—every muscle in the body is playing its part!

The brutal realities of the real world also tell us we need a fast body, rather than a fast body *part*. In combat, in military exercises, in sports, you gotta move your whole body. You know this is true. It's no good having super-fast fingers from playing Xbox if those fingers are attached to a rusted up ton of crap. You can skip those specialist "speed" exercises some athletes love, like flipping and catching cards, or quickly grapping coins flipped off the elbow. There's no carry-over. Skills like these—or even juggling, which some boxers used to do—are too specialized. They will not give you speed in any other area.

The best way to train for explosive power and speed is to pick only those exercises which work the *entire body*. You need to work as many muscles as possible to get the biggest bang for your buck. Sure, in this manual I advise some exercises which seem to work some body parts much more than others—*clap pushups* might seem to work the upper-body, *pogo jumps* might seem to work the lower legs—but as you advance beyond basic conditioning you'll find that the exercise chains in this book work your *entire body* as a unit: the power pushups lead to advanced exercises which also involve the legs, and the jump series quickly recruits the arms and waist to add power. The same is true for all the movements in here.

Total body exercises also have the benefit of building *integrated power*. The body is a true *gestalt* entity—the total is more than the sum of its parts. An athlete who tried to work each body area (in isolation) for power could never be as fast or fluid as the athlete who trained these areas to work as a team. If you are familiar with hardcore strength training you'll understand full well that the strongest men and women in the world are the ones who train their bodies with exercises which work *everything at once,* so they can maximize their system's potential. Training for power and speed is no different.

FOCUS ON A SMALL GROUP OF EXERCISES

This principle follows on from the last one. If you are focusing on exercises which to some degree work the entire body, you don't need to do very many of them—it'd be a waste of time, you'd be needlessly repeating yourself.

If you really want to build monstrous power, speed and agility in the shortest space of time possible, I advise you to stick to only a handful of movement-types which you get better and better at in a measurable way (this is *progression*, and it's the principle up next). Since even *total body* exercises work the body in slightly different ways, I advise my students to pick a handful of classic calisthenics/acrobatic movements to cover all bases. Don't waste your time with inferior exercises—go for the BIG movements which require maximum athleticism!

I personally feel that for the ultimate in hardcore explosiveness training, *six* movements are ideal:

- A jump – to teach posture, explosive leaping, tucking skills and landing
- An explosive pushup – to condition the arms and shoulders for high velocity movements, to improve upper-limb reflexes
- A kip-up – to build high levels of speed/power in the waist and to develop basic agility
- A front rotation – to teach the body to revolve forward at optimal speed
- A back rotation – to teach the body to revolve backwards at optimal speed
- An up-and-over – to teach the body to pull itself upwards with maximum power and skill

(I'll break these six types of movement down a little more in the next chapter.)

Of course, you can tinker with the number "six". You might prefer to work with four movements, or seven. (Some athletes will want to add side-rotations, or twisting movements. I personally think it's safer and easier to add lateral and twisting movements after the athlete gains some basic proficiency.*) Just remember that anything less than six movements and some key speed-power skill gets missed; anything more than this and you risk overkill and loss of focus.

Of course, you can tinker with the number "six". You might prefer to work with four movements, or maybe seven. (Some athletes will want to add side-rotations, or twisting movements. I personally think it's safer and easier to add lateral and twisting movements *after* the athlete gains some basic proficiency.*) Just remember that anything less than six movements and some key speed-power skill gets missed; anything more than this and you risk overkill and loss of focus.

BE PROGRESSIVE

Finally, we reach the essence of true calisthenics—the principle of *progression*!

Again, this principle follows on from the last one. If you are working with a handful of movements, it's no good doing the same old techniques over and over, again and again. Your goal (over time, as you gain power) should be to progress to *harder and harder variations* of those movements. Otherwise, how the hell will you know that you're getting better?

The question is—*how do I make explosive movements progressive?* Part II of this book will give you all the keys you need to understand this area of training, but we'll briefly look at one example now. Let's take *backwards rotation* as an example. If you are working on becoming very explosive in backwards rotation, there is one coveted expert technique you'll need to eventually master—the back flip. In a true back flip, you stand on solid ground and jump up, rotating backwards 360 degrees to land on your feet in exactly the same spot a fraction later. (Your hands help you swing but you don't touch the floor with them at any time.)

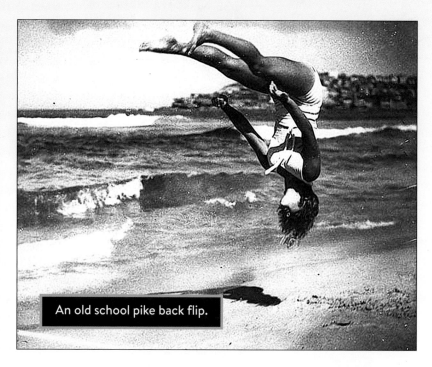

An old school pike back flip.

If you asked most out-of-shape people if they could learn a difficult bodyweight skill like the back flip, most would answer *no*—they'd see it as an impossibility. In one sense, they'd be correct—attempting this technique in one "mouthful" would indeed be impossible. However, if they

*See *round-offs* (page 166) and *cartwheels* (page 167).

broke the backflip into a series of stages—beginning with very easy techniques and moving to harder efforts—they could, in fact, learn this movement. In reality, I could teach pretty much any deconditioned individual how to perform a back flip using this method. This is the essence of progression; techniques which lead to more difficult versions of an exercise are called *progressions*. (Easier versions of a specific technique are called *regressions*.)

If an athlete is new to calisthenics, they must begin with some basic bridging exercises to mobilize and strengthen their spine, shoulders and limbs. Once they've benefited from those basics, the progressions can begin. We start with simple, easy *backward rolls*. Who can't perform a basic roll? As you get used to rolling, you move to a more advanced variation; rolling using the hands. By now, your brain, spine and joints will be used to rotating, so we move to *kick-overs* from a bridge position:

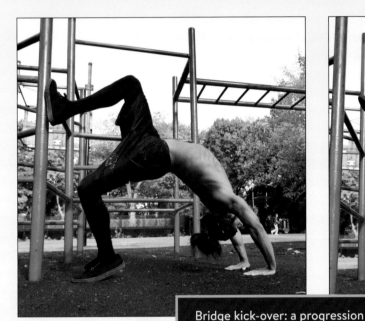 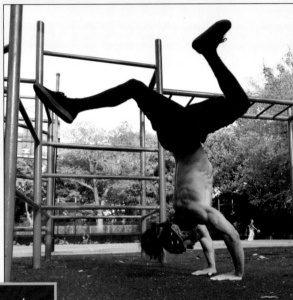

Bridge kick-over: a progression to back flips.

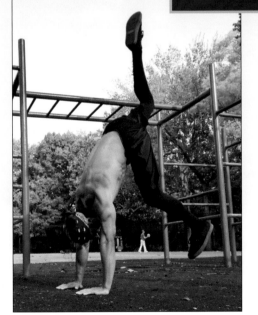

Once these become second nature, you move on to variations of the *monkey flip*—an easy spin/flip which allows you to learn to rotate backwards by approaching the movement side-on. There are several progressions of the monkey flip, and by the time you get to the final one, you'll be ready for the *back handspring*, where you jump and rotate over on your hands. After spending some time training with handsprings, you can explore some transitional exercises which finally lead you through to the *back flip*.

Like anything which seems impossible, the key to victory is to take things step-by-step. Bear in mind that you are not meant to just *try* each progression, then race to the next one if you can do it—that would just lead to failure. At the heart of this method is learning to love each progression—master and milk it for all its worth. You don't become a better athlete by moving up through the progressions you can't do very well. You become a better athlete by taking the time to practice the progressions you *can* do well.

LIGHTS OUT!

A vanishing percentage of people who work out ever even *attempt* to unlock their body's inherent power and speed. That's nuts. In the real world, these qualities are the pinnacle of athleticism and survival ability! And yet, folks stick to the same old slow training, or boring cardio on machines.

Almost none of this tragic negligence has to do with the body. It's all down to attitude. Psychology. How many people who train avoid incredible feats like the back flip because, in their mind, they are *impossible*? Too many trainees are of the opinion that there are just "some people" who are naturally gymnastic, and these are the kind of people who go on to learn these feats—it's beyond the safe reach of the average Joe or Jane. I've spoken to athletes who thought they were "too old" to learn explosives, or "too weak", or "too heavy", or whatever. These athletes don't understand that their bodies are *fully capable* of performing incredible feats of power—they just need to be programmed the right way: using the five principles in this chapter. As soon as these self-doubting trainees see and begin to *understand* the progressions I've included in the following pages, something "clicks" within them...and they realize that they too can achieve the elite, super-impressive explosive moves in this book.

And so can you!

EXPLOSIVE CALISTHENICS

3

How to Use This Book
CORE CONCEPTS AND ANSWERS

I know—you're raring to get to the meat and potatoes of this book—the exercises! Good on ya. But woah yer horses there, Hoss. I've slipped in this chapter to give you an overall view of the entire manual. I also want to make sure you are grounded in the key terms used in my system, terms like the *Explosive Six*, the *Ten Steps, Master Steps* and so on.

We'll be at the exercises soon—they're up in Part II, which begins in the very next chapter. Just for now, let's use our smarts and get ourselves an overview of this beast we're about to tame.

THE EXPLOSIVE SIX

If you read **Convict Conditioning**, you'll know I based the techniques in that book around six different movement families: the "Big Six". These were:

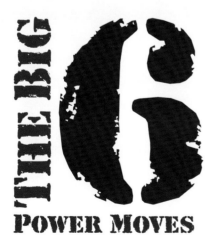

1. **PUSHUPS**
2. **SQUATS**
3. **PULLUPS**
4. **LEG RAISES**
5. **BRIDGES**
6. **HANDSTAND PUSHUPS**

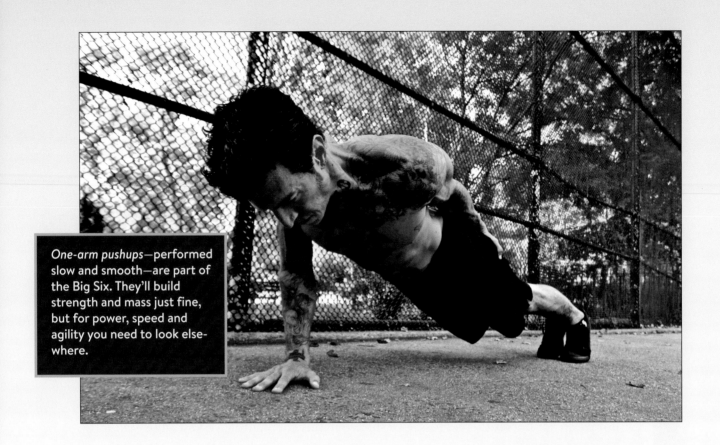

One-arm pushups—performed slow and smooth—are part of the Big Six. They'll build strength and mass just fine, but for power, speed and agility you need to look elsewhere.

FAQ: HOW FAR ADVANCED SHOULD I BE IN *CONVICT CONDITIONING* BEFORE TRYING EXPLOSIVES?

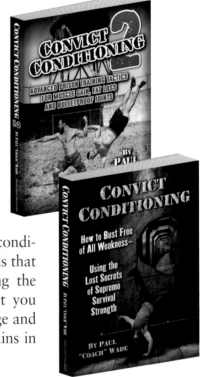

You *don't* need to own *Convict Conditioning 1* or *2* to use this book—at all. But you *should* have some basic bodyweight strength under your belt before attempting high-velocity calisthenics. High-power work can injure sedentary or overweight individuals who are not ready for it. Bodyweight strength training (when performed correctly) is the *very best* way to condition the joints and adequately prepare them for the loads that explosives place on them. If you have been following the *Convict Conditioning* strength system, I'd advise that you reach at least step 5 on the pushup, squat, pullup, bridge and leg raise movements before exploring the explosive chains in this manual.

Just as the Big Six represent the finest calisthenics movements for *strength* and *muscle-growth*, the Explosive Six are the best possible movements you can perform for *explosive power* and *body-weight speed*. Hard work on just one of the Explosive Six will add speed, agility and explosive power to your entire body. If you manage to tackle *all* of them, you'll become something akin to a *ninja* genetically-spliced with a *jungle cat*.

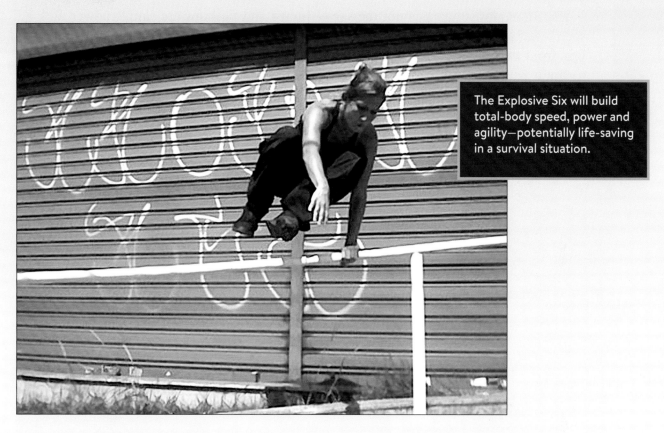

The Explosive Six will build total-body speed, power and agility—potentially life-saving in a survival situation.

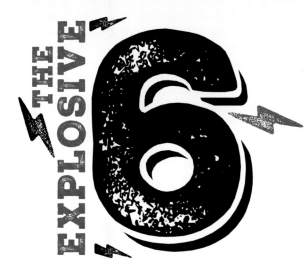

THE EXPLOSIVE 6

1. **JUMPS**
2. **POWER PUSHUPS**
3. **KIP-UPS**
4. **FORWARD ROTATIONS**
5. **BACKWARDS ROTATIONS**
6. **EXPLOSIVE (UP-AND-OVER) BAR WORK**

FAQ: DO I NEED TO LEARN THE EXPLOSIVE SIX IN ANY PARTICULAR ORDER?

Yes. All explosive work is not the same! **Jumps** and **pushups** are simple power and speed exercises which condition the joints and build basic movement proficiency. **Kip-ups, front flips, back flips** and **muscle-u**ps are also "skill" exercises. I advise all athletes to begin working with the jump chain and the power pushup chain to strengthen the joints and build power and speed. Once you are comfortable with these two—to at least step 5 of each—feel free to begin working with the other movements!

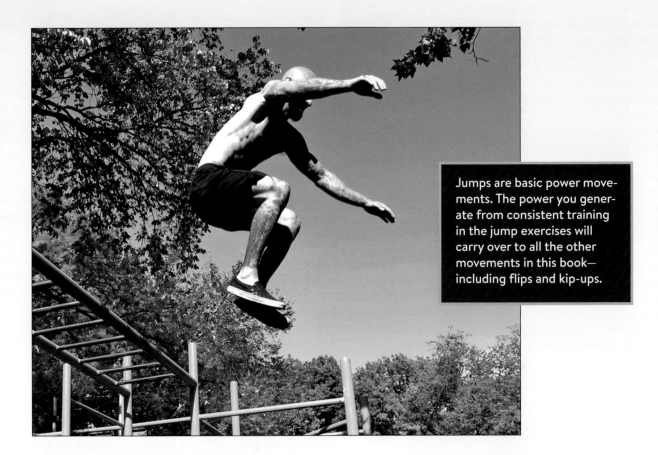

Jumps are basic power movements. The power you generate from consistent training in the jump exercises will carry over to all the other movements in this book—including flips and kip-ups.

THE TEN STEPS

In *Convict Conditioning* and this book, I've split the major six movement-types into *ten* different exercises. These are called the *ten steps*. Step 1 is the easiest, and should be do-able by most reasonably fit athletes. In progressive calisthenics, a series of progressively harder techniques is called a *chain*; from step 1 on, each technique gets progressively harder till you reach the ultimate step. Step 10 is the hardest exercise: the *Master Step*.

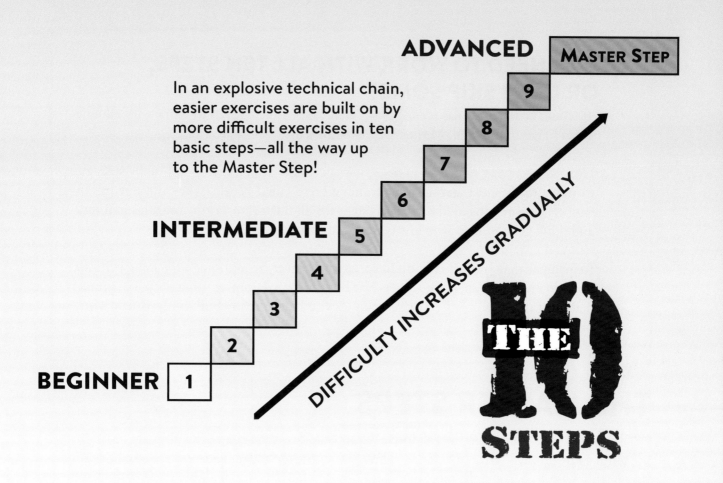

ADVANCED · MASTER STEP

In an explosive technical chain, easier exercises are built on by more difficult exercises in ten basic steps—all the way up to the Master Step!

INTERMEDIATE

BEGINNER

DIFFICULTY INCREASES GRADUALLY

THE 10 STEPS

TEN STEPS FAQ:
Q. WHY TEN STEPS? WHY NOT MORE, OR LESS?

A. The answer is simple: ten is a digestible number for human beings. We typically get ten fingers, ten toes, ten eyes. No, wait. Not ten eyes. But we do have a decimal number system based on tens. And Ten Commandments. I could have easily cut out exercises, and used eight steps; or added more and had twelve steps.

Q. DO I HAVE TO START WITH STEP 1,
OR CAN I JUMP IN ANYWHERE?

A. I would advise athletes to begin at **step 1** with all chains. Doing so will protect your joints, help develop body wisdom and build training momentum.

As in all things, you should use common sense. If you have been an acrobat half your life, then you probably don't *really* need to begin at step 1. That said, even then, how would it hurt you to spend a few sessions exploring the earlier steps? You may even learn something. Relearning the basics is never a mistake.

Q. DO I NEED TO WORK WITH ALL TEN STEPS, OR CAN I SKIP SOME?

A. It would be flat-out false for me to say that every athlete needs to work with all nine steps to get to the final, Master Step. Not all will.

However—having said that, in my experience most athletes who eventually struggle to move to the next step in their training have failed because they did not put in enough time **milking** all the previous steps for all they were worth. Bear this in mind, and don't get obsessed with always moving up to the higher steps.

Remember that you actually **build** speed and power by *working with steps you can do well*. Moving up a step does NOT build speed, power or agility—it simply **demonstrates** how many of these qualities you have already built with patient work on the earlier steps.

THE MASTER STEPS

The goal of your training in the Explosive Six techniques is to achieve the ultimate movement—the tenth step—in each of the six chains. These six tenth-step movements are called *Master Steps*. If you truly wish to become the most explosive athlete your DNA will allow, your goal must be to attain all of the Explosive Six Master Steps. They are:

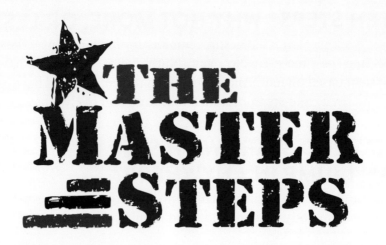

EXPLOSIVE SIX MOVEMENT-TYPE	MASTER STEP	THE MASTER STEPS
JUMPS	SUICIDE JUMP	
POWER PUSHES	SUPERMAN	
KIP-UPS	NO-HANDS KIP-UP	
FRONT ROTATIONS	FRONT FLIP	
BACK ROTATIONS	BACK FLIP	
UP-AND-OVER	MUSCLE-UP	

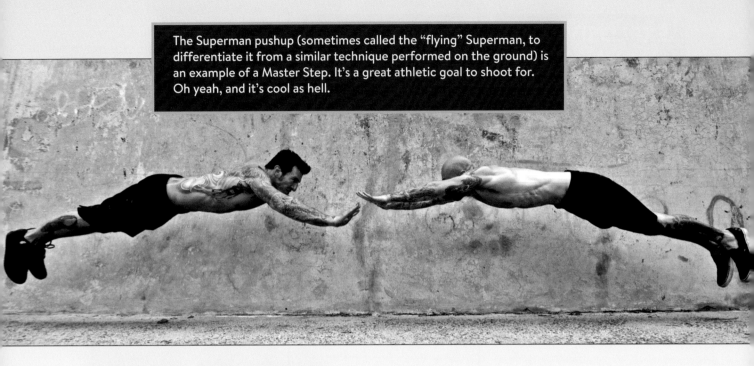

The Superman pushup (sometimes called the "flying" Superman, to differentiate it from a similar technique performed on the ground) is an example of a Master Step. It's a great athletic goal to shoot for. Oh yeah, and it's cool as hell.

GOING BEYOND— SUPER-ADVANCED TECHNIQUES

Attaining the Master Steps of each chain can turn even stiff, sluggish athletes into lightning-like speed machines. But does that mean you can't—eventually—reach an even higher level of mastery...? No way!

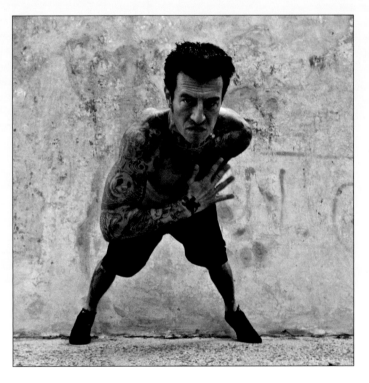

There is really no *end point* in any of the bodyweight arts. No matter how explosive—or strong, or flexible—you become, there are always further advanced techniques to explore; more elite variations you can experiment with. For this reason, you should see the Master Steps in this book as superior goals to *guide* your bodyweight training. They do not represent the "end" of anything. When you achieve the greatness that I know is in you and actually reach a Master Step, you will aspire to even greater bodyweight feats. I've included some ideas for you to take your training even further in the *Going Beyond* section that follows each of the Master Steps.

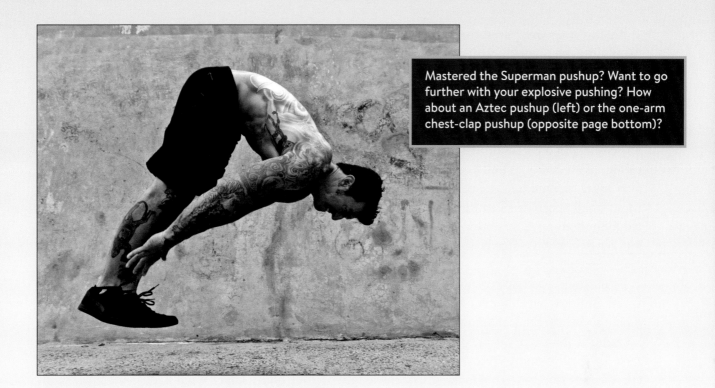

Mastered the Superman pushup? Want to go further with your explosive pushing? How about an Aztec pushup (left) or the one-arm chest-clap pushup (opposite page bottom)?

SMALL SPACE DRILLS

After the *Going Beyond* section of each exercise chapter, I include a handful of my favorite ancillary drills for you to explore, if you choose to. The bulk of these techniques have been drawn from prison experience, and represent the kind of hardcore, low-tech methods we used in our cells to build agility, elite reflexes and Nth-level swiftness over a short space.

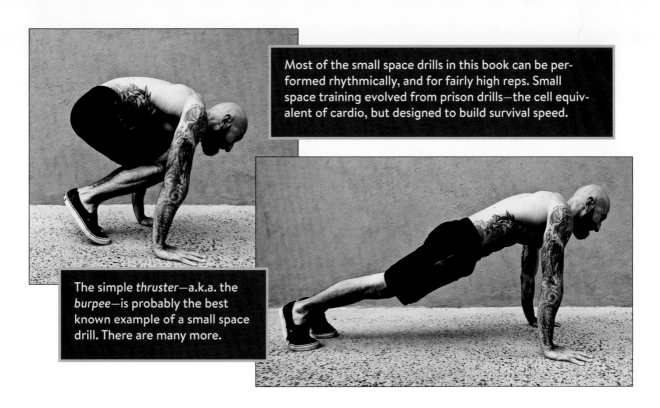

Most of the small space drills in this book can be performed rhythmically, and for fairly high reps. Small space training evolved from prison drills—the cell equivalent of cardio, but designed to build survival speed.

The simple *thruster*—a.k.a. the *burpee*—is probably the best known example of a small space drill. There are many more.

Because they are based on prison workouts, the drills I show you require virtually no equipment—maybe a sturdy wall at most. (I'm betting you can find a wall, right?) Certainly nothing expensive or specialized. I've grouped the cell training drills together with the most appropriate chapters I could—for example, the drills in the jumping chapter will help leg speed and responses; the drills in the muscle-up chapter will help aspects like arm extension speed, etc. But—because the drills mostly work the entire body, to some degree—this way of grouping should be considered a loose one, not a catch-all. It's more helpful to think of the small space drills as a grab bag of interesting, fun techniques that you can apply to *any t*raining session for variety and freshness. They are also great for building reflexes, coordination and overall spatial awareness. As a bonus, many of these small space drills can be performed *rhythmically*, and/or for high reps (think about aiming for a hundred reps, or setting a timer to perform drills for a minute, non-stop.) Suddenly you have a potential cardio element, if you need it. There's TONS of crossover to be had here.

I still think, even on the outside, that this *small space* training is an interesting way to train for speed and dexterity. Think about it; most guys on the outside train for speed by doing things like running sprints. Sure, that makes you fast over, say, a hundred meters. But in a survival situation in a cramped jail—like a riot, or physical combat—fast movements over a hundred meters are *useless*. To survive and excel, you gotta be fast over a fraction of that distance...faster-than-the-eye speed over distances like arm length, or the length of your body. That's what keeps you alive, keeps you on top.

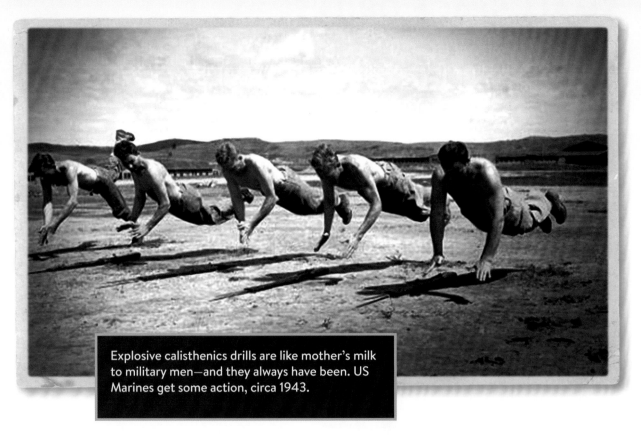

Explosive calisthenics drills are like mother's milk to military men—and they always have been. US Marines get some action, circa 1943.

You don't need to be a cell athlete to train this kind of way. I've spoken to plenty of military guys who apply this species of drill to keep sharp and stay the best at what they do. Navy men are a great example of athletes who apply this "small space" training in cramped conditions, even smaller than cells. If it works for them, it will sure as hell work for you!

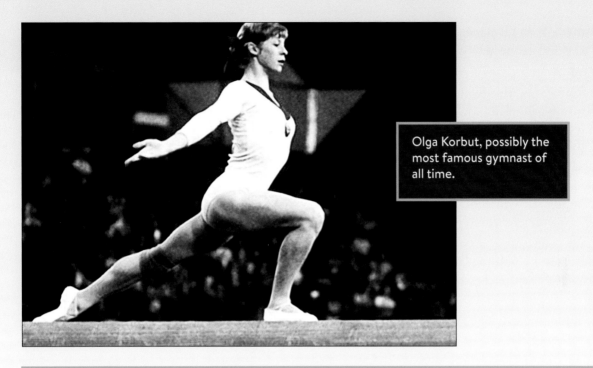

Olga Korbut, possibly the most famous gymnast of all time.

FAQ: ISN'T THIS JUST GYMNASTICS?

Although some of the movements in this book—for example, front and back flips (called the front and back *tuck*, in gymnastics) look very similar to movements in gymnastics, *this is not a book about gymnastics*. This manual is about building **raw power**, **speed** and **agility**, **alone**, and with **zero special equipment**. Gymnastics is a specialist **sport** based on judgement of qualities like **balance** and **aesthetic movement**—in the same way dance is. Gymnasts typically employ plenty of **special equipment** in training, including foam blocks, matting, cables, rings, specially surfaced flooring, wedges, etc. Gymnastics is generally also taught using highly-trained **spotters** to assist with the movements. I respect and admire gymnasts, but **explosive calisthenics is not gymnastics**. Don't expect it to be!

PART III: PROGRAMMING

Please, *don't* just flick through this book and start playing with exercises. There are serious moves in here, and that's a good way to get hurt. That's no way for a true athlete to roll.

Be smart, kid. Take your training seriously. Get a program. Part III of this book has got everything ya doggone need:

- **Chapter 10** will introduce you to the PARC principle, which will tell you how to progress from step-to-step

- **Chapter 11** will explain the difference between training with simple *power* exercises (jumps and power pushups), and *agility* exercises which should be treated as a *skill*

- **Chapter 12** will cover power building, and explain the *Rule of Three* and the *Rule of Six*, which you can use to govern your training volume

- **Chapter 13** will explain the methods of *time surfing* and *consolidation training*, which are excellent approaches to skill training

- **Chapter 14** will give you some great *program templates*

LIGHTS OUT!

The Master Steps in this manual are incredible expressions of human ability—requiring speed, power, agility and a perfectly functioning physique. Many athletes are strong in static movements like the deadlift or bench press, but total-body explosive movements like *backflips* and *muscle-ups* really separate extreme athletes from the stiff, strong-but-unathletic Frankensteins in most gyms. I don't care how rusty, injured, weak or unathletic you *think* you are. If you are under the age of 70 and have four limbs, then you *can* achieve all of these Master Steps. Folks have achieved them with less going for them, trust me!

I'm your coach now. I'm here for ya, gorgeous. Take my hand and follow these methods, and we got this thing *owned*, together. You can take this explosive training just to the level you are happy with, or—if you want—you can take it all the way.

In fact...how can you fail?

PART II

THE
EXPLOSIVE

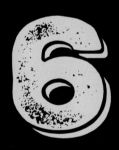

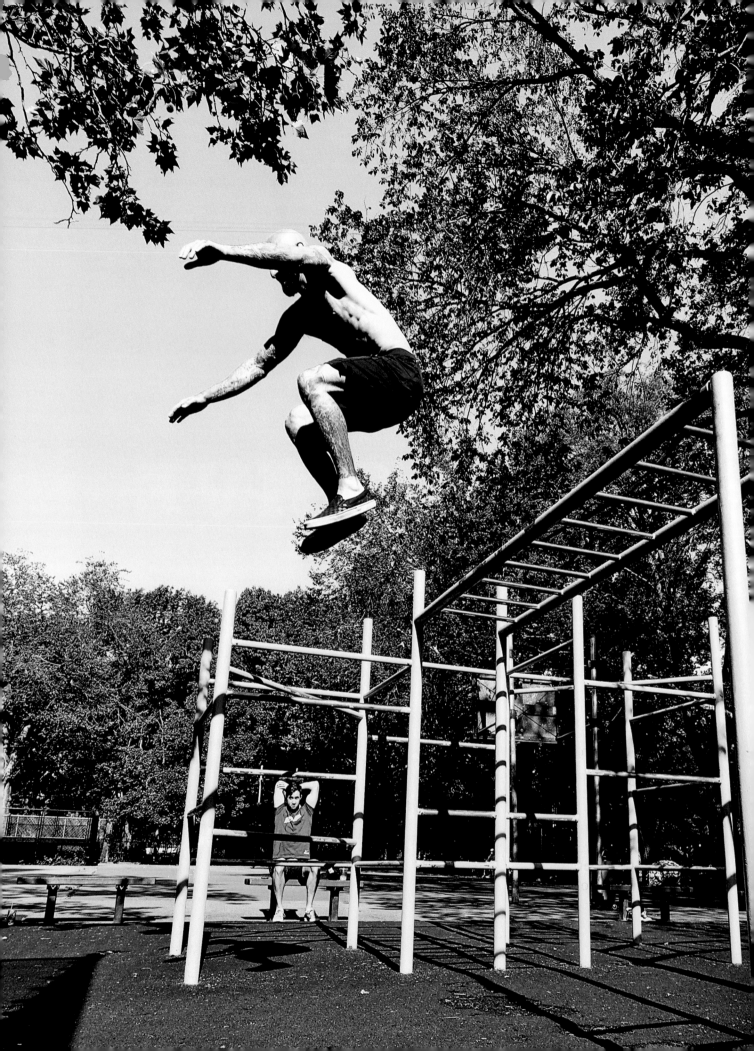

4
POWER JUMPS
ADVANCED LEG SPRING

If you speak to most coaches and athletes about *true* power training—moving force at the highest possible speeds, as opposed to the heavy-load work of weight-lifting—then most of them will immediately think about *jumps*: those explosive leaps—upwards or horizontal (a.k.a. *bounds*)—using the body's own weight as resistance.

There are some real compelling reasons why so many coaches make jump training central to any explosiveness program: powerful, fast legs are pretty much useful for everything sports or movement related. The Ancients believed that the leg "spring" was the source of a man's youth and athleticism, and—as ever—they were right. Without explosive power in the legs, running is impossible. High power acrobatic movements—flips, rotations, dives—all depend on getting *height*, which can only happen through optimal leg power. Basketball, football, hurdling, soccer, martial arts, parkour—it's pretty tough to name a sport which doesn't hugely depend on having springy legs.

A lot of guys talk about gaining leg "power" through exercises like heavy squats, or even deadlifts, but this is a fallacy. True power is *strength x speed*, and adding a load like a big barbell effectively kills the athlete's ability to move at faster-than-normal levels. For maximum power, bodyweight is the only way to go. It's also just more *realistic* to stick to bodyweight—can you think of any sports when you need to *jump* while carrying hundreds of pounds?

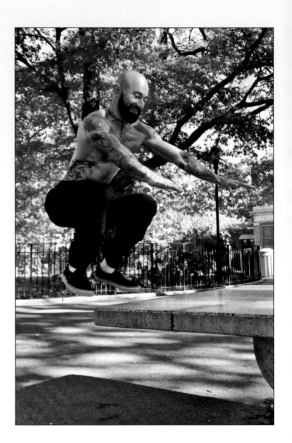

DECONSTRUCTING POWER JUMPS

Jump training has seen an interesting resurgence in the last ten or twenty years. These days, it's tough to go into a commercial gym without seeing someone jumping up and down onto some kind of over-priced box. A lot of this has happened as the "functional" movement has invaded gyms, previously monopolized with slow, un-natural looking movements on machines. Some of it has been to do with the dominance of *CrossFit* as a training method.

Whatever the source, I think it's mostly a good thing that athletes are jumping again. But I would add two provisos to this. First up, athletes and coaches should understand that simply *jumping up and down* on a box must not become the be-all end-all of this kind of training. (You don't need a box—or anything at all—to jump, but people do love their equipment, don't they?) As a second point, I would add that correct bodyweight jump training is about *more* than just gaining height over time. *As well as* gradually building linear power—in the form of jump *height*—all jump training should include drills which develop the following four basic skills:

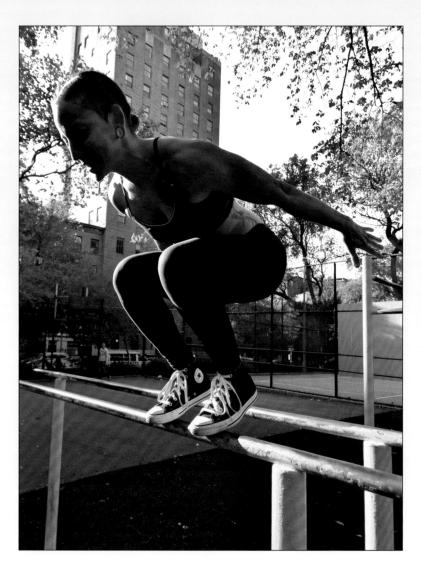

LAUNCHING

Most athletes don't know the optimal way to squat *down* (you have been performing your bodyweight squats, haven't you?), let alone how to explode *up* for height. The keys are body symmetry, leading with the hips (as if *sitting* down, rather than *bowing* down) and exploding up using total-leg and hip power. The best way to acquire these qualities are by lots and lots of thoughtful reps on the basic jumps.

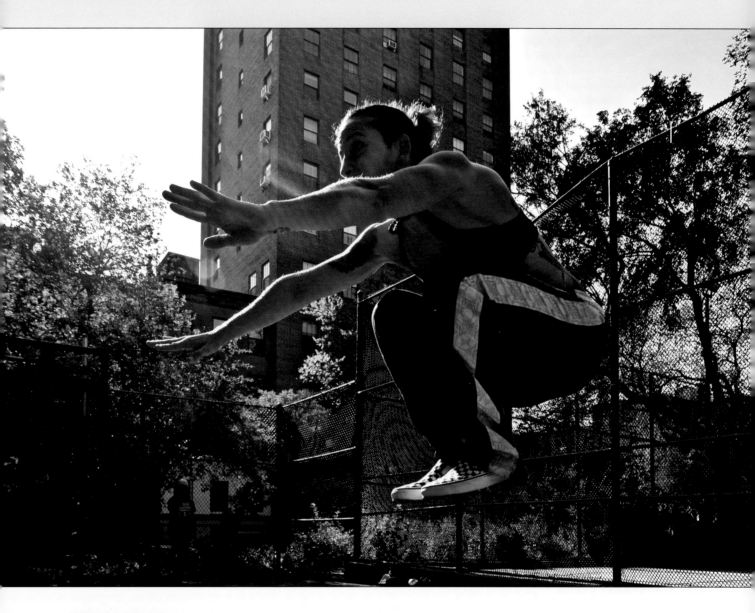

TUCKING

A correct jumping course must teach the athlete how to *tuck* correctly—that is, to pull the knees up (and, ultimately, into the chest). In real-life, tucking is an essential part of *functional* jumping—imagine jumping on, or over something—you need to bring your knees up, right? This is difficult without powerful hip flexors, but the steps in the power jump chain will get you there gradually.

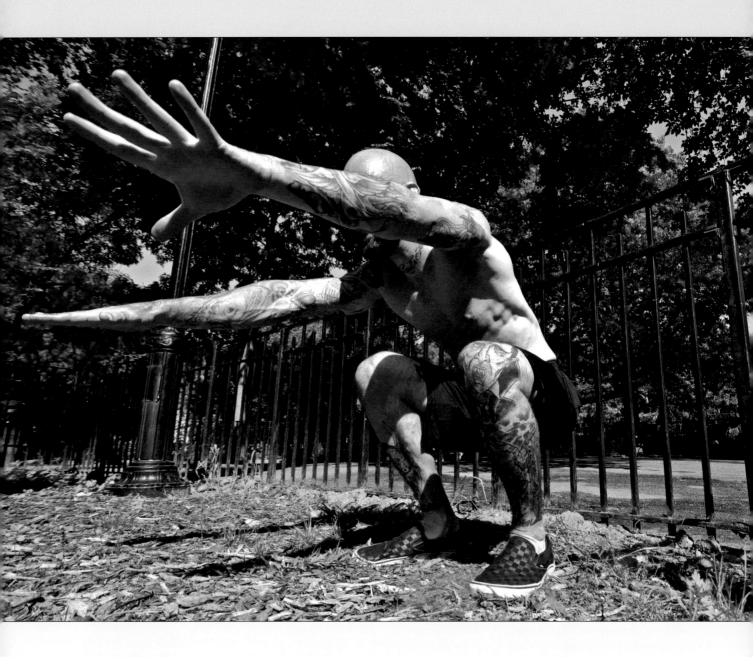

LANDING

It's ironic that *landing* is something many coaches give little or no thought to—they only see the jump as the "up" part. It's ironic because so many athletes—especially newbies, the overweight, older athletes or those with joint injuries—find landing the most difficult and intimidating aspect of the exercise. You can learn to be a truly great jumper despite these factors; you just have to *teach* your body how to land. As with launching, the keys are symmetry, a hip-led squat bend, and the absorption of force with the entire leg and body, not just the feet and ankles. Beginning slowly with small jumps (and hops) will also condition the soft tissues well.

MYOTATIC REBOUND

One of the reasons that our tendons possess some strong elasticity is to allow them to absorb and redirect forces. We see this turned up to the max in the huge leg tendons of a kangaroo; these beasts leap, and on landing the elasticity in their legs makes the next jump easier. This phenomenon also involves the nervous system making the stretched muscles contract at *just* the right time to support the elastic effect, and this is called the *myotatic reflex*—it is the myotatic reflex which is at the heart of modern "plyometric" training (which is not the same as explosive training—see: *Utilize the Plyometric Edge!* On page 315). Learning to exploit this skill is easy, in the case of jumping: *don't pause in between jumps.* The second you land, allow yourself to "bounce" back up, rhythmically. This technique can be employed with most steps in the chain. (It also works in some of the small space drills peppered around this manual. Experiment.)

Athletes who wish to explore more dynamic, acrobat movements should also be looking at building a fifth jumping skill:

BLOCKING

Blocking involves the transformation of horizontal momentum into vertical momentum. If you watch an acrobat preparing to perform a flip, you'll notice that they take a little run-up first, followed by planting the feet together and jumping up. This run/foot-plant maneuver—which most athletes perform instinctively—is called *blocking*. Performed correctly, it also exploits the myotatic rebound.

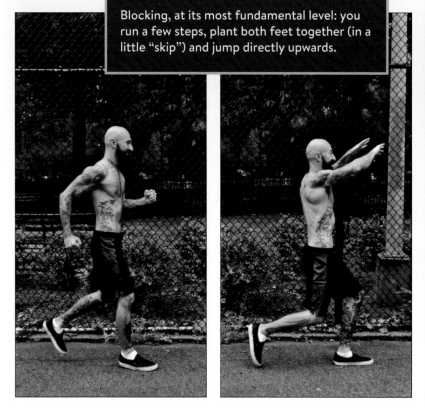

Blocking, at its most fundamental level: you run a few steps, plant both feet together (in a little "skip") and jump directly upwards.

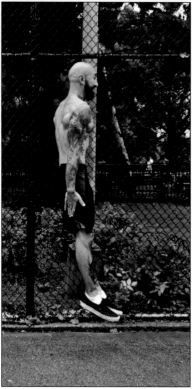

All these skills are essential if you wish to progress to the back and front flip chains. It might be obvious to non-athletes why *launching*, *landing* and *blocking* may be essential to perform a flip—but in fact *tucking* is even more important. It is so central to the techniques, that gymnasts still call the front and back *flip* the front and back *tuck*. So there.

THE POWER JUMP CHAIN

Careful, intelligent progress through all the steps of the jump chain will impart all five of the above essential jumping skills. It will also develop joint integrity and ensure that the athlete has enough raw *power* to get a good level of height—the Master Step (the *suicide jump*) is impossible without a high level of launch power.

Athletes begin with the simplest, easiest of all jumping drills: the *straight hop* (step 1). Hopping requires no space, and develops the elastic rebound of the lower legs, without placing much stress on the knees and back. The hop also teaches good foot and ankle positioning for landing.

The next step is to integrate the knee and hip joints into the jump pattern. The *squat jump* (step 2) strengthens the knees and begins to build more rounded power. Once this movement has been mastered, the arms are trained to come into play with the *vertical jump* (step 3). Vertical jumps teach the athlete to coordinate lower and upper-bodies for increased power and momentum. Once static vertical power has been established, the athlete adds in a run-up and works with *block jumps* (step 4), exploring *blocking* (turning horizontal momentum into vertical momentum). As mentioned earlier, this is an essential skill for any would-be acrobat to nail.

The next four steps are devoted to mastering a proper tuck (see page 39). The tuck requires strong hip flexors to bring the knees up into the chest. We start gently with *butt-kick jumps* (step 5) which teach good height and leg speed—you need to get high enough to kick your butt with your heels, and fast enough to whip your legs down before gravity forces you down. Because (in a correctly performed butt-kick) the knees are brought up a little—but still below the level of the waist—this exercise is also the perfect means to begin conditioning the hip flexors for the harder tucks to come. Next up are *slap tuck jumps* (step 6), where your slap your knees during the jump. This involves a higher tuck than before—around waist level. The process continues in regular *tuck jumps* (step 7), where the knees are bought even higher, as close to the chest as possible. *Catch tuck jumps* (step 8) represent a good basic mastery of the tuck—you have to fully pull your knees into your chest in mid-air (you may have seen Olympic divers do this).

The *thread jump* (step 9) is a unilateral "trick" jump where the athlete holds their own foot and jumps over it. It's challenging for most people, but it shouldn't pose a problem for any athlete who has attained the previous steps—it's really just a neurological warm-up to help athletes approach the next, and final step. The tenth step—the Master Step—of the jump chain is the *suicide jump*, so called because you jump over a bar or broomstick which you are holding—and if you screw up, a faceplant is a serious possibility. If you can perform this Master Step, you'll have achieved a great level of height, leg speed, and impressive tension-flexibility in the hips, enough to make tucks second nature. You are now a master jumper.

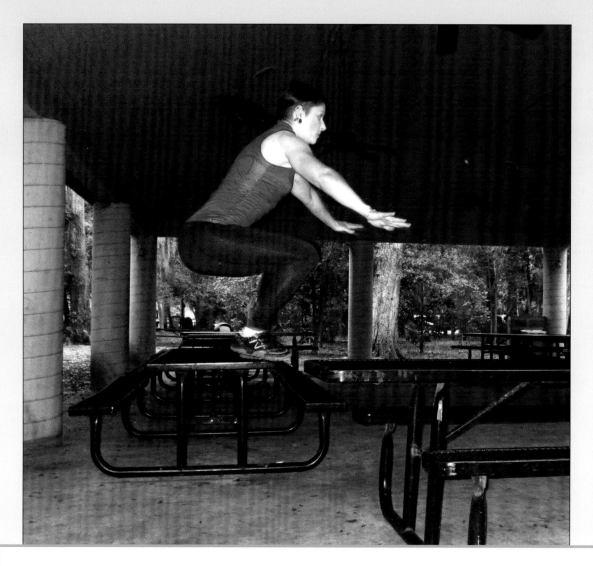

DO YOU NEED PLYO BOXES?

Many athletes begin their jump training by jumping up onto something. Gym boxes are the most popular choice. In fact, I'd say 90% of jump training in gyms is done on those damn boxes!

Box jumps are great, but I think using them exclusively is a mistake. I advise my students to begin their training with free-standing jumping drills, to build important skills like bounding, tucking and catching. *Free-standing* work also allows athletes to unlock and express maximum power without worrying about tripping over anything. If you want to explore box jumps as a variant once you have the basics under your belt, go for it. But always remember, you don't really *need* a box (or any plyometric gym equipment) to become super-explosive. There were incredibly explosive athletes—tumblers, acrobats, martial arts masters—for *centuries* before metal boxes were manufactured and placed in gyms.

STEP ONE: STRAIGHT HOP

PERFORMANCE

- Stand with feet around shoulder-width, with your body flexed for action.

- Dip down slightly. (You only want a slight flexion in the knees—less than a quarter squat position).

- Without pausing, explode upwards, using the power of your lower legs plus all the total-body spring you can muster.

- "Pull" up with the shoulders, but keep the arms reasonably neutral.

- Land softly, catching most of your weight on the balls of your feet.

- Use the elastic rebound to immediately repeat the technique.

EXERCISE X-RAY

Simple hops should be the first phase of any explosive jump training, particularly for neophytes. Hops teach take-off and landing patterns, and strengthen the ankles and knees in preparation for more intense jump work. Due to the limited movement at the knee, jump height is naturally limited, making for an excellent, safe, foundation drill.

REGRESSION

This is one of the easiest basic jumping exercises. Making it less vigorous is done simply by jumping less intensely. Keeping the body "loose" rather than "flexed" (coiled like a spring), will also lessen the difficulty.

PROGRESSION

Make the hops total body movements by swinging the arms up with the hop, and bending slightly more at the knee. Don't bend too much though, or you will be performing *squat jumps* (step 2).

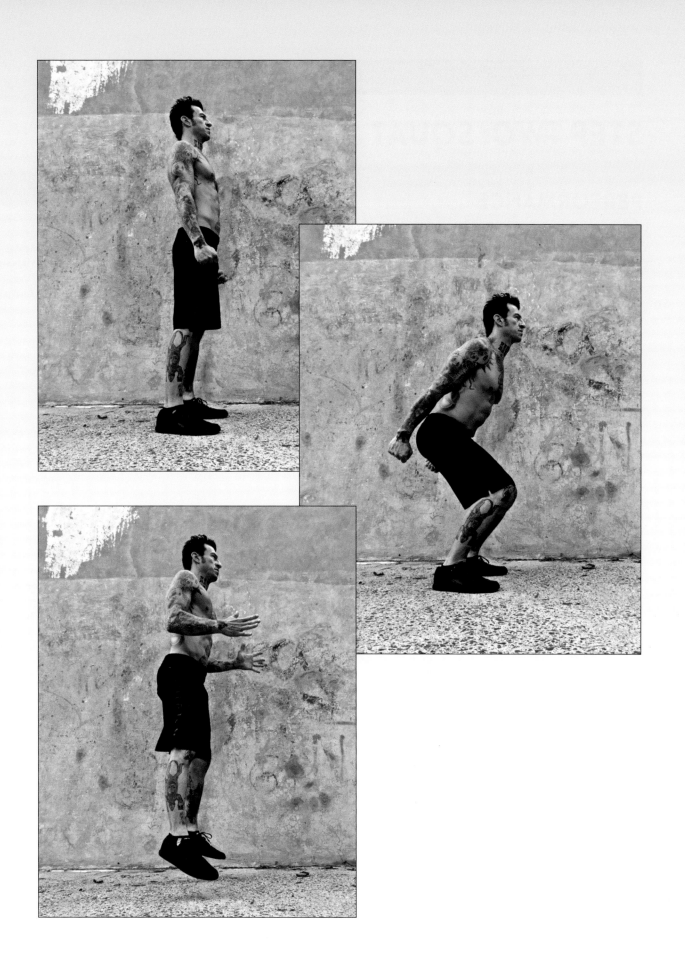

STEP TWO: SQUAT JUMP

PERFORMANCE

- Stand with your feet a little wider than shoulder-width, with your body flexed for action.

- Dip down into a squat. For most people, the peak knee-bend for maximum height will be not quite a half squat—around a third of the way down. Stronger athletes can explore greater depth, dipping until the thighs are parallel to the ground (*see photos*).

- Explode upwards, using the power of your lower body plus all the total body spring you can muster.

- Try to keep the arms reasonably neutral at first.

- After take-off, let the legs move naturally; don't pull them up or thrust them down.

- Land softly, catching most of your weight on the balls of your feet.

- Use the elastic rebound to immediately repeat the technique.

EXERCISE X-RAY

The *squat jump* is the cornerstone of all jumping techniques. Ask a novice to "jump" and this is what they will instinctively do. Due to the knee-bend, greater height is achieved, and this results in more work for the knees on take-off, and for the knees and ankles on landing.

REGRESSION

A less acute bend of the knees will make this exercise easier. Focus on *quarter* squat jumps as a mini-step between *pogo hops* and *squat jumps*.

PROGRESSION

To work the knees more, you can bend to below parallel. This will strengthen the knees and gluteal muscles, but beware that bending the knees too acutely will reduce your explosive potential. Using a closer stance will also make most jump drills tougher.

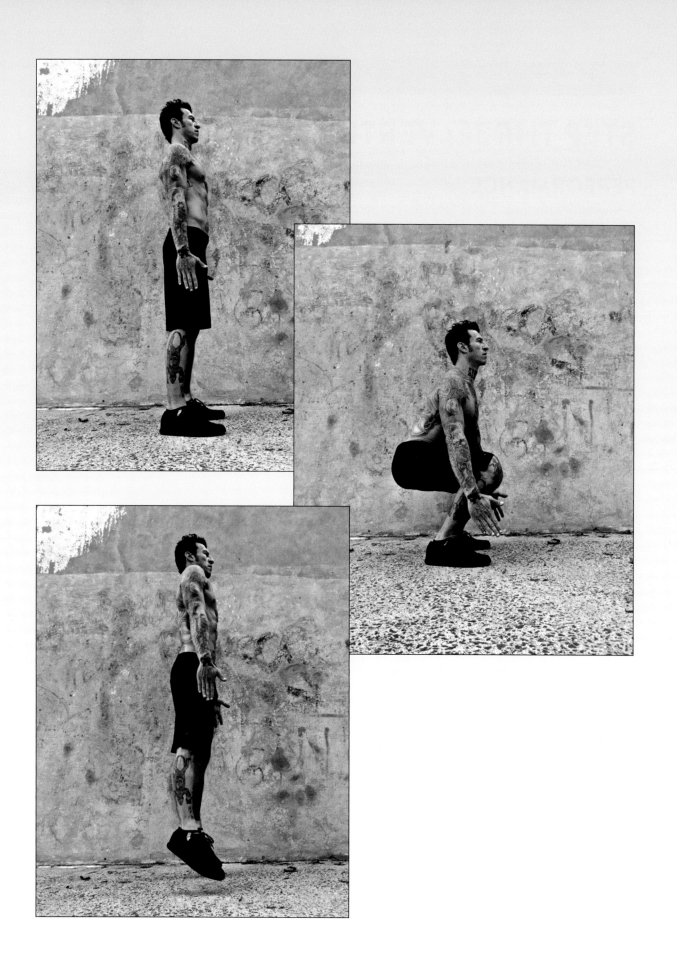

STEP THREE: VERTICAL LEAP

PERFORMANCE

- Stand with your feet a little wider than shoulder-width, with your body flexed for action. Keep your arms by your sides.

- Dip down into a squat. For most people, the peak knee-bend for maximum height will be not quite a half squat—around a third of the way down. Stronger athletes can go deeper.

- Explode upwards, using the power of your lower body plus all the total body spring you can muster.

- As you lift off, swing your arms up above you for maximum momentum.

- After take-off, let the legs move naturally; don't pull them up or thrust them down.

- Land softly, catching most of your weight on the balls of your feet. Allow your arms to fall by your sides again.

- Use the elastic rebound to immediately repeat the technique.

EXERCISE X-RAY

Hops teach athletes to unlock the natural elastic forces inherent in the feet and ankles, a major fundamental of jumping ability through all mammal species. *Squat jumps* combined that with the power of the hips, legs and knees. With *vertical leaps*, you bring the *arms* into the mix, also. Many high-level agility movement patterns require optimal arm explosiveness to complete—look at front and back flips, and you'll see what I mean.

REGRESSION

Begin this exercise slowly, with moderate swinging movements of the arms. Over time swing your arms to the fully overhead stretch position.

PROGRESSION

The *vertical leap* is a favorite of athletics coaches because you can easily record progress over time by measuring reach height.* This can be done as simply as reaching for a chalk-line on a wall.

*To learn more about this kind of measuring protocol, Google *Sargent Jump Test*.

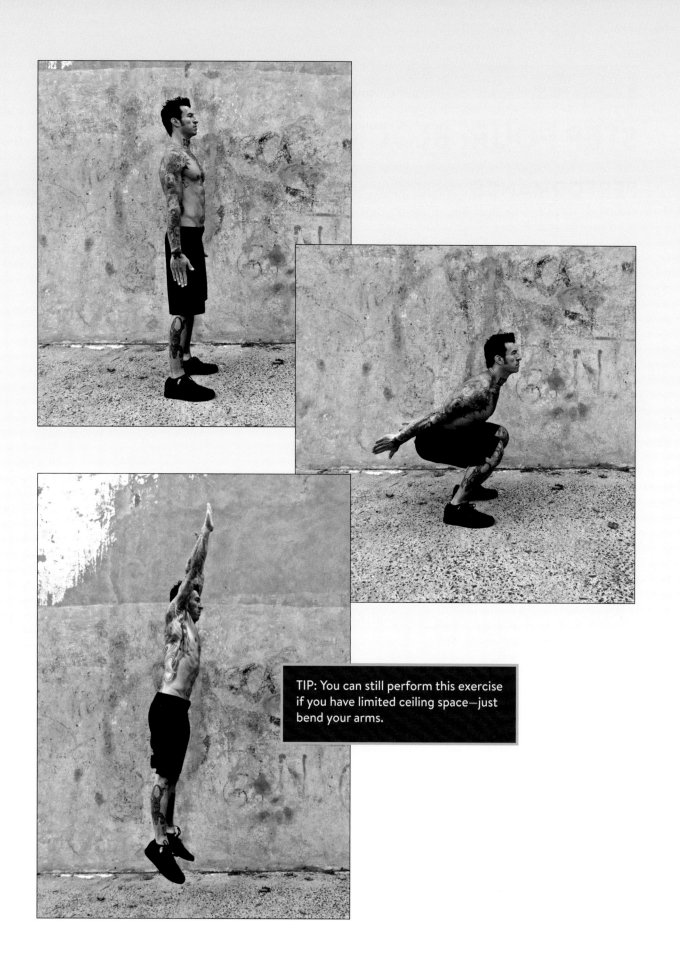

TIP: You can still perform this exercise if you have limited ceiling space—just bend your arms.

STEP FOUR: BLOCK JUMP

PERFORMANCE

- Take a short run-up—a handful of steps is better than too many.

- Swing your arms up and take one big step, then plant both your feet together.

- Your knees can bend a little as you dip down then immediately use your total body to "punch" down through the floor with both feet; swing down with your arms as you go.

- This "punching" down is designed to transfer your momentum into the floor, to push you up.

- Take off vertically, extending the body as you jump as high as you can.

- Land softly, catching most of your weight on the balls of your feet. Allow your arms to fall by your sides again.

- Reposition and repeat the technique.

EXERCISE X-RAY

Once an athlete has built a good level of ability in the basic *vertical leap* (step 3), it's time to master the skill of *blocking*. Blocking involves taking horizontal momentum—generated from running a few steps—and turning it into vertical momentum—an upwards jump. (You "block" your running momentum by punching the floor with your feet, hence the term "blocking"). This kind of force-transference is useful in developing a good level of ability and explosive strength, and blocking specifically is an essential skill pattern to absorb if the athlete wishes to explore more advanced explosive drills such as *front flips*.

REGRESSION

An athlete can learn this drill slowly. Begin with only a couple of steps and master the feet-together transition at low speed first. It might help to think of the final big step before the block as a *skip*.

PROGRESSION

Instead of jumping into a linear air-position, advance by jumping into a *tuck* position (step 7) or a *catch tuck* (step 8).

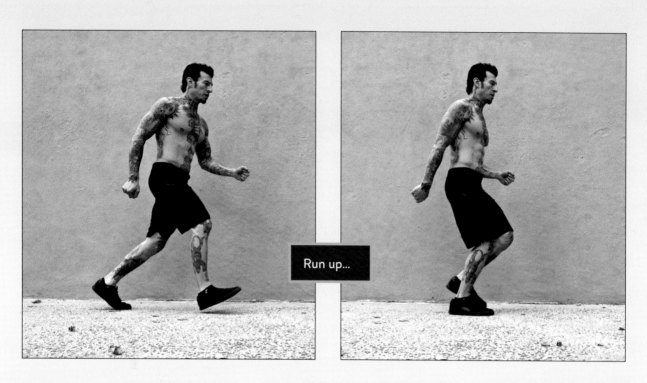

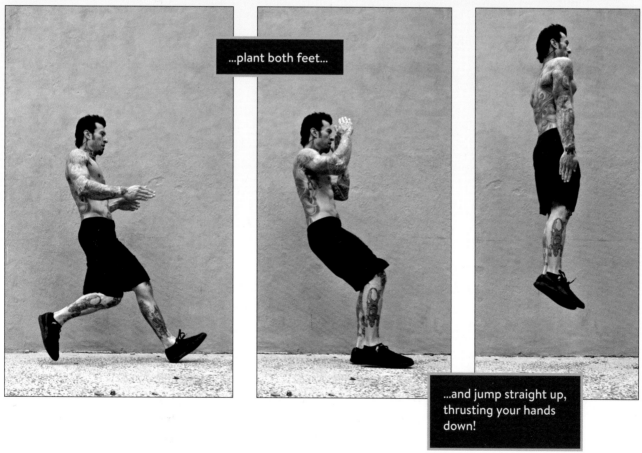

STEP FIVE: BUTT-KICK JUMP

PERFORMANCE

- Stand with your feet around shoulder-width, with your body flexed for action.

- Dip down into a squat, as for *squat jumps* (step 2).

- Explode upwards, using the power of your lower body plus all the total-body spring you can muster.

- At the peak of the jump, explosively bend your legs, driving your heels up and back, kicking yourself in the butt.

- After the kick, throw your legs back down for landing.

- Land softly, catching most of your weight on the balls of your feet.

- Use the elastic rebound to immediately repeat the technique.

EXERCISE X-RAY

Although your goal is to kick your glutes with your heels, the *butt-kick jump* is the first drill in the chain which requires you to lift your *knees* during airtime. If you look at the photos, you'll see that the knees are pulled slightly forward by the hips. This will condition the hips to allow you to perform even more explosive tuck jumps, which come next in the chain. This is also the first step which places *objective performance criteria* onto the athlete: if you don't jump to a certain height, or move with enough leg speed, you will not be able to kick your butt and release your legs in time for landing.

REGRESSION

Some athletes just can't find the speed to kick their backside—at least, at first. They either can't jump high enough, or can't contract their hamstrings with enough force. It can help to begin *unilateral butt-kick jumps*: jump, but only kick yourself with one leg.

PROGRESSION

As ever, the arms can help with explosive momentum—taking them out of the picture will make this technique tougher. Place your hands behind your head—but keep the fingers loose and remember not to pull on your neck.

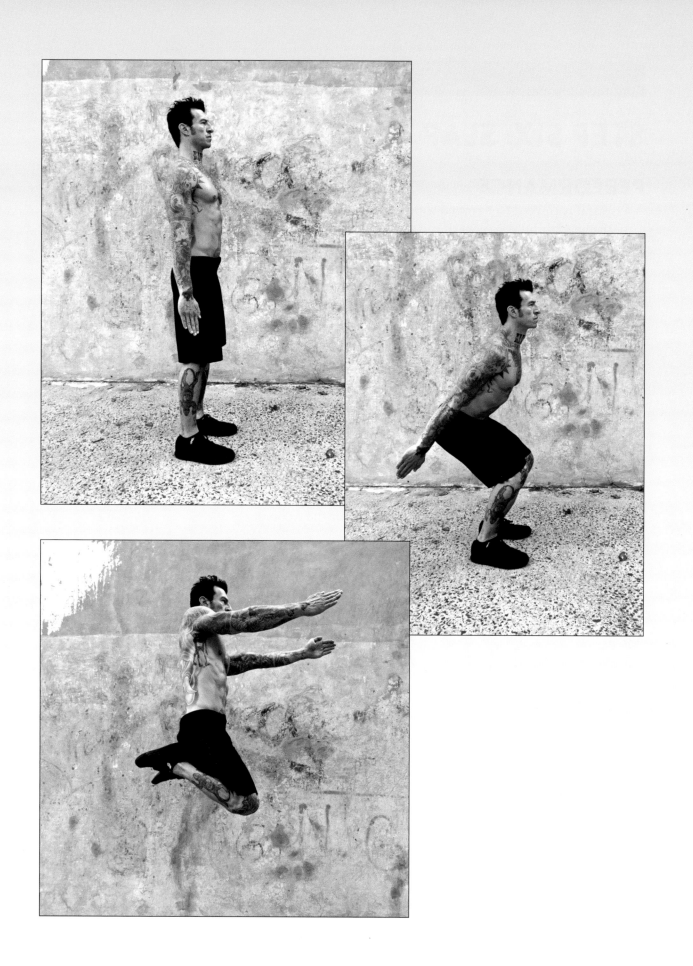

STEP SIX: SLAP TUCK JUMP

PERFORMANCE

- Stand with your feet around shoulder-width, with your body flexed for action. You can place the hands a little in front of the chest, palms down, or keep them by your sides *(see photos)*.

- Dip down into a squat, as for *squat jumps* (step 2).

- Explode upwards, using the power of your lower body plus all the total body spring you can muster.

- At the peak of the jump, explosively draw up your knees up to slap your hands. (If you began with your hands by your sides, you'll have to move them even quicker than your legs.) If you do it right, your knees will be about level with your hips at the top of the movement.

- After the tuck, throw your legs back down for landing.

- Land softly, catching most of your weight on the balls of your feet.

- Use the elastic rebound to immediately repeat the technique.

EXERCISE X-RAY

The *slap tuck jump* is an important step in learning a true tuck (bringing the thighs close to the chest) while jumping—which is beyond the abilities of the average athlete. The best way to learn any difficult bodyweight movement pattern is *gradually*. In step 4 (*butt-kick jumps*) you learned to lift your knees slightly during jumps. In this step, you'll be lifting your thighs to about parallel, to touch your hands. In the next step you will learn to go beyond even that. Step-by-step progressions are always the way to go.

REGRESSION

This is an easy drill to regress—if you can't raise your knees to the level of your hips, drop your hands to slap your knees at a lower point.

PROGRESSION

If slapping the knees is easy, you can explore harder variations with greater hand/arm movement, such as slapping the side of the calves, the insteps or your feet.

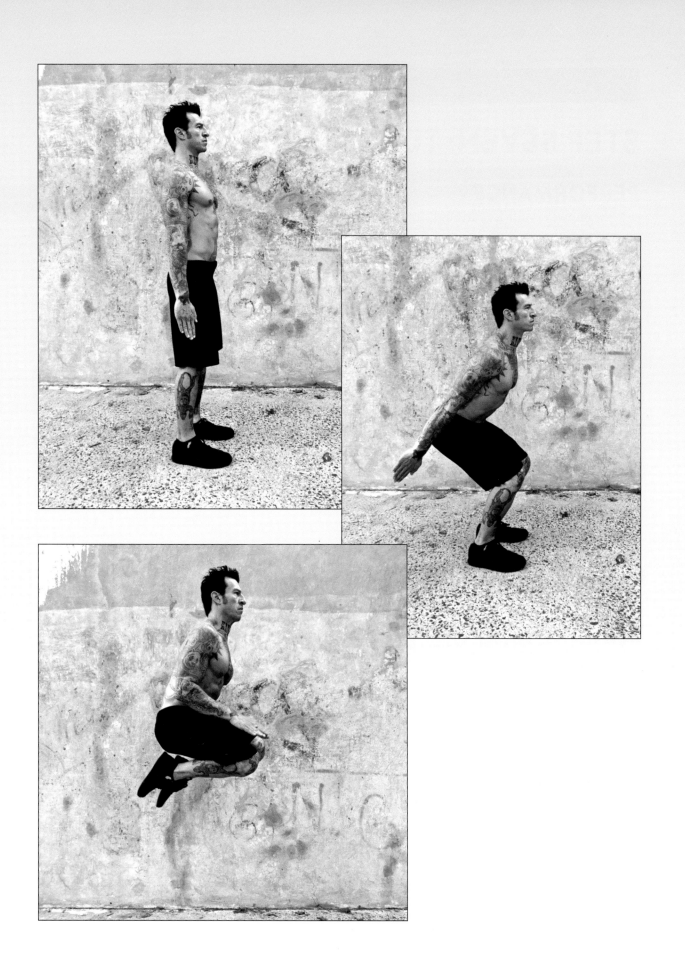

STEP SEVEN: TUCK JUMP

PERFORMANCE

- Stand with your feet around shoulder-width, with your body flexed for action.

- Dip down into a squat, as for *squat jumps* (step 2).

- Explode upwards, using the power of your lower body plus all the total-body spring you can muster.

- At the peak of the jump, explosively draw up your knees as close to your chest as you can. (This is called a *tuck*.) Your trunk will naturally lean forward, but try not to bend over excessively.

- After the tuck, throw your legs back down for landing.

- Land softly, catching most of your weight on the balls of your feet.

- Use the elastic rebound to immediately repeat the technique.

EXERCISE X-RAY

Tuck jumps confer some serious explosive power to the lower body. The calves and ankles, glutes, thighs and even the lower back need plenty of crisp speed to reach the height required for the movement, and the hips and abdomen must have great explosiveness to pull the knees up horizontally during the jump. Tuck jumps may seem simple, but they are an *essential* movement skill for more advanced explosive feats. Simply put, if you can't tuck properly, you can forget becoming *really* fast.

REGRESSION

Form is everything on tuck jumps. If you can't get your knees up close to your chest, try at least bringing them up to hip level. Increased knee height will come with practice.

PROGRESSION

If regular tuck jumps are no problem, increase your height. The classic way to test this is by adding a hand clap under your hamstrings at the peak of the movement. This also accentuates midsection involvement, and builds in some hand speed.

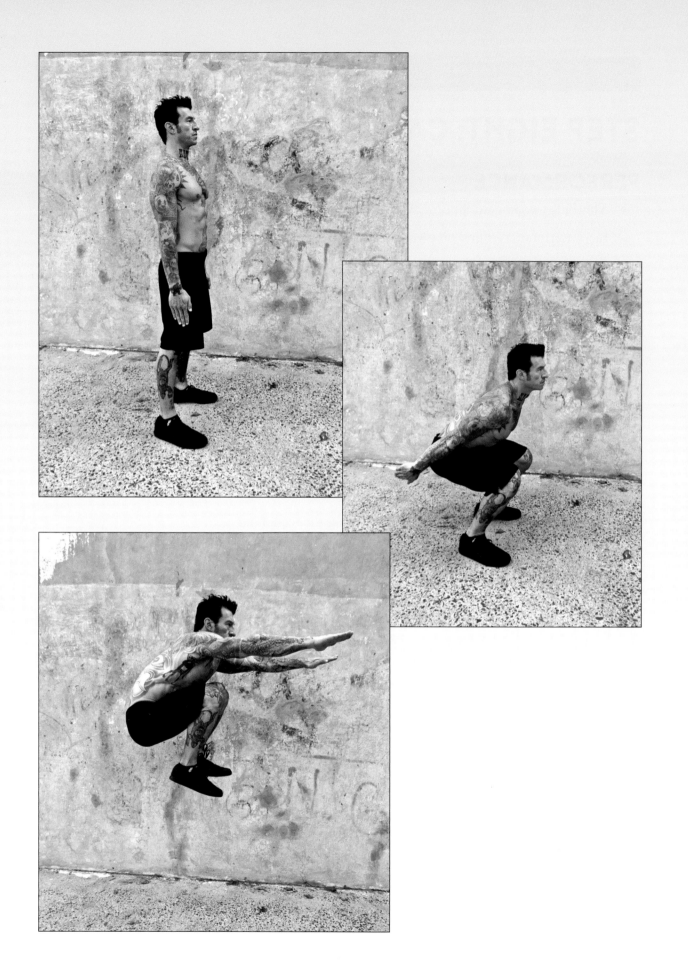

STEP EIGHT: CATCH TUCK JUMP

PERFORMANCE

- This bullet-point description is wrong. It has been drawn from the previous exercise. The correct description is found on p64 of my manuscript, and should read:

- Stand with your feet around shoulder-width, with your body flexed for action.

- Dip down into a squat, as for squat jumps (step 2).

- Explode upwards, using the power of your lower body plus all the total-body spring you can muster.

- Explosively draw up your knees as close to your chest as you can.

- At the peak of the jump, pull your shins into your body with your hands. Your thighs should be completely compressed against your chest at this point.

- Release your shins and, throw your legs back down for landing.

- Land softly, catching most of your weight on the balls of your feet.

- Use the elastic rebound to immediately repeat the technique.

EXERCISE X-RAY

Tuck jumps (step 7) require explosive power in the legs and hips to bring the knees up high. To be able to perform the Master Step of this chain—*suicide jumps*—an athlete also requires some forward power generated by the trunk, to really compress the legs into the abdomen tightly. Mastery of this exercise will develop this quality. "Pulling in" the legs with the arms during a tight tuck is also a very useful pattern in more complex explosive movements, like front and back flips. You may have seen gymnasts performing flips this way.

REGRESSION

At first don't try to pull the tuck too tightly—just perform the best tuck you can, and try to get your arms to meet beyond the legs. Over time, wrap the arms around the legs, and finally pull the legs in tightly with the arms.

PROGRESSION

Once your tuck is tight—with a strong hug of the arms—focus on bringing the knees higher and higher, until they are under the chin.

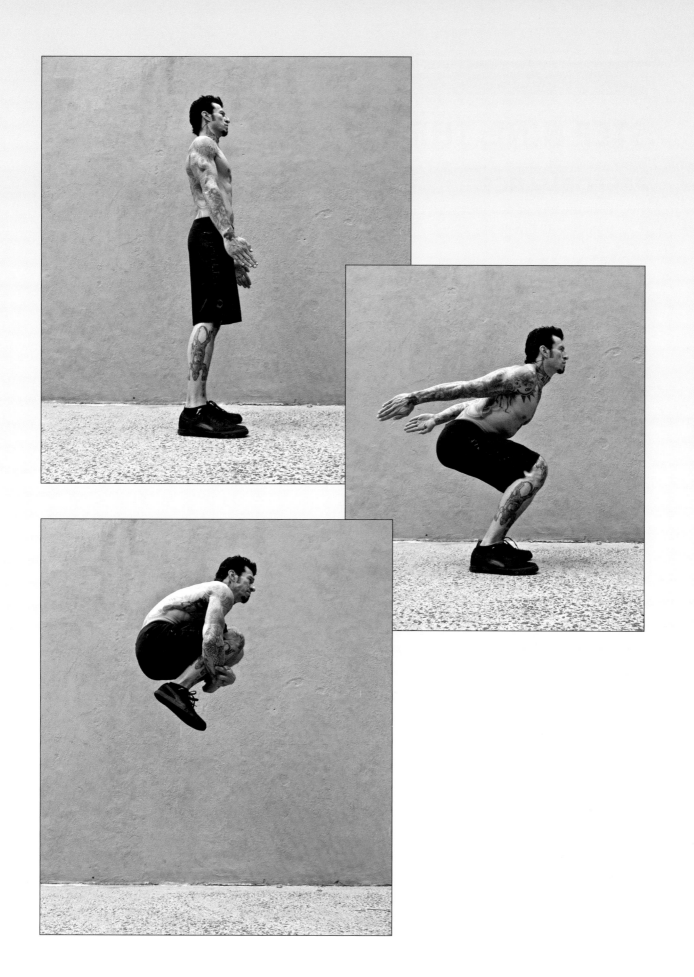

STEP NINE: THREAD JUMP

PERFORMANCE

- Grip the end of one foot with the opposite hand. Keep your standing leg straight, and your trunk as upright as you can.

- Dip slightly with the loaded leg, and explode upwards with that leg, tucking the knee as high, and close to your chest, as you can while staying upright.

- At the peak of the leg movement, whip your linked hand and foot under your jumping foot, so it's behind you. Many athletes go wrong by trying to jump their *foot* through the hole; this is incorrect—you should lift your jumping leg up, and then pull the *hole* back.

- After the thread, throw your leg back down for landing.

- Upon landing, catching most of your weight on the ball of your foot.

- Reposition and repeat the technique, or immediately perform a *reverse thread jump*.

EXERCISE X-RAY

The term *thread* comes from breakdancing; you might even recognize the move from an old hip-hop video. It's pretty obvious why it's called what it is—you thread your foot through the gap like you'd put *thread* through the eye of a needle. This is a great unilateral way to safely prepare for the technical demands of *suicide jumps*. If you screw up, you can just release your foot and land safely.

REGRESSION

Always begin exploring this exercise with a very loose grip around your foot, in case you have to bail quickly. You should begin with a wider-angled hole by gripping the very end of your toes, but if you really need to you can sling a slim towel or belt around your ankle and hold that instead of your foot. That's more forgiving to thread through as you learn the move.

PROGRESSION

Gripping the *outside* of your foot instead of the *toes* makes this move tougher. An even harder version of the thread jump involves beginning with your linked hand/foot *behind* your jumping leg. You then jump up and pass your hand/foot *forward* as your jumping leg threads through (the *reverse thread jump*). Eventually you will be able to perform the front and back thread versions back-to-back.

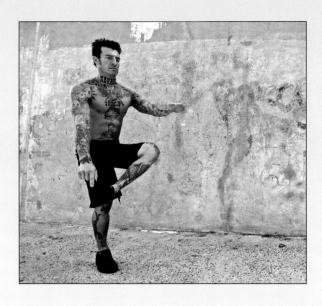
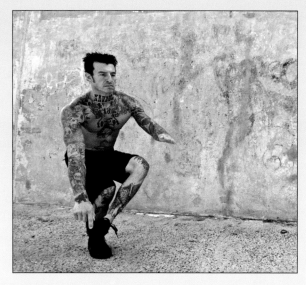
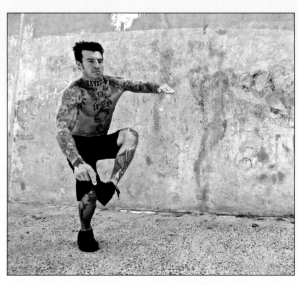
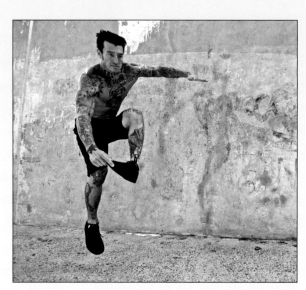
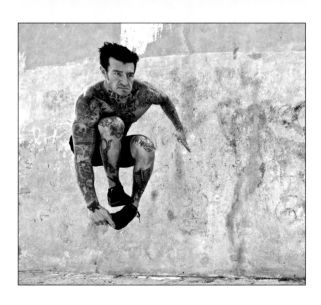
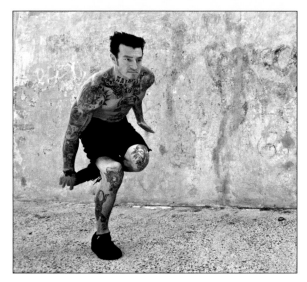

EXPLOSIVE CALISTHENICS

MASTER STEP: SUICIDE JUMP

PERFORMANCE

- Stand with feet around shoulder-width, with your body flexed for action. Hold a length of dowel (a broomstick works well) with a wide grip, in front of your hips. (If you are scared of falling at first, you can use a lightly-gripped rope or belt in place of the stick.)

- Stand up straight. (Beginners seem to think that bending/squatting to hold the bar lower will help. It won't!)

- Dip down slightly. You only want a slight flexion in the knees—less than a quarter squat position.

- Without pausing, explode upwards, tucking your knees up to your chest.

- At the peak of the leg movement, whip the bar under your jumping feet, so it's behind you.

- After the thread, throw your legs back down for landing.

- Upon landing, catching most of your weight on the balls of your feet.

- Reposition and repeat the technique, or immediately perform a *reverse suicide jump* (See page 64).

EXERCISE X-RAY

Any athlete can practice simple jumps—like steps 1-3—to build maximum jumping power. This chain is designed to give you more than that. From step 5 (*butt-kick jumps*) onwards, you will have been gaining the strength, power and technique to *tuck* perfectly—to jump up, bringing the knees up to the chest. *Suicide jumps* represent the *ultimate* tucking drill: if you can't bring your knees very high—and quickly—it's impossible to pass the bar. The exercise also requires mastery of all the basic components of explosive jumping; a powerful lift-off, hip and waist integration, the capacity to quickly throw down the feet (faster than gravity), and expert force-absorption upon landing. Once this drill is second nature to you, more impressive explosive techniques—kip-ups, but also the front and back flips, in particular—will come much easier than you would otherwise imagine.

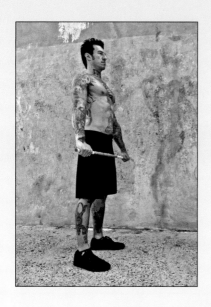
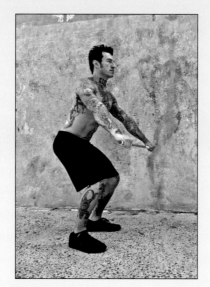
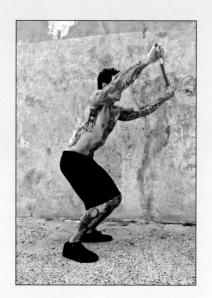

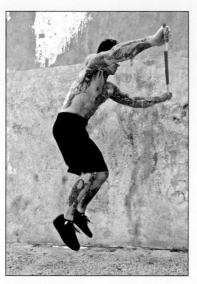
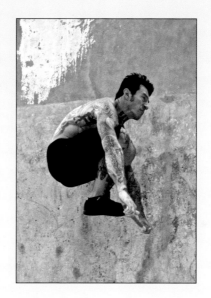

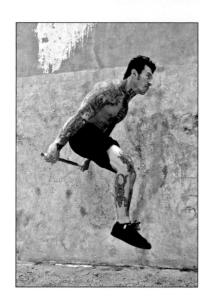
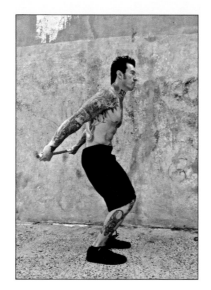
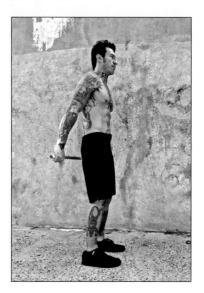

GOING BEYOND

Once an athlete can consistently perform smooth, clean *suicide jumps*, he or she will have—by necessity—developed the skills of *launching*, *landing*, and especially *tucking* to a high level. These are the most important abilities required to excel in more complex explosives, flips in particular. That doesn't mean your time performing power jumps is over. Jumps are an essential movement to build—and *maintain*—power in the lower body. Just like a karate master must continue performing their basic forms in order to drill the fundamentals, so all athletes desiring power must keep working with jumps.

So where do you go, once the suicide jump is easy? First things first—the suicide jump is *easy*, right? Simple way to tell—do it backwards! Hold the bar behind your back, and jump up, pulling the bar under your feet in mid-air, and in front of you.

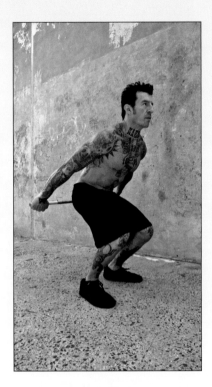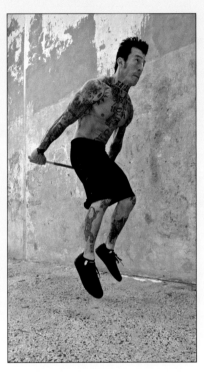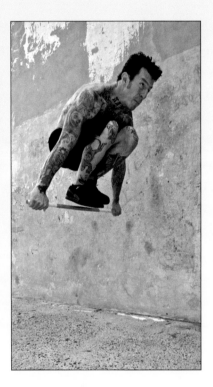

In fact, I'm teasing. The *reverse suicide jump* is much, *much* harder for most athletes than the basic suicide jump. The awkward position of the bar, combined with the fact that humans almost never jump *backwards* over an object, makes this version very tricky. But if you're really looking to master the suicide jump, this is a must-do. Try it, at least—but be careful not to crash!

As ever, you can increase difficulty with calisthenics movements simply by manipulating *leverage*. In a tuck, for example, the knees are *bent*, transmitting less load to the hip flexors and midsection—*extending* the legs will increase the workload, and the challenge. You can do this by gradually decreasing your knee-bend until the legs are locked, or you can start with your legs locked, and increase the angle of your legs. This second method is shown below; start with the *angled pike jump*, and move to a *full pike jump*, where the straight legs wind up parallel to the floor.

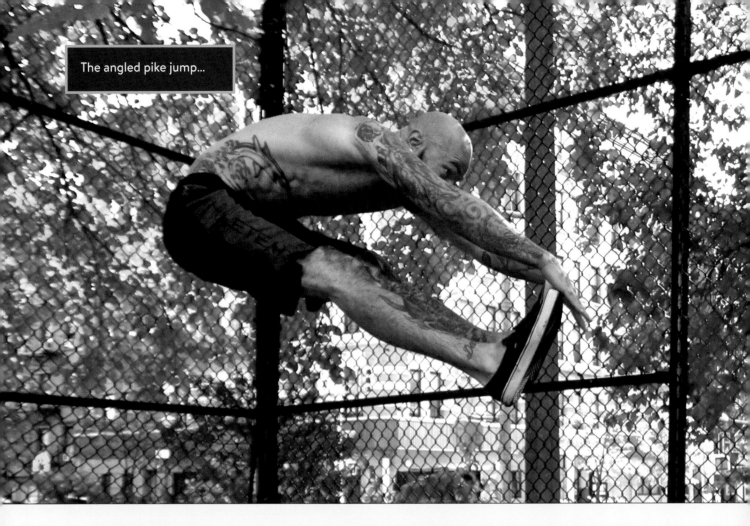

The angled pike jump...

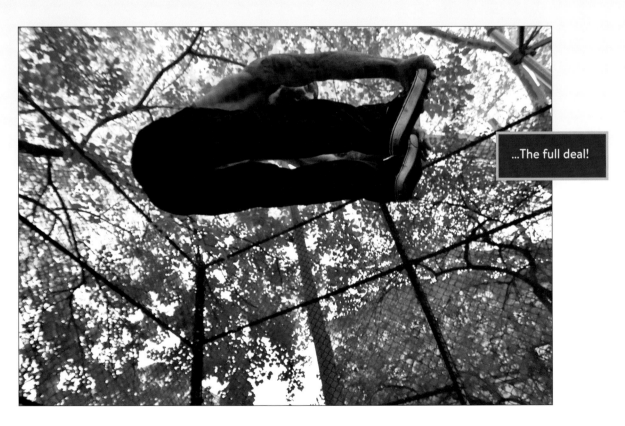

...The full deal!

An alternative way of moving forward in your jumping ability is to perform more explosive mid-air stunts, requiring more height and total-body power. Of course, this is exactly what you are doing by moving onto the *front* and *back flip* chains in this manual: what is a *standing front flip* if not one of the hardest *jumping* techniques you can perform?

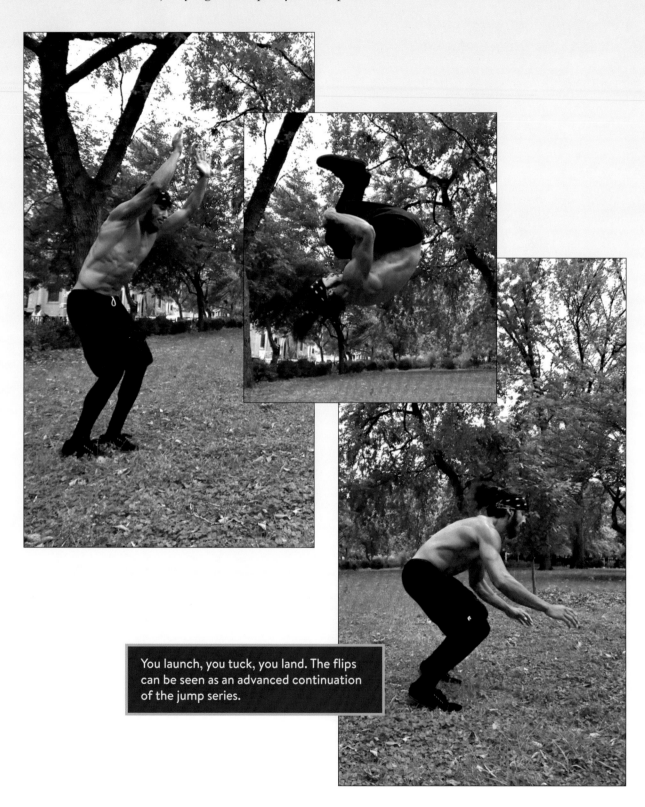

You launch, you tuck, you land. The flips can be seen as an advanced continuation of the jump series.

It could be argued that if you are at a high level on the back or front flip chain, you no longer need to perform simple jumps to build power, as the flips themselves require power-jumping. I personally think that retaining some basic training on jumps is a great idea; simply because flips and similar techniques require a lot of energy to focus on agility, equilibrium and coordination. Basic up-and-down jumps require very little—all your energy and focus can be devoted to power and height (or length), making jumps more efficient for building base power. Many athletes begin their jump training with box jumps, but I am convinced that if you're going to explore jumping up onto objects, this is best tackled after some basic proficiency. Box jumps add variety and also allow for height measurement. They also require a different mindset than regular jumps. Remember though, as long as the object you jump onto is dry and sturdy, you don't need a gym plyo box. Take a tip from those parkour guys...they use anything. Now *that's* functional jumping!

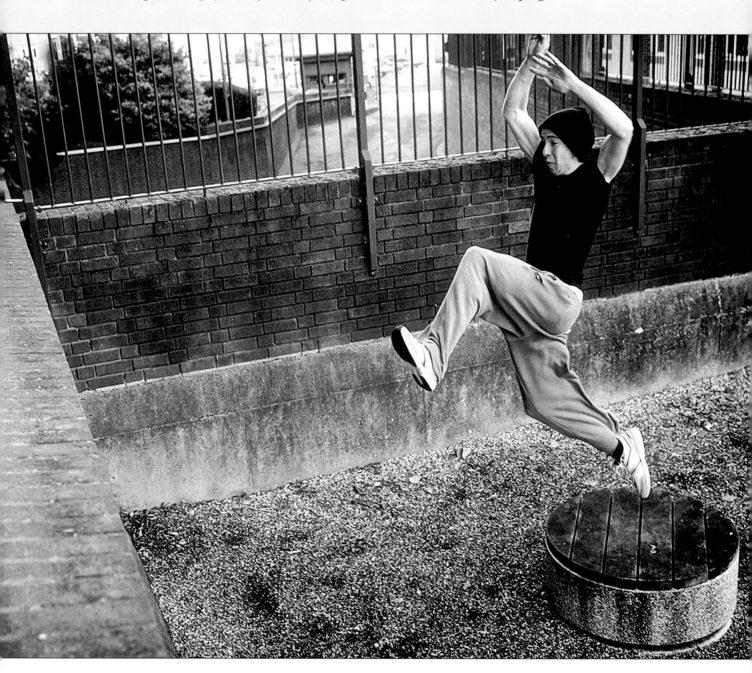

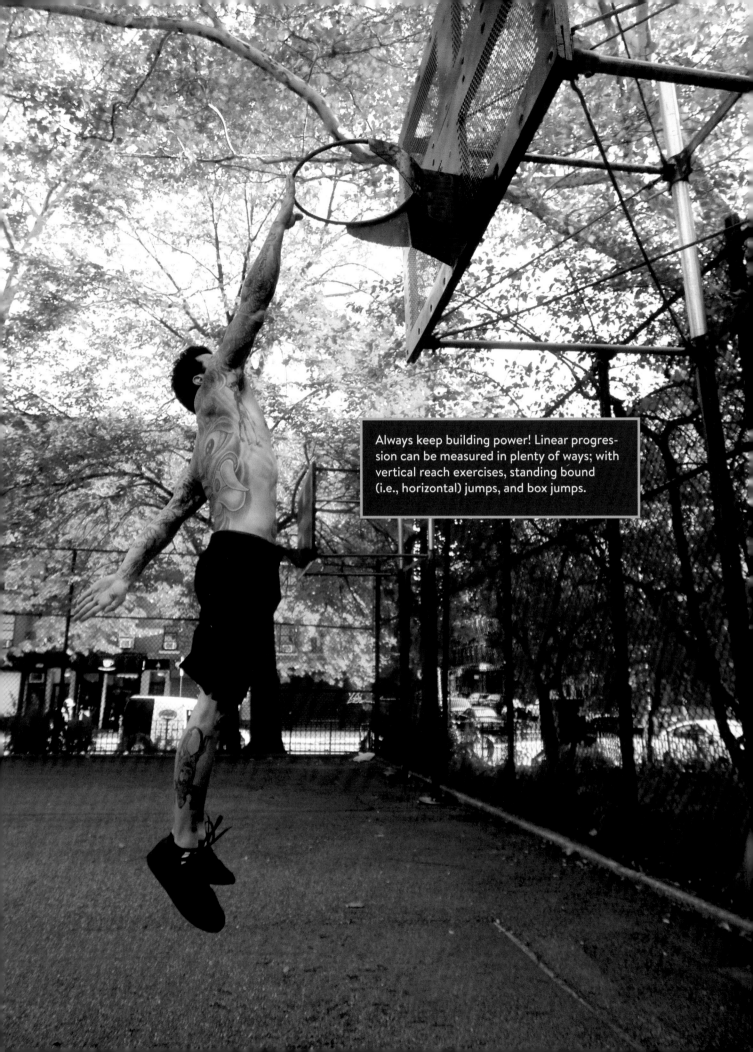

Always keep building power! Linear progression can be measured in plenty of ways; with vertical reach exercises, standing bound (i.e., horizontal) jumps, and box jumps.

SMALL SPACE DRILLS

Following are three useful speed and power techniques you can utilize in your routine for variety, as ancillary work or to train your muscles from different angles. They are all solo drills, and they require zero equipment. Unlike the progressive exercises in the chains, most of the following drills can be performed rhythmically for higher reps, and can work well when used with any of the chains in this book. In this sense, they can also work as warm-ups or finishing exercises in an explosives session.

COSSACKS

Jump training tends to build power in a shallow range of motion. To power-up the knees, hips and ankles *on the stretch*, you need *Cossacks*. Named after the traditional dance of the Cossack people, assume a low stance and bob up and down slightly, stretching your legs out in an alternate manner. Also builds tension-flexibility (*supple strength*) and balance.

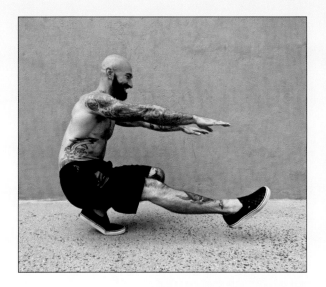
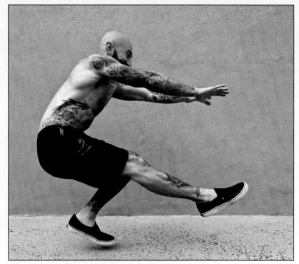
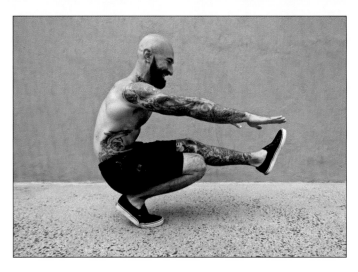

WIDE-TO-CLOSE POP-UPS

Fast legs must be paired with fast arms to unlock total-body power. From a close pushup position, dip and explode your body up so that your hands leave the floor. Quickly spread them so that you "catch" yourself in a wide pushup position. Without pausing, dip down and repeat for reps.

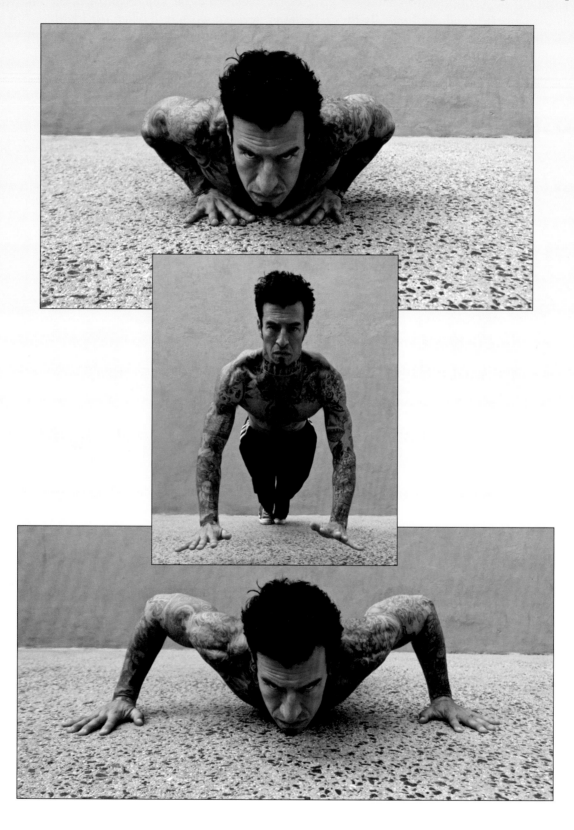

WALL THREADS

This one's similar to the two threads in the preceding chain (Step 9 and 10), so it works well with jumps, although like all these drills you can mix and match. Place one foot on a sturdy vertical base, and jump over it, keeping the foot in place as long as you can. Awesome for fast feet.

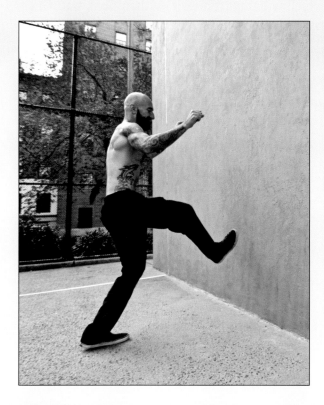
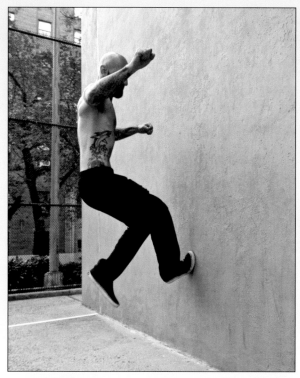
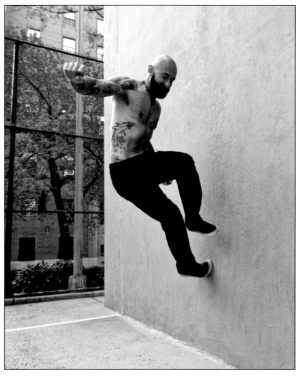
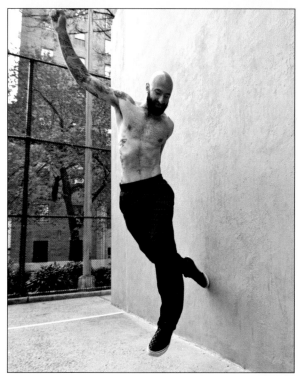

LIGHTS OUT!

If you really want to become explosive, your legs are the source of it all—and the best way to train them is with progressive *power jumps*. Weights or slow movements just won't do it. All athletes should learn the five basic skills of jumping, which will impart power on their own, but which are indispensable if the athlete wishes to move forward in acrobatics.

Although I talk about the "skills" required in jumping, these skills are simple and easy to learn, and are very closely connected to simple power (*strength x speed*). For this reason—although there is some overlap—jumps should be primarily thought of as a basic *power* movement, rather than a complex *skill* movement (like a *kip-up*). The different types of drills must be approached differently, as I explain in Part III of the manual.

When utilized correctly, the jump chain will build maximum speed-power in the hips and lower body. To round out a basic power training regime, the athlete should pair up *jumps* with a movement chain which performs a similar job for the upper-body and arms. The best drills for this are *power pushups*: they're up next.

5

Power Pushups
STRENGTH BECOMES POWER

I t's always been kinda ironic to me that when sports coaches think *explosive*, they immediately turn to *lower-body* work—box jumps, broad leaps, and the like. When I was in jail, convict-athletes were much more dedicated to *upper-body* explosive work...power pushups, pop-ups, behind-the-back pushups and triple claps were the order of the day. These moves gave those men arms like freaking jackhammers. It skyrocketed their power levels, maximized their speed, and also added slabs of muscle to their torsos and guns. This prison approach still makes a lot more sense to me. I'm not disrespecting lower-body work—*you need to do those jumps!*—but the upper-body needs survival power at least as much. Punching, blocking strikes, throwing, pushing—these techniques all require optimal power if they are gonna be devastating. If you want to knock someone out, your punch has to be explosive, and so does your upper-body. If you get attacked in a backstreet, nobody cares how high you can jump.

There's a tasty bonus to having an explosive upper-body. Speed-power training is essentially training the nervous system and joints to handle greater loads. The more power you have in your arms, chest and shoulders, the *stronger* they become. And the stronger they become, the harder you can work them and the *bigger* they get. Calisthenics athletes who only ever perform their exercises in a slow gear can get pretty big, but a guy who mixes in high-speed work will definitely gain an edge in strength, and size too.

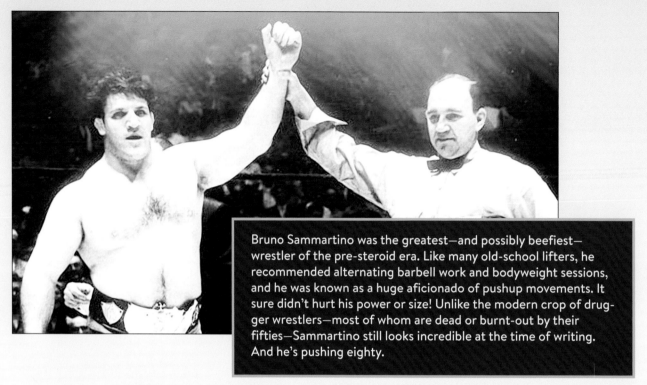

Bruno Sammartino was the greatest—and possibly beefiest—wrestler of the pre-steroid era. Like many old-school lifters, he recommended alternating barbell work and bodyweight sessions, and he was known as a huge aficionado of pushup movements. It sure didn't hurt his power or size! Unlike the modern crop of drugger wrestlers—most of whom are dead or burnt-out by their fifties—Sammartino still looks incredible at the time of writing. And he's pushing eighty.

Perhaps part of the reason why athletes on the outside are jumping over ribbons and zig-zagging through cones is that there's a lack of knowledge when it comes to upper-body explosives. Yes, you sometimes see brothers throwing medicine balls around, but this is an inferior method—it has always been an inferior method. The balls are too damn light to trigger true changes in power. Sure, you can use heavy barbells explosively—push presses, jerks and what have you—but these methods typically focus on such high loads that speed is badly compromised, and true power is lost. Bodyweight pushups also prepare the athlete excellently for the open-hand springing-type movements (*front handsprings, back handsprings*) which are such crucial elements of acrobatics. There is also the fact that the heavy external lifts are definitely gonna wreck your shoulders over time. (Not to mention your wrists, elbows, upper back...etc). As ever, the best way is the *natural* way. Use your body, dude.

DECONSTRUCTING POWER PUSHUPS

It can be difficult to describe the perfect power pushup, because so many of the techniques vary. But we can discuss a few of the principles that cover the majority of moves in the technical chain which follows:

ELBOW POSITIONING

This is the first consideration. Where you put your *hands* is crucial, because the elbows follow the hands in closed chain exercises like pushups; and the shoulders follow the elbows. The secret, as ever, is found in what feels *natural*. Avoid extra-wide hand positions—they will not generate optimal power, and they place the shoulder joint in a vulnerable position. At the other end of the spectrum, always using a real close position can be too hard on the wrists, forearms and elbows if you are going explosive. Find somewhere in the middle that feels right to you. For regular pushups, I like a shoulder-width hand position, or slightly closer, to allow my elbows to brush my lats. For explosive pushups, most people find that slightly wider than shoulder width allows them to spring back hardest, allowing the elastic tendons of the shoulder girdle to absorb a little more force than the elbows.

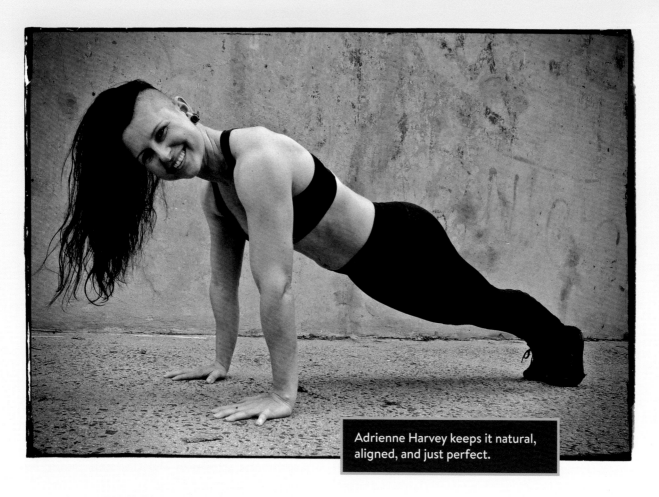

Adrienne Harvey keeps it natural, aligned, and just perfect.

HAND POSITIONING

A few pointers on how to use the hands. Some guys with banged up wrists perform pushups on their knuckles—even the back of their hands. Trust me, trying this with explosive pushups is a recipe for a quick fracture. Even if your knucks are karate-strong, one bad rep can "turn" your hand on its side—like an ankle can turn during running—leading to a broken wrist. Keep your palm flat on the floor and spread the fingers a little; spread fingers act as shock absorbers, saving stress on the wrists and forearms; endeavor to spread the force as much as you can through the hands.

ALIGNMENT

This third point is a biggie. When you do pushups, you need to keep your body *aligned*—your thigh-bones, hips and torso must form a straight line. Your hips shouldn't sag down, and—listen to me, brethren—*your butt shouldn't come up.*

Now, most serious athletes seem to understand this fact when they are demonstrating standard pushup form. But when they start performing power pushups, it all goes out the window. Even on strong guys, the butt shoots up as soon as they push themselves up! This ungodly habit is called "worming" (sometime called the "caterpillar") because it's evocative of an inchworm pushing his little body up as he crawls along.

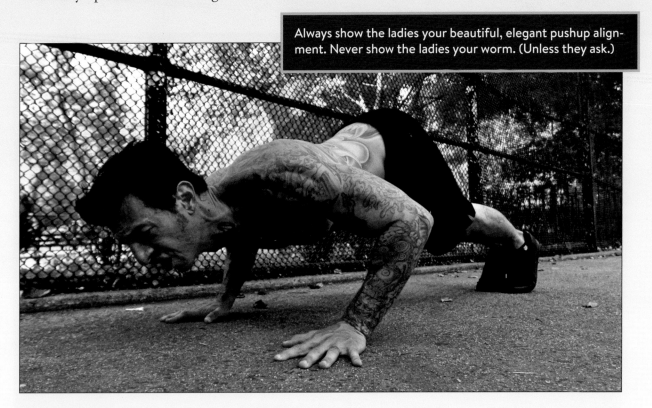

Always show the ladies your beautiful, elegant pushup alignment. Never show the ladies your worm. (Unless they ask.)

There's a reason why this habit is associated with explosive pushups. It improves leverage and increases "airtime" (for claps, say) making all exercises much easier. Unless you are deliberately performing *pike, jackknife* or *Aztec*-style pushups, worming is a form of cheating and should be avoided. Never forget that you are performing your exercises to *build* freakish levels of power—not to *demonstrate* that power. Yes, to the untrained eye, worming may make it look like you can clap more times in between pushups. But you are only fooling the foolish. Strict form and an aligned body will build greater levels of explosive strength, faster.

Why would you cheat yourself outta gains?! I won't have it—your training is too important to me.

STANCE

For slow, strength-based pushups, I always recommend a close stance—because close legs prevent cheating by *twisting*, so commonly seen in one-arm work. Explosive pushups are a different animal. For one, the higher speeds mean you need a more secure base; for another, asymmetrical exercises are much rarer in explosive work (they don't exist in the power pushup chain at all), therefore twisting, and similar cheating methods, aren't such a problem. For this reason, you do not need to keep your legs close together.

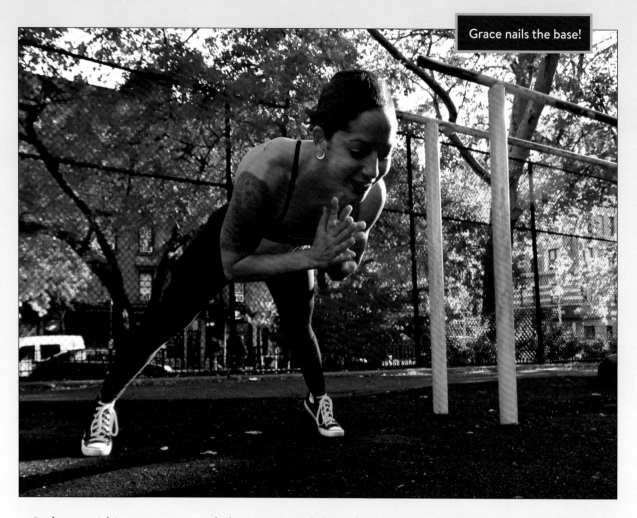
Grace nails the base!

In fact—within reason—a wide base is a good thing for explosive pushups. Somewhere between just beyond shoulder width and twice shoulder-width is going to be perfect for just about everyone. More advanced athletes—with superior balance—can apply a close stance. Experiment, Edison.

DEPTH

Another difference between standard speed and power pushups is *depth*—how far your chest descends on the negative. For regular pushups, a "full" range of motion is advisable—that means descending until your sternum is about a fist's width from the floor. For power pushups, you don't need to go that deep—you are looking for maximum strength-speed, and going too deep will slow you down. To train the joints and nervous system to maximum explosiveness, you really only need to go a few inches; maybe one-third of the way down. Think in terms of your arms "dipping" you down, rather than *lowering* you for a full negative. Experiment; if you don't dip far enough, you won't get enough spring to bounce back as high as you can; dip too low, and your tendons elastic force goes out of its comfort zone.

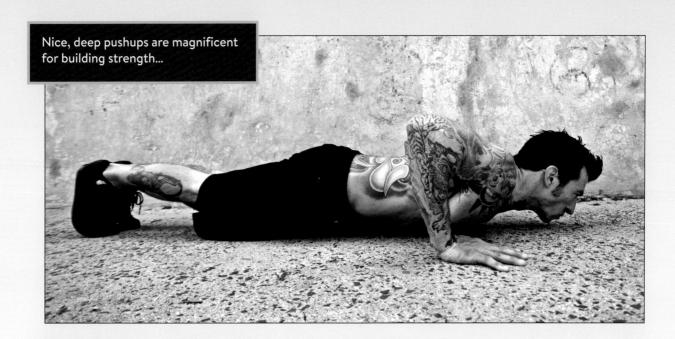

Nice, deep pushups are magnificent for building strength...

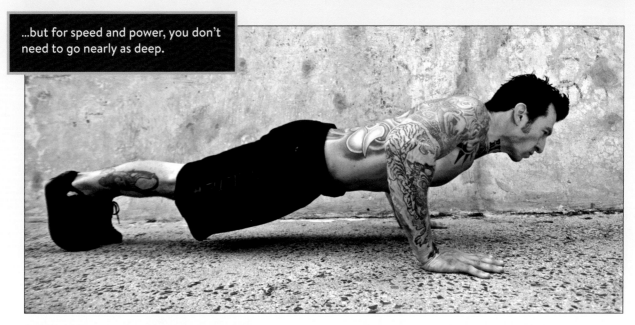

...but for speed and power, you don't need to go nearly as deep.

MYOTATIC REBOUND

When you are performing slow pushups, a pause at the bottom is ideal—it generates huge strength and muscle. But if it's power and speed you are working for, *don't pause at the bottom*. Quickly dip down under the pull of gravity, and immediately blast back up, as fast as you can. Doing so will utilize the capacity of your tendons to express elastic force; it will also allow you to make the best use of your *myotatic reflex*. (For more on applying plyometrics, see page 315). Don't think of this quick reversal as "bouncing"—think of it as "applying rebound".

THE POWER PUSHUP CHAIN

The chain begins with the simplest, safest, explosive pushing exercise; *incline pop-ups* (step 1). The athlete can perform ballistic presses while in a semi-standing position. Once this becomes easy, we move to *kneeling push-offs* (step 2). These are much more explosive, yet require scaled down arm and chest power—plus less midsection strength—due to the leverage of the kneeling position.

With *flat pop-ups* (step 3), the athlete moves to the floor, continuing the basic pop-up movement learned in step 1. When pop-ups (which involve pushing a few inches off the floor with the hands) become easy, the athlete is ready to add a clap to the movement: the classic *clap pushup* (step 4).

Once the clap pushup has been mastered, the athlete should build to longer hand movements during "airtime", which will necessitate a more powerful launch. Once the hands can be clapped easily, the next step is to slap the *chest* with the hands (step 5), then the *hips* (step 6). The most difficult variation is to clap the hands *behind the back*, as in *convict pushups* (step 7).

The next two steps prepare the athlete for the demanding *Superman pushup*, where the hands are thrown out in front, and the feet are lifted behind you, as if you were flying—hence the name. You begin by mastering the hands-out-front position with *half-supers* (step 8), then you learn to lift the legs off the floor at the *top* of the movement, a drastic variation which requires great strength in the trunk, plus total-body explosiveness. This is called a *full-body pop-up* (step 9). Once the half-superman and the full-body pop-up are developed well, the athlete can slot these two techniques together, lifting the legs off the ground with the hands thrown in front; this comprises the Master Step, the *Superman*.

This variation requires vastly more power and speed than regular clap pushups, which is the level most athletes stall at. Not you, though.

STEP ONE: INCLINE POP-UP

PERFORMANCE

- Find a solid, secure base that is around chest height.

- Place your hands on the base, at around shoulder width.

- Place your feet as wide as you feel you need to, for balance.

- Keep your legs, hips and torso aligned and slightly inclined towards your pushing base.

- Bend arms and shoulders, bringing your torso to a point several inches from the base.

- Immediately push explosively off the base, straightening your arms.

- Push hard enough to allow your hands to leave the base by several inches.

- As gravity reverses your movement, "catch" the base with your hands again.

- Use the elastic rebound to immediately repeat the technique.

EXERCISE X-RAY

Inclines are a perfect way to gently condition the shoulders, elbows and wrists for the harder work to come.

REGRESSION

A novice could begin explosive pushups at an even easier level, by pushing off a vertical wall; however since athletes should have some joint conditioning work under their belts before exploring explosive training (see page 24), this isn't really necessary.

PROGRESSION

In all incline pushup work, the lower the base you push off—that is, the lower the hands and the more inclined your body—the harder the exercise. You can make things tougher by using a lower surface over time; begin with a table or work surface, then graduate to a bunk or bed, then a box, etc. A great way to make this exercise progressive is to use the bottom portion of a set of stairs or steps—use lower steps over time. Whatever equipment you use, you need to ensure it's real sturdy; that applies to all explosive work.

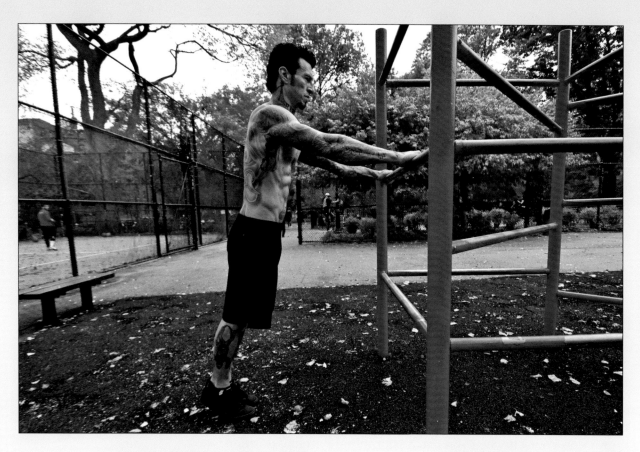

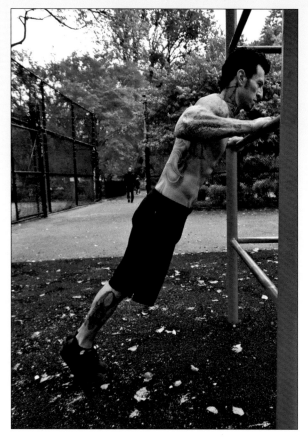

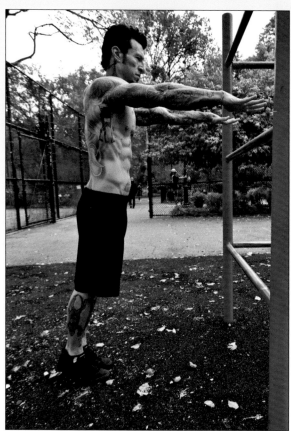

STEP TWO: KNEELING PUSH-OFF

PERFORMANCE

- Kneel on the floor, with your thighs and trunk upright. Place your arms out in front of you, and keep them braced.

- Lean forward until your torso begins to fall; keep your thighs, hips and trunk aligned.

- Touch down with your palms at around shoulder width or slightly wider.

- Bend your arms and shoulders, dipping your torso closer to the floor. Stronger athletes can dip down all the way to the ground (*see photo*).

- Immediately push explosively off the base, straightening your arms.

- Explode upwards as hard as you can, keeping your thighs hips and trunk aligned.

- Stop yourself when you reach your initial kneeling position.

- Repeat the technique.

EXERCISE X-RAY

This movement requires a big jump up in the power stakes—believe it or not, some strong guys have trouble with kneeling push-offs at their first attempt. It's not that they lack strength—it's because they just don't have the speed to turn that strength into *power*.

REGRESSION

It's really cheating, but bending at the hips is one way to approach this exercise if you just can't manage it. A better way is to incline your body by placing your hands on a base. Some athletes have found that it can help to get this "feel" of this technique by spending some time just performing the *negative* phase—falling to the ground onto the hands.

PROGRESSION

Once your speed kicks in, you'll find that this exercise is achievable *unilaterally*—pushing off one arm. This is an exceptional way to build punching force. Some athletes can even perform this exercise (with two arms) in the classic pushup style—using their feet/toes as a pivot, rather than the knees. That should considered an extreme variation, however.

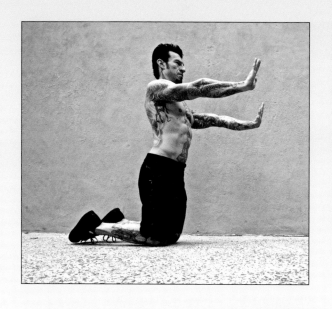
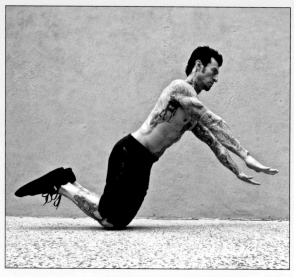
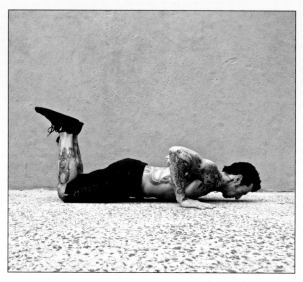
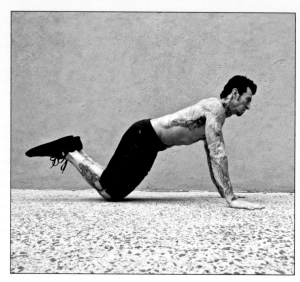
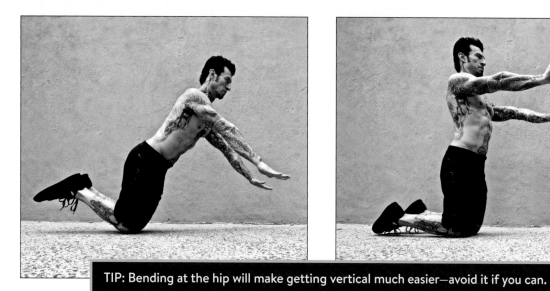

TIP: Bending at the hip will make getting vertical much easier—avoid it if you can.

EXPLOSIVE CALISTHENICS

STEP THREE: POP-UP

PERFORMANCE

- Squat down, place your palms on the floor and stretch your legs out behind you.

- Your palms should be below your shoulders, spread at shoulder width or wider.

- Place your feet at whatever width you are comfortable with; beginners should use a wider base, experts can go closer.

- Keep your legs, hips and torso aligned and horizontal.

- Bend your arms and shoulders, dipping your torso towards the floor.

- Immediately push explosively off the floor, straightening your arms.

- Push hard enough to allow your hands to leave the floor.

- As gravity reverses your movement, "catch" the floor with your hands again.

- Use the elastic rebound to immediately repeat the technique.

EXERCISE X-RAY

Pop-ups are a near-magical preliminary exercise for those brothers and sisters who want to get better at *clap pushups* (step 4, next). Many athletes are directed to perform clap pushups to gain upper-body power...and fail miserably, often crashing into the floor in the process. Pop-ups serve as a wonderful bridge towards the more difficult clapping version.

REGRESSION

This exercise is the basis of almost all explosive pushups, and the transition between regular (slow) pushups and power pushups (via *pop-ups*) is very simple. Just begin trying to increase pressing speed when you can. Eventually your hands will leave the floor for a tiny distance.

PROGRESSION

Pop-ups are a perfect exercise to begin generating the airtime that athletes need to be able to master harder plyometric variations, and this is how you should approach them—really use them to build height over time. In the early days, your hands will barely get clear of the ground; but with a little practice, you'll be flying upwards.

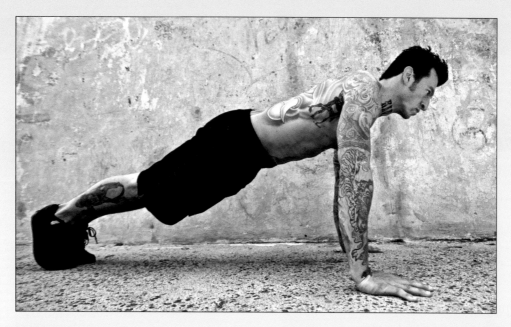

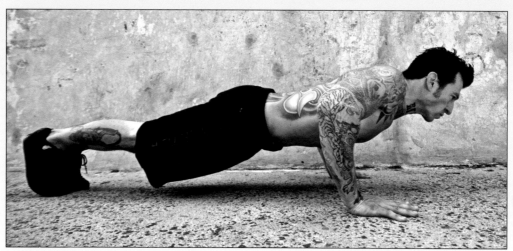

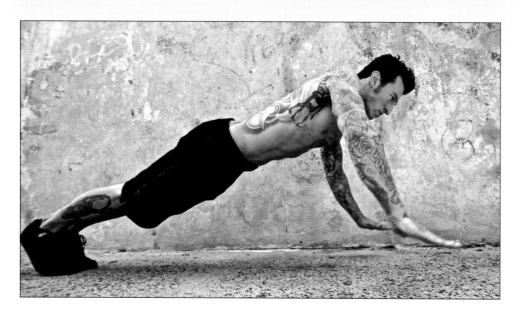

STEP FOUR: CLAP PUSHUP

PERFORMANCE

- Squat down, place your palms on the floor and stretch your legs out behind you.

- Your palms should be below your shoulders, spread at shoulder width or wider.

- Place your feet at whatever width you are comfortable with; beginners should use a wider base, experts can go closer.

- Keep your legs, hips and torso aligned and horizontal.

- Bend your arms and shoulders, dipping your torso towards the floor.

- Immediately push explosively off the base, straightening your arms.

- Explode upwards as hard as you can, and while you are in mid-air, quickly clap your hands together—the clap should be audible.

- As gravity reverses your movement, return your palms downwards to "catch" the floor with your hands again.

- Use the elastic rebound to immediately repeat the technique.

EXERCISE X-RAY

Clap pushups are probably considered the classic upper-body exercise for explosive pushing power—and with great reason. Boxers, martial artists and football players have always known that this exercise build great levels of torso power and quick hands, whilst toughening the arms and shoulders.

REGRESSION

Begin with the hands close together and they travel less distance.

PROGRESSION

There is a pretty classic linear way to improve your clap pushups, once your form is impeccable. You know what I'm gonna say, right? Add more claps before landing! Many guys get so fast with their hands that they can do half a dozen claps, but this is more of a trick than anything—the hands look like they're *fluttering* rather than *clapping*, and the airtime required typically encourages *worming* (see page 76). You are better off focusing on good, strong pushes and building up to a nice, audible double, and even triple clap. Beyond that point, focus on striking the body with the hands.

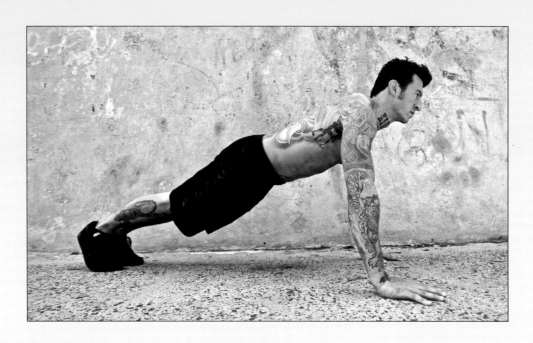

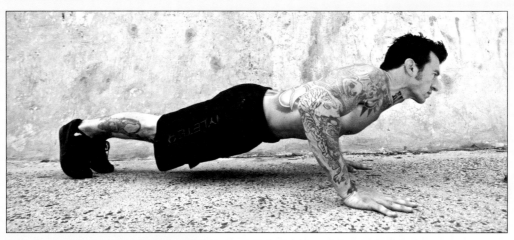

TIP: With all legs-extended pushups, a good way to increase intensity is to put the feet up on something. The higher your feet, the greater the proportion of bodyweight going through your arms.

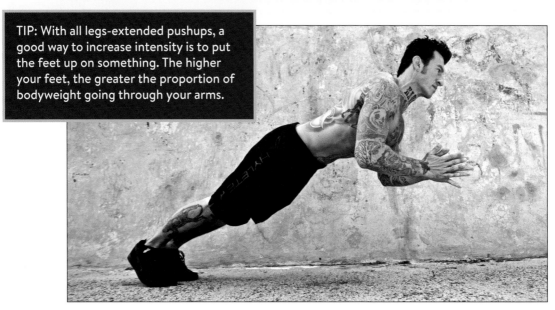

STEP FIVE: CHEST-STRIKE PUSHUP

PERFORMANCE

- Squat down, place your palms on the floor and stretch your legs out behind you.

- Your palms should be below your shoulders, spread at shoulder width or wider.

- Place your feet at whatever width you are comfortable with; beginners should use a wider base, experts can go closer.

- Keep your legs, hips and torso aligned and horizontal.

- Bend your arms and shoulders, dipping your torso towards the floor.

- Immediately push explosively off the floor, straightening your arms.

- Explode upwards as hard as you can, and while you are catching air, whip your hands vertically upwards to slap your chest with your palms.

- As gravity reverses your movement, return your palms downwards to "catch" the floor with your hands again.

- Use the elastic rebound to immediately repeat the technique.

EXERCISE X-RAY

The degree of hand movement during the airtime portion of a power pushup is a great way to measure the amount of airtime you can get—and, likewise, the amount of airtime you can get increases in direct proportion to your upper-body explosive pushing power. This is why chest-strikes represent a significant step upwards in ability from simple *clap pushups*; the hands cover a greater distance. The biceps are also involved, and are forced to fast-twitch with lightning speed to *snap* the palms upwards.

REGRESSION

Begin by just lifting the hands *towards* the chest, before "catching" the floor. In time you'll be able to slap your pecs.

PROGRESSION

It's simple to progress from *chest-strike pushups* to *hip-strikes*. Once you have mastered the chest touch, move to touching your ribs; when that's easy touch your obliques at the top of the rep. From there it's not far to the hips.

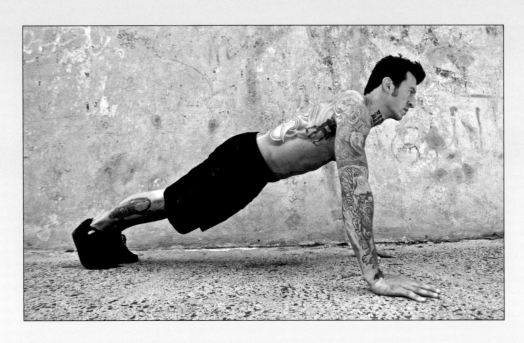

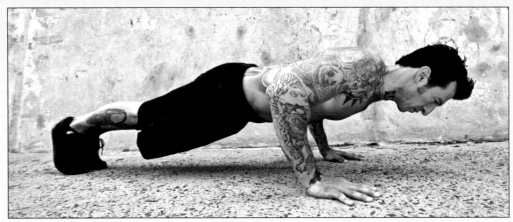

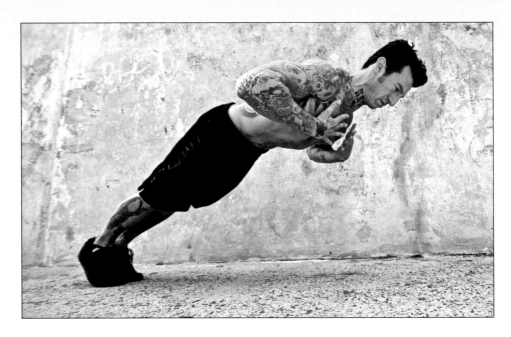

STEP SIX: HIP-STRIKE PUSHUP

PERFORMANCE

- Squat down, place your palms on the floor and stretch your legs out behind you.

- Your palms should be below your shoulders, spread at shoulder width or wider.

- Place your feet at whatever width you are comfortable with; beginners should use a wider base, experts can go closer.

- Keep your legs, hips and torso aligned and horizontal.

- Bend your arms and shoulders, dipping your torso towards the floor.

- Immediately push explosively off the floor, straightening your arms.

- Explode upwards as hard as you can, and while you are catching air, whip your hands back to slap your hips.

- As gravity reverses your movement, return your hands in front of you "catch" the floor with your hands again.

- Use the elastic rebound to immediately repeat the technique.

EXERCISE X-RAY

Even powerful athletes, who can perform *clap pushups* fairly easily, can get their asses kicked when they try clapping their hands *behind their backs* during their plyo pushups. *Hip-strike pushups* are a killer bridging exercise between clapping in front of the body, and clapping behind the back (step 7).

REGRESSION

If you can't reach the hips just yet, split the difference between the chest and hips and attempt to strike your belly.

PROGRESSION

The jump from *hip-strikes* to *convict pushups* (step 7) can be a pretty big one for some athletes. As ever, the key to making *impossible* calisthenics feats *possible* lies in multiple small steps. Once you can strike your hips, inch your hands back a tad farther over time, until you can touch the sides of your thighs. From there, work on throwing your hands up *behind* your hips—almost like a straight-arm kickback. Once you can get the hands up behind your back on each rep, bringing them into contact (*convict pushups*) will not seem quite so overwhelming.

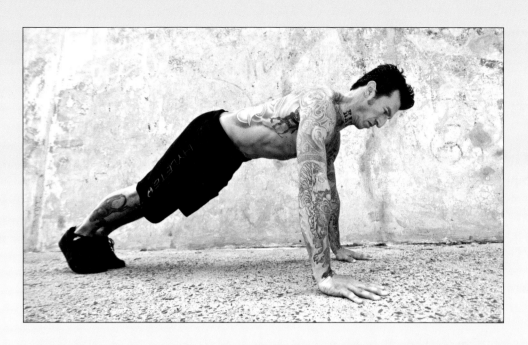

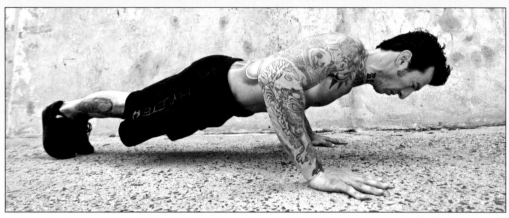

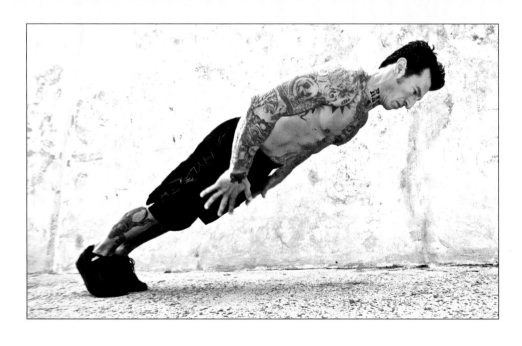

EXPLOSIVE CALISTHENICS

STEP SEVEN: CONVICT PUSHUP

PERFORMANCE

- Squat down, place your palms on the floor and stretch your legs out behind you.

- Your palms should be below your shoulders, spread at shoulder width or wider.

- Place your feet at whatever width you are comfortable with; beginners should use a wider base, experts can go closer.

- Keep your legs, hips and torso aligned and horizontal.

- Bend your arms and shoulders, dipping your torso towards the floor.

- Immediately push explosively off the floor, straightening your arms.

- Explode upwards as hard as you can, and while you are catching air, whip your hands back and clap them together behind your back.

- As gravity reverses your movement, return your hands in front of you "catch" the floor with your hands again.

- Use the elastic rebound to immediately repeat the technique.

EXERCISE X-RAY

Convict pushups were considered a pretty staple power exercise in many jails. I've never heard this term on the outside, but behind bars we would sometimes call this exercise "convict" pushups because when you clap behind your back, your hands are (briefly) in a standard handcuff position. (If you don't like the term, just think of them as *behind-the-back clap pushups*.)

REGRESSION

Don't fall flat on your face when trying this the first time, brother. To get used to the unique rear clap technique, I'd advise trying this exercise kneeling first, in the manner of step 2 (page 82).

PROGRESSION

Some guys inside practically worship this exercise. I once knew a dude who could do a front clap, then a rear clap—twice—with great form, all in the same airtime! It's even possible to add a fifth clap (to the front) before landing, but you need to be a pushup genius to make that happen. *Quintuple clap pushups*, anyone?

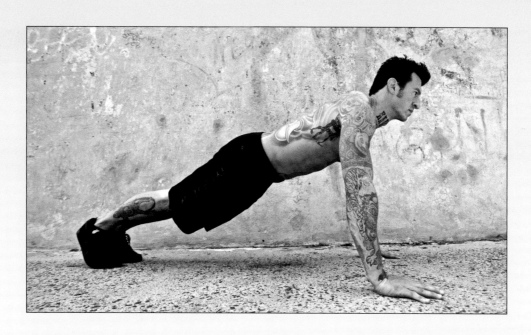

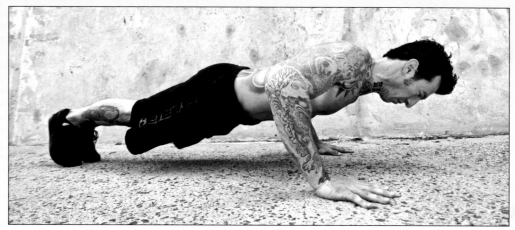

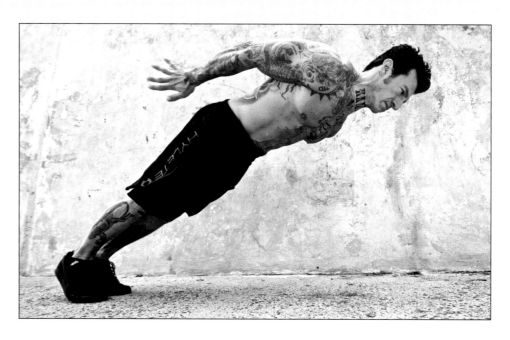

EXPLOSIVE CALISTHENICS

STEP EIGHT: HALF-SUPER

PERFORMANCE

- Squat down, place your palms on the floor and stretch your legs out behind you.

- Your palms should be below your shoulders, spread at shoulder width or wider.

- Place your feet at whatever width you are comfortable with; beginners should use a wider base, experts can go closer.

- Keep your legs, hips and torso aligned and horizontal.

- Bend your arms and shoulders, dipping your torso towards the floor.

- Immediately push explosively off the floor, straightening your arms.

- Explode upwards as hard as you can, and while you are catching air, thrust your hands directly out in front of your body.

- As gravity reverses your movement, return your hands in front of you "catch" the floor with your hands again.

- Use the elastic rebound to immediately repeat the technique.

EXERCISE X-RAY

Half-supers are named that way because if you do them right, half the body—the upper-half—achieves the "Superman" position (see opposite). Once you have nailed the *Superman* position with just the upper-limbs, the next step is to be able to nail the position with just the lower limbs—that's step 9, *full body pop-ups* (page 96). From there, you just work on putting the upper and lower-limb actions together. Because the arms shoot out forwards, beyond the head, this exercise builds high levels of pure shoulder speed—useful for all you martial artists out there.

REGRESSION

I'd advise athletes to initially try this technique with just *one* hand out in front, on each side. When this is easy on both sides, experiment with the full version. You can also explore the kneeling version as preparation.

PROGRESSION

A harder variation involves clapping the top of the head *after* throwing both arms out front, when they are on the return journey prior to quickly catching the floor again.

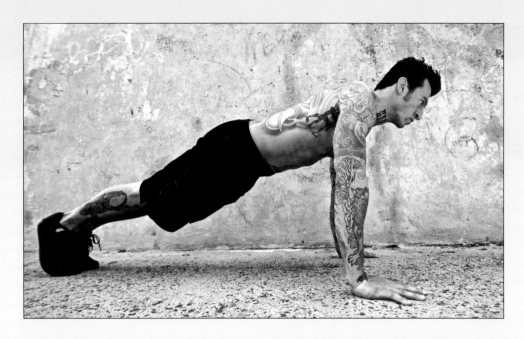

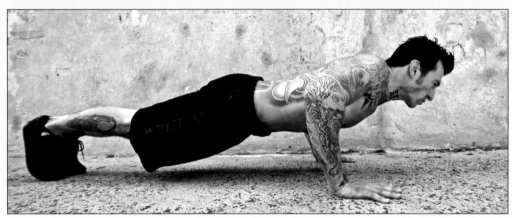

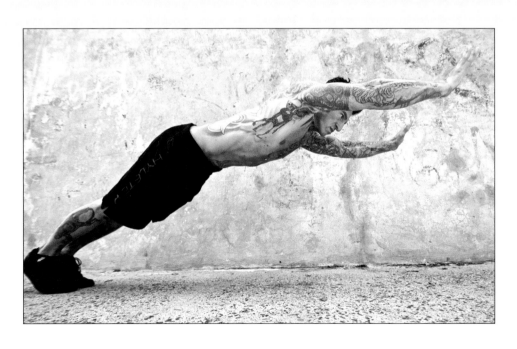

STEP NINE: FULL BODY POP-UP

PERFORMANCE

- Squat down, place your palms on the floor and stretch your legs out behind you.

- Your palms should be below your shoulders, spread at shoulder width or wider.

- Place your feet at whatever width you are comfortable with; beginners should use a wider base, experts can go closer.

- Keep your legs, hips and torso aligned and horizontal.

- Bend your arms and shoulders, dipping your torso towards the floor.

- Immediately push explosively off the floor, straightening your arms.

- Simultaneously kick your legs out and up behind you, trying to keep your body aligned as you go.

- Explode hard enough with all four limbs to allow your hands and your feet to leave the floor at the same time.

- As gravity reverses your movement, "catch" the floor with your hands and feet again.

- Use the elastic rebound to immediately repeat the technique.

EXERCISE X-RAY

In step 3, you learned to pop your upper limbs off the floor in the pushup position; now it's time for something much harder—popping *all four* limbs off the ground. It's true that some previous steps (such as *convict pushups*) force the upper-body to push more explosively than this exercise, but full body pop-ups are an essential prerequisite skill to learn if you want to master the *Superman*—that's why they've been placed as step 9.

REGRESSION

Begin by popping only three limbs off the floor—vary *which* limbs.

PROGRESSION

This exercise is much easier to do when *worming* (see page 76). The hardest way is to keep your body perfectly aligned. As you improve at the technique, keep pushing off higher and higher—check out how high Danny's hips are in the final photo opposite.

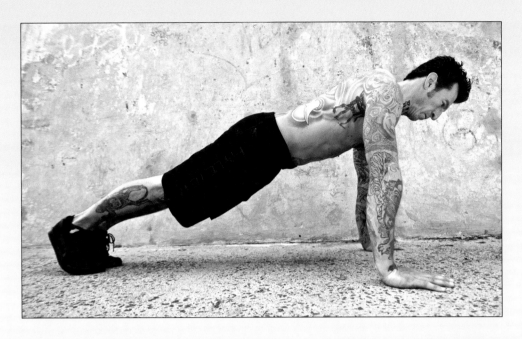

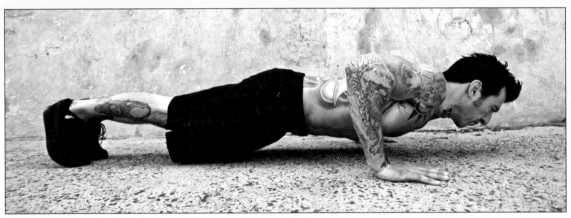

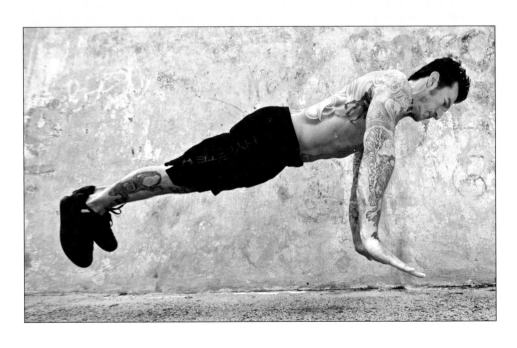

MASTER STEP: THE SUPERMAN

PERFORMANCE

- Squat down, place your palms on the floor and stretch your legs out behind you.

- Your palms should be below your shoulders, spread at shoulder width or wider.

- Place your feet at whatever width you are comfortable with; beginners should use a wider base, experts can go closer.

- Keep your legs, hips and torso aligned and horizontal.

- Bend your arms and shoulders, dipping your torso towards the floor.

- Immediately push explosively off the floor, straightening your arms.

- Explode upwards as hard as you can, and while you are catching air, thrust your hands directly out in front of your body.

- Simultaneously kick your legs out and up behind you, trying to keep your body horizontal as you go.

- Explode hard enough with all four limbs to allow your hands and your feet to leave the floor at the same time.

- As gravity reverses your movement, "catch" the floor with your hands and feet again.

- Use the elastic rebound to immediately repeat the technique.

EXERCISE X-RAY

Sure, it looks as cool as hell. Sure, it's a bodyweight feat virtually no athletes in a gym can replicate correctly (without giving themselves a hernia, at least). But the *Superman* is much, much more than a wicked-looking move. All true explosive exercises work the whole body—not just one or two areas—and the Superman is no different. Whereas regular pushups strongly work the *anterior* chain (the abs, hips and quads), to stop the hips sinking, the Superman also works the *posterior* chain (the spinal muscles, glutes, and hamstrings) to blast the feet off the ground. What's more, it works both chains explosively, and in conjunction with the upper-body pushing muscles (the chest, triceps, shoulders) which become kung fu powerful and robust as a gorilla's. If God has handed us a "perfect" explosive upper-body exercise, it might be this one, boys and girls. Go master it!

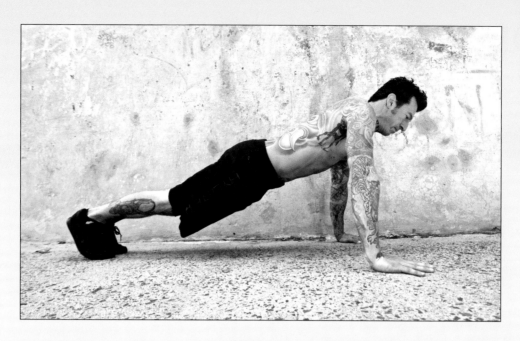

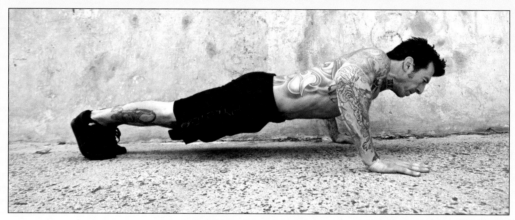

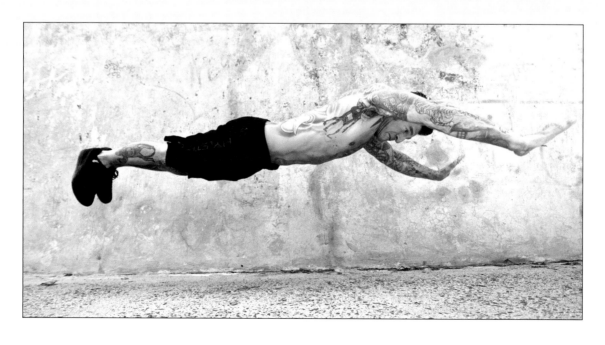

GOING BEYOND

Like jumps, athletes can choose to increase *linear progression* in power pushups; you just clap more often, or push up higher. Some athletes can push all the way from the floor into a standing position—although I've never seen this done with a perfectly aligned body. Most athletes—if dedicated, and not too heavy—should be able to master the negative, or eccentric version of this movement, which involves dropping down into a pushup position from standing (see page 316).

One simple way to add a twist to the *Superman pushup* is to spread-eagle the arms and legs at the top: this is sometimes called the *X-jump pushup*. This requires greater limb movement, therefore more airtime, but also more hip activation.

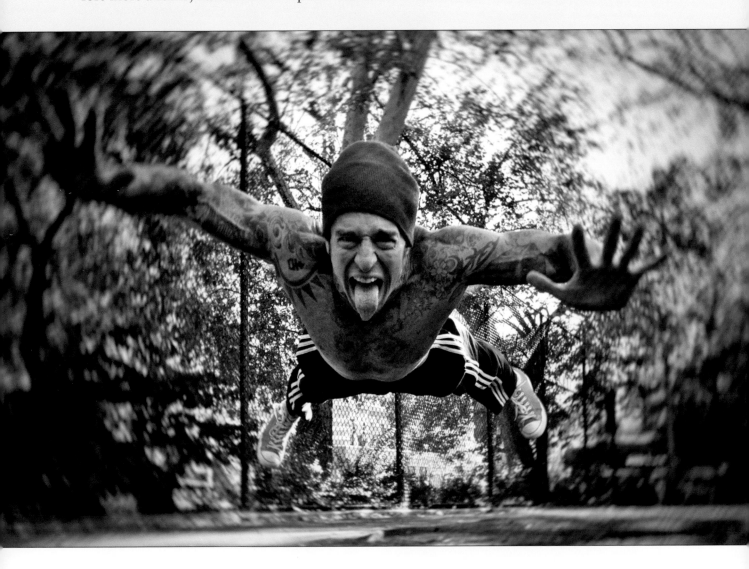

This is just one way of adding variety to the Superman. You can also explore hybrid versions, perhaps striking the chest mid-air, clapping behind your back, or even placing the hands behind your head. Once you've mastered the Superman, a whole plethora of ice cold power pushups open up to you.

THE AZTEC PUSHUP

Even tougher than the *Superman* is the legendary *Aztec pushup*. This involves propelling your hips so high that you can perform a toe-touch pike in the top position. It's an incredible exercise but to my mind it's less of a pure pushup, because it's as much about waist power as upper-body snap.

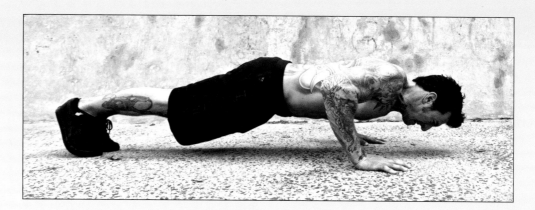

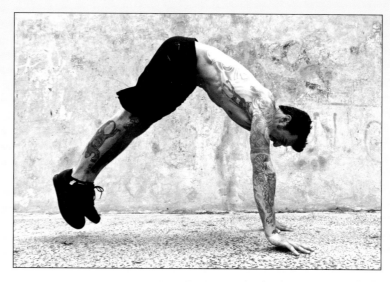

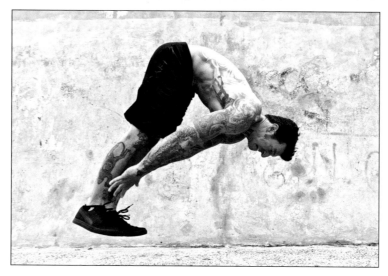

THE CROSSING AZTEC PUSHUP

If the *Aztec* is too easy (what are you, a mutant?) you can increase the coordination requirements by touching your opposite hand and foot in the top position. This is the *crossing Aztec pushup*.

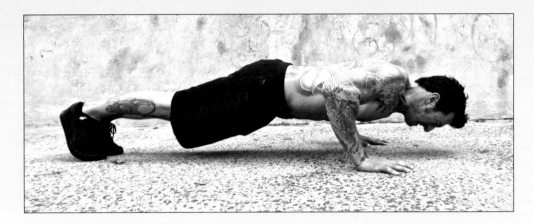

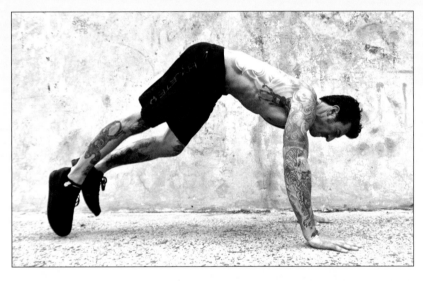

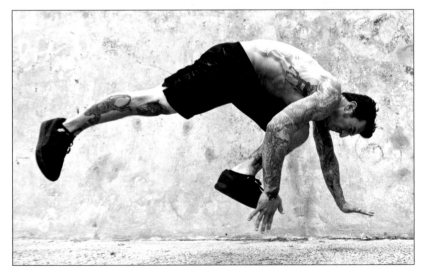

EXPLOSIVE CALISTHENICS

All progressive bodyweight masters understand that one of the best routes to maximize ability is to go unilateral—use just one limb! I know that for many a *one-arm clap pushup* (striking the *chest*, since the other hand is missing!) may seem impossible to some. Not so. If you're Al Kavadlo, the impossible is always in reach!

For even more upper-body power, I'd also advise athletes to explore *handsprings*—front (page 156) and back (page 156) when they are ready. These really are high force (due to momentum) and high speed movements which will radically increase arm and shoulder power. But pushups should be your base!

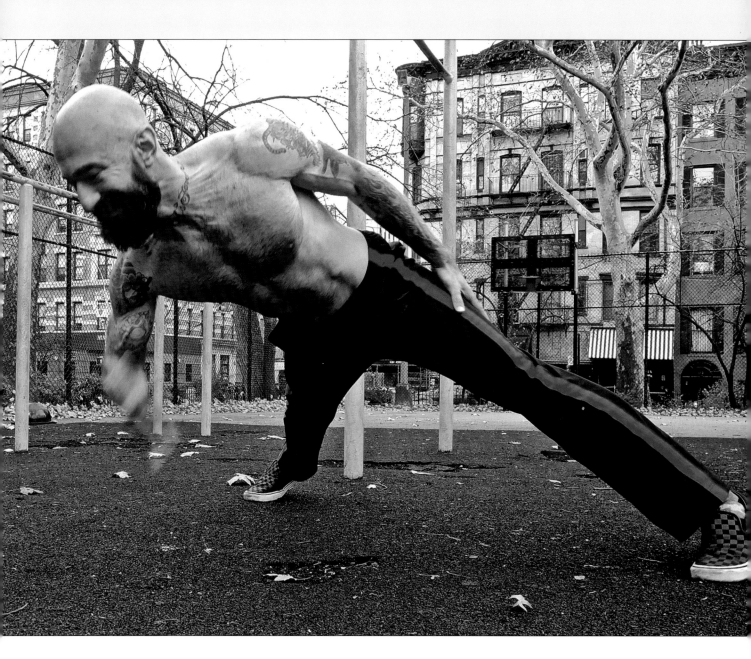

SMALL SPACE DRILLS

Following are three useful speed and power techniques you can utilize in your routine for variety, as ancillary work or to train your muscles from different angles. They are all solo drills, and they require zero equipment. Unlike the progressive exercises in the chains, most of the following drills can be performed rhythmically for higher reps, and can work well when used with any of the chains in this book. In this sense, they can also work as warm-ups or finishing exercises in an explosives session.

PUSH GET-UP

From the pushup position, dip down and explode up, bringing your legs in so that you finish in a standing position. A great upper-lower body exercise, plus a brilliant preliminary drill for *Aztec pushups*, the *push get-up* is also the coolest possible way to get back on your feet after performing your pushups.

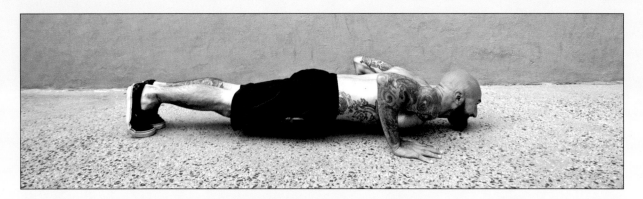

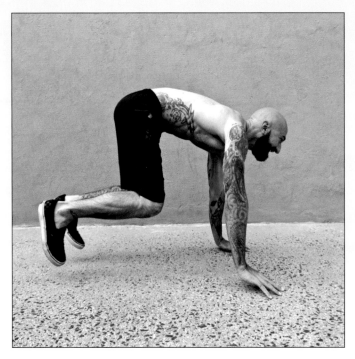
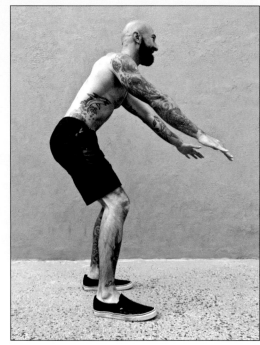

ROUND-THE-CLOCK PUSHUPS

This one's a great move for building explosive endurance in the upper-body. Assume the pushup position, dip and explode up, but land with your hands about a foot to the side. Using your feet as a pivot point, continue this rhythmically—no pausing—until you've gone a full 360 degrees. You can do this clockwise, counter-clockwise, or mix and match.

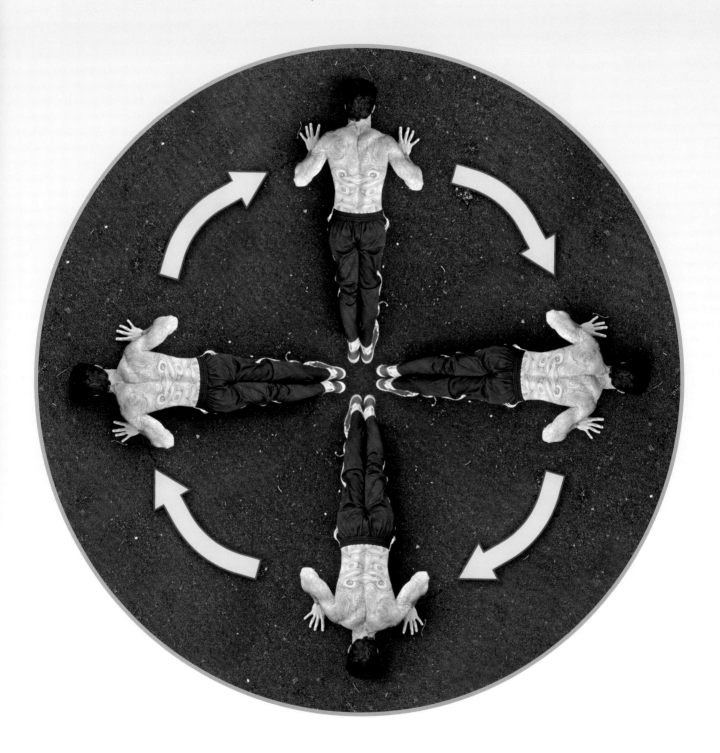

360 JUMP

Fast hands and fast feet go together like biscuits and gravy! The 360 jump is simple and effective. Jump and spin, landing back where you started. If that's too tough, start with 180 degrees (jump and spin facing the other way) and build up. Always remember to master both directions.

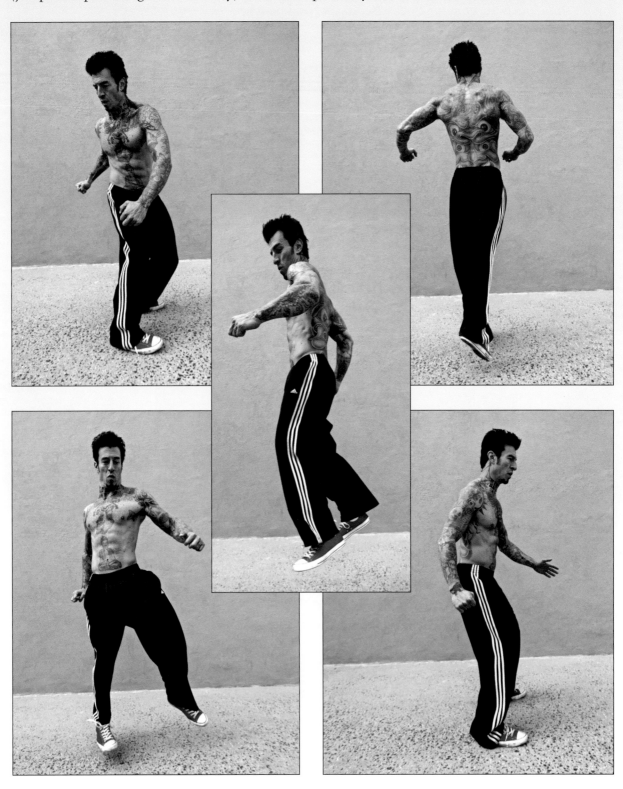

LIGHTS OUT!

Mastery of progressive calisthenics is like building an arsenal full of weapons. With the jump chain, you have everything you need to build superlative lower-body power. With the power pushup chain that followed, you've got the upper-body equivalent. These exercises will super-charge your nervous system, improve your reflexes, ramp up your speed and power, and strengthen your shoulders, hands, wrists, elbows, and even bones, turning you from a slow, clumsy "normal" into a lightning-powered cyborg, more than capable of approaching the advanced acrobatic moves necessitated by the remaining Explosive Six chains.

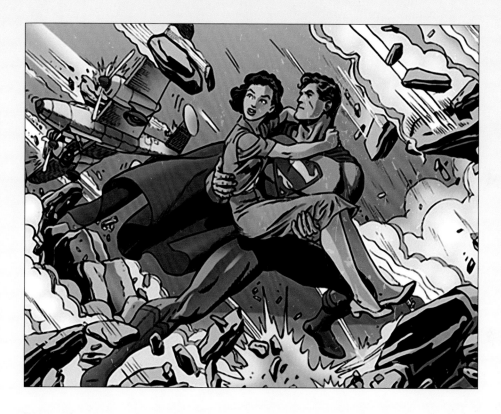

With time, effort and patience, the *Superman* is waiting for you. Now get to it, and go save Lois Lane.

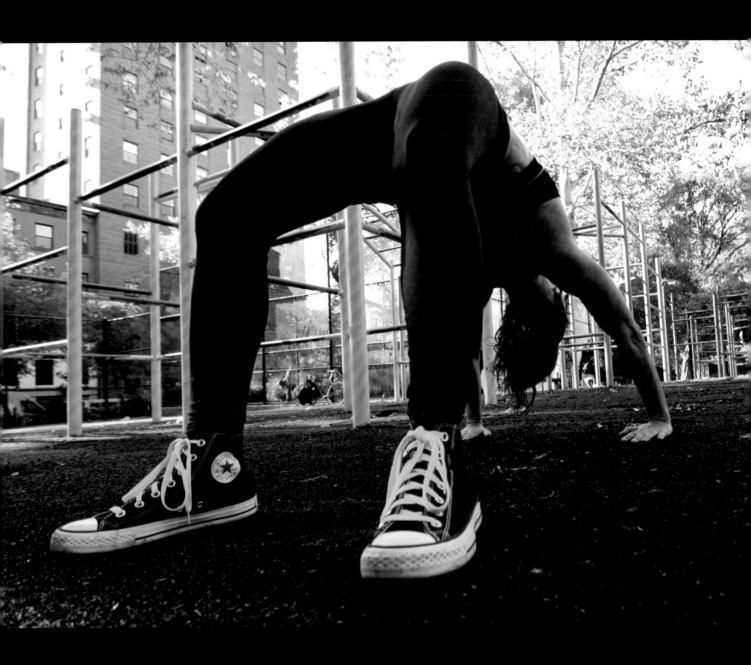

6

KIP-UPS
KUNG FU BODY SPEED

Very few athletes have seriously attempted a *muscle-up*, but you'd be pressed to find a teenage dude today who hasn't done his damndest to pull off a *kip-up*. For those few of you who aren't aware of the movement (or the name: it's sometimes called a *nip-up*), the kip-up is the most explosive way of getting up off your back: you "roll up" your body and spring your legs out and down. It's not difficult to understand the allure of the kip-up. It's a mesmerizing movement—one second you're on your back, the next you're up on your feet, like magic. And they seem to be everywhere. Kip-ups are part of tricking and street dance styles; and you see them in pro wrestling all the time. Possibly the crown for most epic wrestling kip-up of all time goes to The Rock. With a silent speed, he'd effortlessly roll up, and— *thwip*—he was suddenly on his feet, graceful as a cat. He got so good the old-fashioned way: practice. Back when he was training in wrestling as a kid, he made it a point to always get up off the canvas via a kip-up. Even if he hit the deck a hundred times in a session, even if he was exhausted, he kipped himself up. When it comes to masters of the kip-up, I have to also give a shout-out to the great Jackie Chan. He was busting out perfect kip-ups back in his earliest movies, and he did 'em so well that you won't find a kung fu movie anywhere today where some master doesn't kip-up.

Is it any wonder this move is so widely attempted?

Unfortunately, just because a lot of folks *try* the kip-up, it doesn't follow that a lot of them can *do* it. I'd estimate that only one in ten kids who try the kip-up actually manage it—and remember, these are teens who are mostly in way better shape than their adult counterparts. Most adults wouldn't even attempt this move. And it's a crying shame, because aside from just looking like a cool "trick", the kip-up is actually a surprisingly useful technique in explosive calisthenics

Why is it "useful"? Because it teaches athletes to push their bodies up explosively, through the hands; it teaches basic balance and equilibrium; and it builds huge levels of high-speed snap into the waist and spine. You will often hear weight-lifters talking about "hip snap". Well, forget about weights—the kip-up will teach you the *gold standard* hip snap. Best of all, these qualities all act as a perfect training ground for athletes who want to move to more sophisticated acrobatic movements, like front and back flips.

For these reasons, I'm convinced that the kip-up should be the very first skill-based explosive chain athletes start working with, after they make some progress with the basic power drills: *jumps* and *power pushups*.

DECONSTRUCTING KIP-UPS

I've already touched on some essential elements of the basic kip-up. The points which require attention typically are:

THE ROLL-UP

Before you can kip-up, you need to explode your legs out in a kick. Super-athletes can do this with minimal telegraphing, but most of us have to coil our bodies up—like springs—to aid with the kick. The *easiest* way to generate the momentum you need is to begin with a full range-of-motion on the roll-up—bring your knees up close to your head. Believe it or not, a proper dynamic roll-up is beyond the abdominal power of most people. I'd advise all would-be kip-uppers to begin with some kind of compound midsection exercise to condition this area. Since you raise your legs in the roll-up, *leg raises* are the obvious choice. Stay away from junk like *crunches* or ab-machines and infomercial gimmicks, as they isolate the abdominals, and thus don't train the muscles which cross the hips (*hip flexors*). They are the key to this kind of real-world stuff.

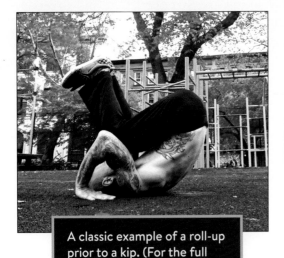

A classic example of a roll-up prior to a kip. (For the full move, check out page 126.)

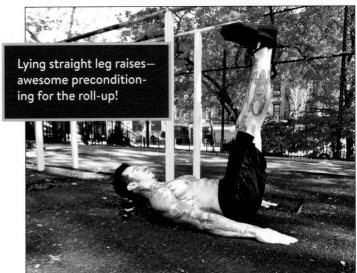

Lying straight leg raises—awesome preconditioning for the roll-up!

HAND POSITIONING

To help with the kick, you need to stabilize your roll-up and assist with your hands. Truly advanced athletes can dispense with the hands altogether, but it's still a key learning stage in the technical chain. The hands need to quickly be placed fingers-down alongside the ears—those of you used to *bridging* (hopefully most of you) will be familiar with this pattern and will pick it up quickly. The arms also assist in the initial push, to get things moving with the kick. This can seem like a strange angle to push from, and if your rotator cuffs are stiff you may have trouble. The steps in this chapter will get you there, but if your body is used to the bridge push-up from *Convict Conditioning*, it'll be a breeze. (See—I told you all that stuff was useful!)

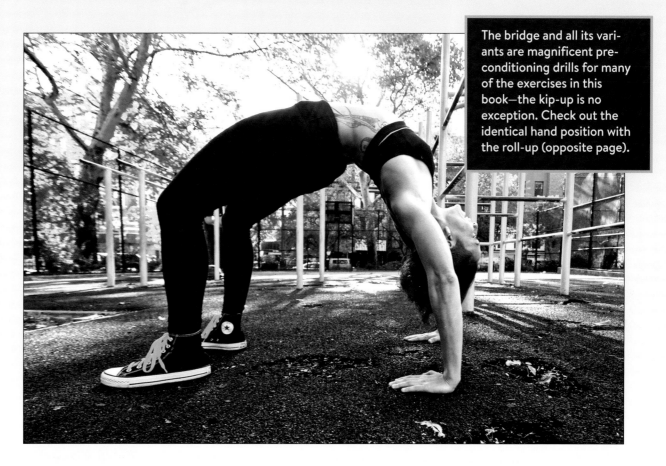

The bridge and all its variants are magnificent pre-conditioning drills for many of the exercises in this book—the kip-up is no exception. Check out the identical hand position with the roll-up (opposite page).

THE KICK

The kick is where the basic kip-up starts to get tricky for most athletes. For a start, it has to be *powerful*; along with the push from the hands, the kick needs to generate enough momentum to counter the body's mass and lift you from the ground. Luckily, if you have been working on your jumps, this will not pose a serious problem. The kick should proceed immediately after the roll-up—you are really "bouncing" up out of the roll. If you leave it too long, the elastic energy of the roll-up will dissipate. Coil and explode! The main mistake most athletes make is trying to kick *out*, or worse, *out* and *down*, to the floor—where they think their feet should wind up. This is an error. What you need is not to get your feet to the floor fast—you need to utilize your leg and body power to gain height. You do this by focusing on kicking *up*. I know what you're thinking—if I'm kicking *up*, how do I rotate?

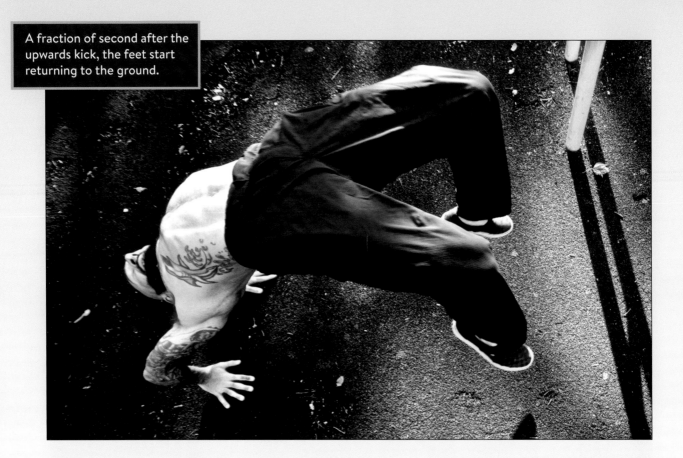

THE ROTATION

It's your hips, upper-body and arms that rotate you—*not* your legs. Bear this in mind: even though you are generating vertical (upwards) power with your legs, your feet won't just fly straight up. They can't. If you have performed a good, deep roll-up, your feet will be *behind you*, so what will actually happen is that your body will spring out like a lock-knife, but real fast. Your waist will be the hinge. At that point, it's not your legs that rotate you, but the continuation of your hand-push into a downwards swing, plus the hip-snap I mentioned earlier—which, essentially, is a lot like a super-fast sit-up. Looking at a point in the far distance above the horizon beyond your feet will keep the head and neck in the right place. The legs kinda take care of themselves at this stage, believe it or not: they naturally arc downwards towards the floor. For most athletes the rotation is the hardest part to master; but it's also the most rewarding, in terms of conditioning. Not only does it build that gold hip-snap and high-speed abs, the partial (90 degrees) rotation also acts as a form of kinesthetic preparation for more demanding rotation acrobatics an athlete might also want to master (such as the front and back flip, both 360 degree rotations).

EXPLOSIVE CALISTHENICS

THE KIP-UP CHAIN

The biggest challenge for most de-conditioned individuals will be the rapid roll-up stage—the abdominal muscles and hips will be too weak. *Rolling sit-ups* (step 1) take care of that by working the midsection in a similar range-of-motion to the classic kip-up. Once the backwards swing of the legs is mastered, the athlete needs to learn the throw his or her momentum *forwards* after that movement; and this is where *rolling squats* (step 2) come in.

The next step is to start working on the vertical momentum; the kick-up with a hand push. *Shoulder pop-ups* (step 3) are a great drill for this, and are used by most coaches in teaching a proper kip-up. With *bridge kips* (step 4) the athlete starts exploding out with the legs, landing on the feet—but only in a bridge position, not standing. The hip-snap—the throwing forward of the waist—is the next skill to be learned, in *butt kips* (step 5) where you throw your torso forward but land on your glutes. The next step, *half kips* (step 6) are a transitional stage, during which you are building momentum to kip up fully on your feet—the classic *kip-up* (step 7).

For most people, the classic kip-up is the only real kip-up style they know. In fact—with practice and dedication—most athletes can achieve even more advanced variations. Keeping the legs straight (step 8) is the basic way of rendering the move tougher: without movement at the knee, the hips and spine have to open at high speed. Another way to make the waist work hard is to take the arms out of the movement; a transitional stage is to make pushing through the hands harder, and you can do this by placing your hands out to the sides. This is the *wushu kip-up* (step 9). The Master Step is attained by taking the hands out of the movement completely: the super-tough *no-hands kip-up* (step 10).

STEP ONE: ROLLING SIT-UP

PERFORMANCE

- Sit on the floor with your knees bent and heels on the ground. You can place your palms on the floor or on your lower legs.

- Roll onto your back, bringing your legs above your body; keep a bend at the knees.

- As you roll up, place your hands palms down by your ears, with the fingers pointing to your feet (the same hand position as used in *bridging*). Take some of your weight through your palms.

- Continue swinging your legs over and back, as you roll up onto your upper-back and shoulders.

- Bring your knees close to your head, being careful not to hit yourself in the face.

- Roll back into the starting position.

- Repeat the technique.

EXERCISE X-RAY

Rolling sit-ups are a fantastic conditioning exercise which strengthen the midsection, hips and back in preparation for the kip-up. They also contain many of the movement patterns essential for the full *kip-up* (step 7); for example: the roll onto the shoulders; the swing back-then-forward of the lower limbs; and the crucial *fingers-facing-feet* hand position. This movement will also prepare the vestibular system for the rapid reversal we find in kip-ups. This drill is also low-impact, meaning you can practice it frequently—essential for all fundamentals.

REGRESSION

If bringing your legs close to your face is too strenuous for now, begin by just swinging your legs up above your head.

PROGRESSION

At the top of the movement, touch your toes to the ground behind your head.

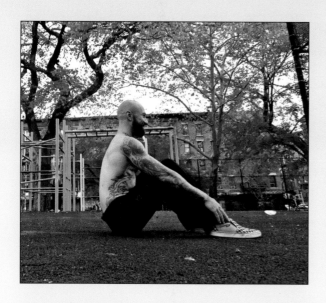
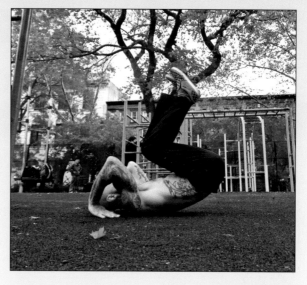
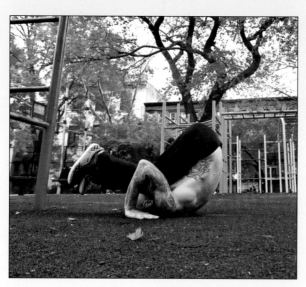
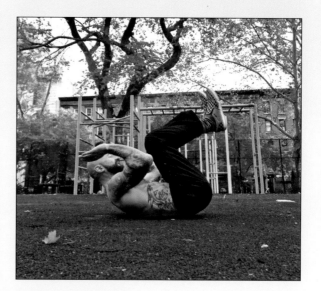
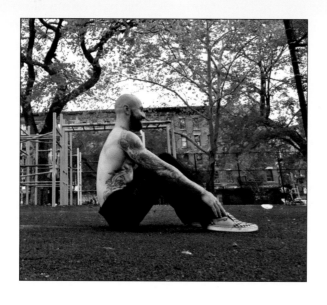

STEP TWO: ROLLING SQUAT

PERFORMANCE

- Sit on the floor with your knees bent and heels on the ground. You can place your palms on the floor or on your lower legs.

- Roll onto your back, bringing your legs above your body; keep a bend at the knees.

- As you roll up, place your hands palms down by your ears, with the fingers pointing to your feet (the same hand position as used in *bridging*). Take some of your weight through your palms.

- Continue swinging your legs over and back, as you roll up onto your upper-back and shoulders.

- Bring your knees close to your head, being careful not to hit yourself in the face.

- Roll back into the starting position, but allow your momentum to push you further forward, until your hips leave the ground. Keeping your arms out in front of you, finish in a low squat position.

- Follow through and extend into a standing position.

- Squat down and roll back, then repeat the exercise.

EXERCISE X-RAY

Rolling squats follow on from *rolling-sit-ups*. The first part of the movement is the same, but you follow it by standing up—this requires the athlete to generate extra forward momentum. (It's the ability to generate forward momentum which really determines whether a full *kip-up* will happen.) For this reason, rolling squats are a great early drill to have under your belt.

REGRESSION

Some beginners have trouble generating enough momentum to get into the low squat position. If this is you, when your glutes touch the ground, place your hands on the floor and push up with your fingers.

PROGRESSION

Folding your arms in front of your chest will take them out of the movement, forcing the legs and waist to generate the required momentum.

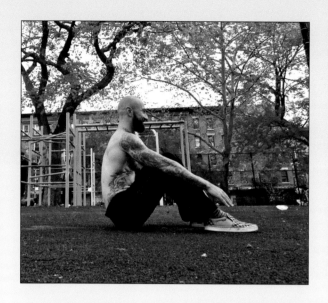
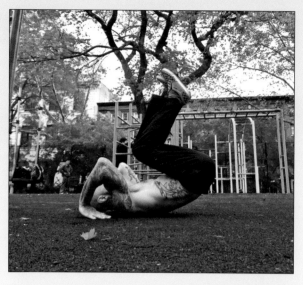
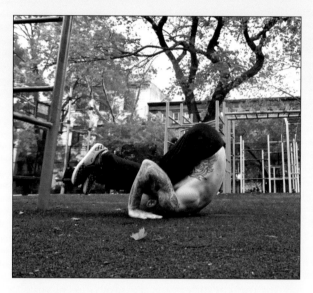
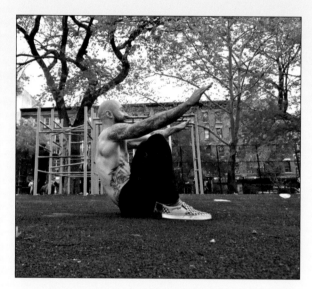
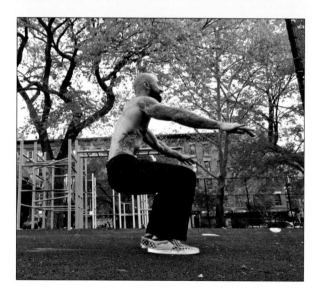
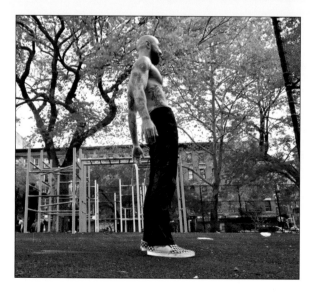

EXPLOSIVE CALISTHENICS

STEP THREE: SHOULDER POP

PERFORMANCE

- Sit on the floor with your knees bent and heels on the ground.

- Roll onto your back, bringing your legs above your body; keep a bend at the knees.

- As you roll up, place your hands palms down by your ears, with the fingers pointing to your feet (the same hand position as used in *bridging*). Take some of your weight through your palms.

- When your feet are above your head, explode your legs straight up, to gain some vertical momentum.

- Simultaneously, push down through your palms, briefly "popping" your shoulders and head an inch or two off the ground.

- Try to cushion the descent of your shoulders as much as possible, using muscular tension in your arms and shoulders (think of them as springs compressing).

- Roll back into the starting position and repeat the exercise.

EXERCISE X-RAY

Steps 1 and 2 taught you how to use your legs and waist to generate some basic momentum. This step begins strengthening and conditioning the wrists and shoulders for the task of explosively pushing the body up, as is required in a classic *kip-up* (step 7).

REGRESSION

If you can't quite lift your shoulders off the floor, just focus on getting your legs above you and kicking *hard*, vertically. In time you'll gain some height.

PROGRESSION

If this is easy, just push your shoulders higher off the ground. (Hand-balancers can push all the way up into a handstand from this position!)

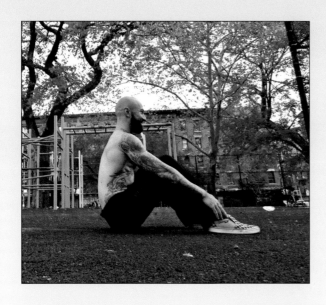 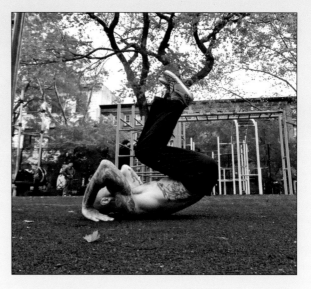

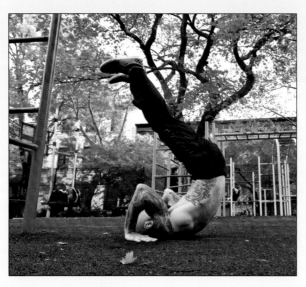 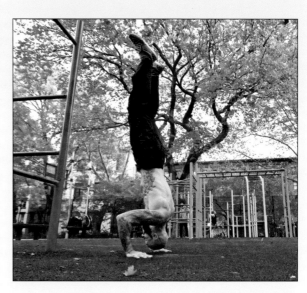

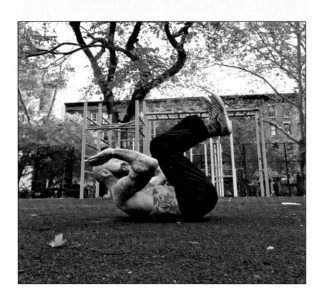 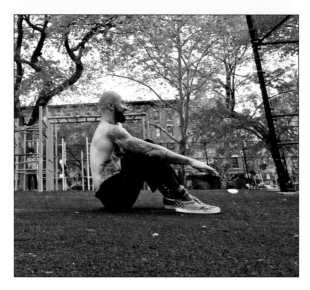

STEP FOUR: BRIDGE KIP

PERFORMANCE

- Sit on the floor with your knees bent and heels on the ground.

- Roll back and swing your legs up as you place your hands in the *bridge* position (by your ears, with the fingers pointing to your feet).

- Roll onto your upper-back and shoulders and squeeze into a tight ball, with your bent knees close to your head (this will give you a better position to spring out from).

- To gain momentum, "unravel" by exploding your legs in an arc, *up* and then *down* towards the ground as you simultaneously push down through your palms.

- Use the momentum to lift your head and upper-back off the floor—push through your arms to help with this. As your feet strike the floor, you should only be supported by your palms and both feet.

- Hold this position—which is essentially a *bridge*—for a moment.

- Lower your body back down and repeat the exercise.

EXERCISE X-RAY

The goal of this step is to learn to generate enough lower-body power to throw the head, shoulders and upper-back off the floor. We don't need them to flip forwards yet—that will come in more intermediate steps.

REGRESSION

If you can't generate the necessary momentum to push your upper-back and head off the ground, you can begin by just practicing kicking up and down in an arc, striking the ground with your feet, but keeping your shoulders/head in contact with the floor. Your head and shoulders will lift if you practice.

PROGRESSION

Develop this movement by improving the quality of the bridge. At first you will only be able to kick out into a semi-bridge, with your head close to the floor; in time you will be able to extend your arms (and legs) more fully.

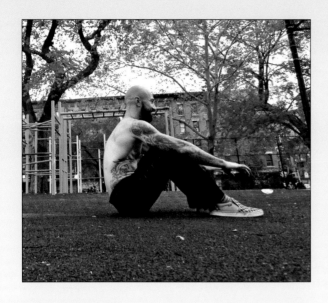

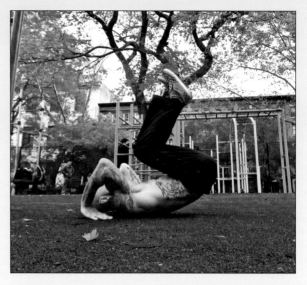

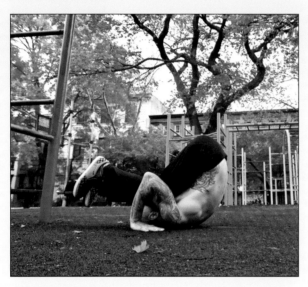

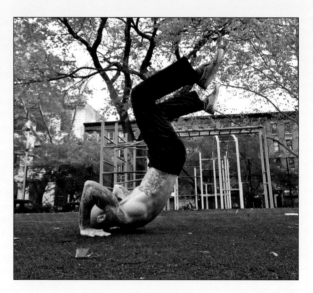

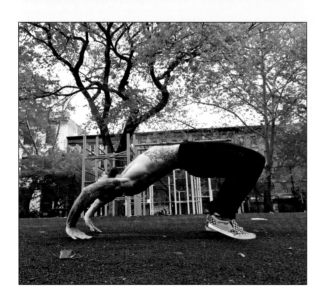

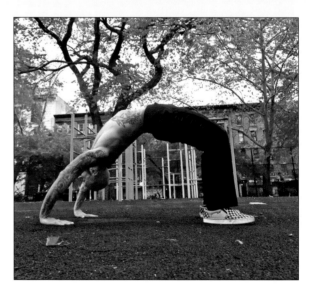

STEP FIVE: BUTT KIP

PERFORMANCE

- Sit on the floor with your knees bent and heels on the ground.

- Roll back and swing your legs up as you place your hands in the *bridge* position (by your ears, with the fingers pointing to your feet).

- Roll onto your upper-back and shoulders and squeeze into a tight ball, with your bent knees close to your head (this will give you a better position to spring out from).

- To gain momentum, "unravel" by exploding your legs in an arc, *up* and then *down* towards the ground as you simultaneously push down through your palms hard enough to lift them off the ground.

- As you kick off, throw your torso and hands forwards, almost like an explosive sit-up.

- Don't try to land on your feet at this stage. Just aim to land on your butt and your feet with your torso upright.

- Lower your body back down and repeat the exercise.

EXERCISE X-RAY

Once you can generate enough power to lift your head and back off the floor (step 4), the next step is to lift the hands off the floor and throw the torso even further forward. If you can use this drill to master the skill of landing on the butt with the torso upright, the next step (6) should come pretty easy.

REGRESSION

You can begin this drill easily, just by kicking in an arc and landing on your butt while bringing the head and back a short way off the floor. In time, you can learn to finish in the upright "sit-up" position.

PROGRESSION

The more momentum you generate, the easier it will be to land on your feet a fraction of a second before you fall back on your butt. When you can do this you have essentially reached step 6, *half kips*.

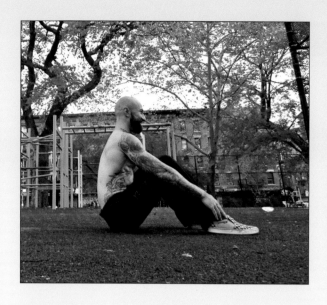
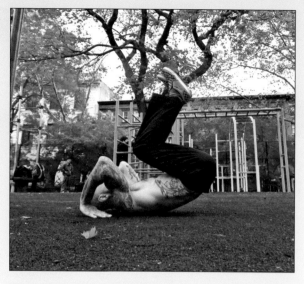
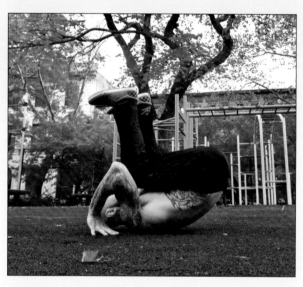
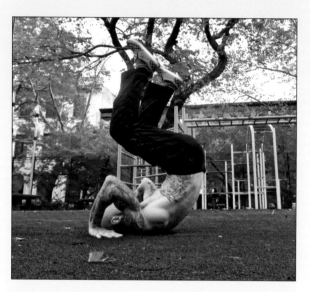
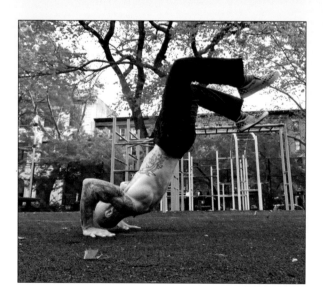
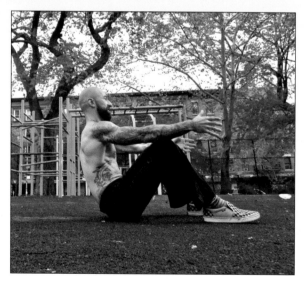

EXPLOSIVE CALISTHENICS

STEP SIX: HALF KIP

PERFORMANCE

- Sit on the floor with your knees bent and heels on the ground.

- Roll back and swing your legs up as you place your hands in the *bridge* position (by your ears, with the fingers pointing to your feet).

- Roll onto your upper-back and shoulders and squeeze into a tight ball, with your bent knees close to your head (this will give you a better position to spring out from).

- To gain momentum, "unravel" by exploding your legs in an arc, *up* and then *down* towards the ground as you simultaneously push down through your palms hard enough to lift them off the ground.

- As your feet touch down, continue throwing your torso and hands forwards.

- Land on both feet, even if only for a fraction of second, before falling back onto your butt.

- Roll back and repeat the exercise.

EXERCISE X-RAY

In step 4 you learned the leg-arc motion; in step 5, you learned to throw the torso forward. Now it's just a matter of fusing these patterns together more explosively until you can propel your center of gravity forwards enough to land on your feet, even if only for a fraction of a second.

REGRESSION

Athletes trying the kip-up for the first time often "discover" this movement by accident. You try to kip up, but you can't throw your center of gravity *quite* forward enough to stay stable in the squat, and you tip backwards. In reality, you are nearly there—all it takes now is a little drill practice.

PROGRESSION

You can use tricks to help you stay upright after the kip—like "catching" a stable object, or a partner's hands. These are really just a distraction from the real job of teaching your body to build the extra power needed to shoot you forward. How do you do this? Drill! Again and again and again!

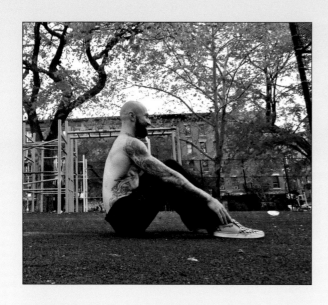
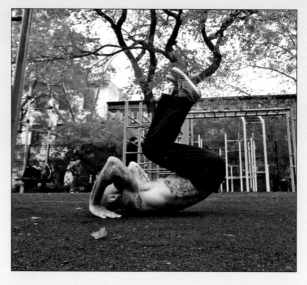
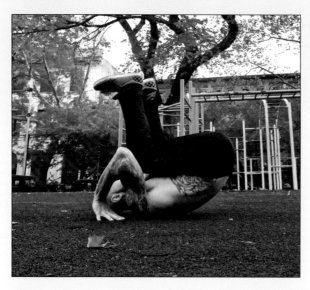
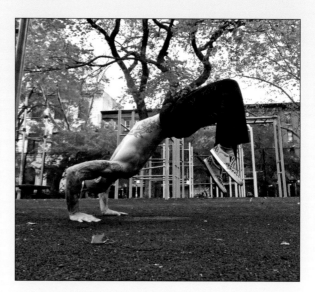
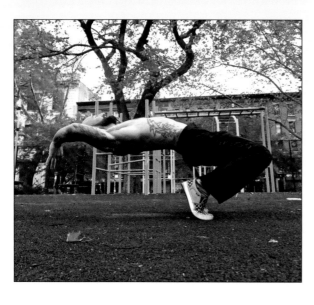
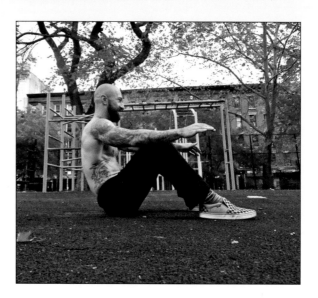

EXPLOSIVE CALISTHENICS

125

STEP SEVEN: KIP-UP

PERFORMANCE

- Sit on the floor with your knees bent and heels on the ground.

- Roll back and swing your legs up as you place your hands in the *bridge* position (by your ears, with the fingers pointing to your feet).

- Roll onto your upper-back and shoulders and squeeze into a tight ball, with your bent knees close to your head (this will give you a better position to spring out from).

- To gain momentum, "unravel" by exploding your legs in an arc, *up* and then *down* towards the ground as you simultaneously push down through your palms hard enough to lift them off the ground.

- As your feet touch down, keep your torso and hands forwards.

- Land on the balls of both feet, into a squatting position. Keep the head and hands forwards until you are stable, and stand upright.

- Squat down, roll back and repeat the exercise.

EXERCISE X-RAY

This is the classic *kip-up*, beloved by martial artists, street dancers and pro wrestlers, to name but a few. Achieving this infamous move is impossible without an explosive waist (hips and lower back), super-fast legs and the total-body agility of a panther. If you have got this far, congrats—you have earned the envy of millions of Bruce Lee fans. Never has getting knocked on your ass been more fun.

REGRESSION

One way of getting your feet under you quicker is to try kipping up into a wider stance. This can work in helping some athletes get their first kip-up.

PROGRESSION

The contrary principle to the regression holds true—the closer your feet are on landing, the more momentum you need. Try keeping your feet together if you want to make those kip-ups harder. (This works for all kip-up styles.)

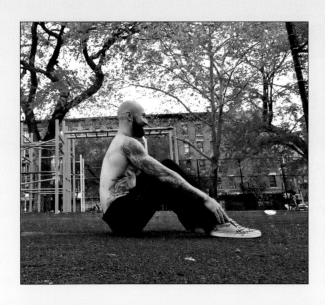
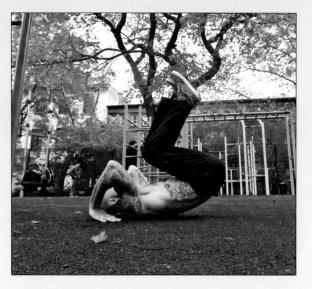
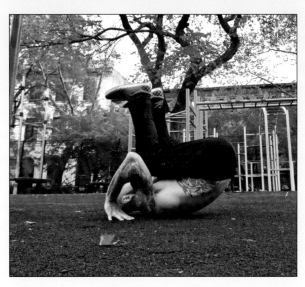
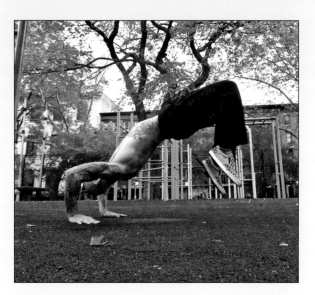
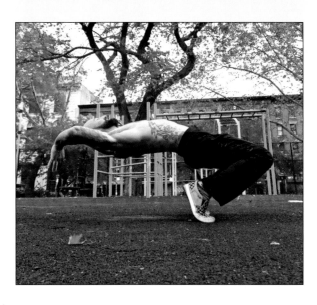
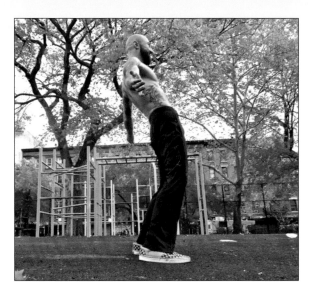

EXPLOSIVE CALISTHENICS

STEP EIGHT: STRAIGHT-LEG KIP-UP

PERFORMANCE

- Sit on the floor with your legs straight.

- Roll back and swing your legs up, keeping them straight, as you place your hands in the *bridge* position (by your ears, with the fingers pointing to your feet).

- Roll onto your upper-back and shoulders and swing your legs over your head, still keeping the legs straight. Your knees should come close to your head.

- Explode your legs up by straightening at the hips as you simultaneously push down through your palms hard enough to lift them off the ground.

- As you take-off, bend the legs and whip them underneath you as you continue the forward motion begun by your torso and arms.

- As your feet touch down, keep your torso and hands forwards.

- Land on both feet, into a squatting position. Keep the head and hands forwards until you are stable, and stand upright.

- Squat down, roll back and repeat the exercise.

EXERCISE X-RAY

If you thought the regular *kip-up* (step 8) was the Master Step of the kip-up chain, think again! Beginning the kip-up with *straight legs* is of a much higher difficulty level. With regular kip-ups, you can use your thighs and glutes to extend your legs, generating extra momentum. With straight legs, the hips and waist are forced to do the work, making the drill much tougher.

REGRESSION

Regressions are simple and continuous for this exercise. Once you can perform a regular *kip-up* (step 7), just try to use less leg bend over time. The greater the knee-bend, the easier the kip-up.

PROGRESSION

To make the exercise harder, don't begin by rolling back from a sitting position—this adds momentum. Begin lying flat on the floor instead. (This progression works with all the steps in this chain.)

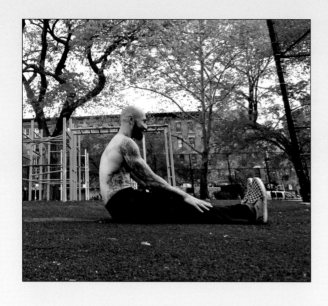
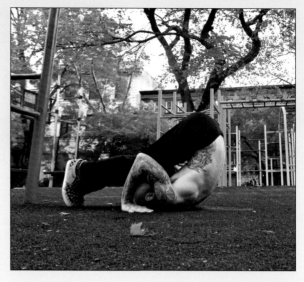
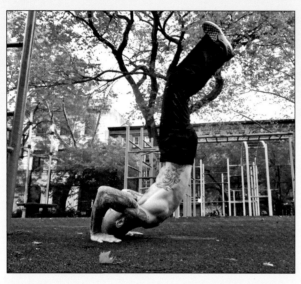
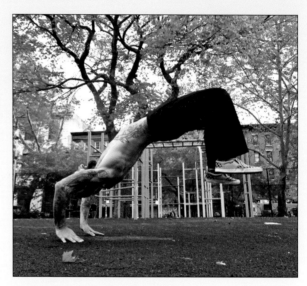
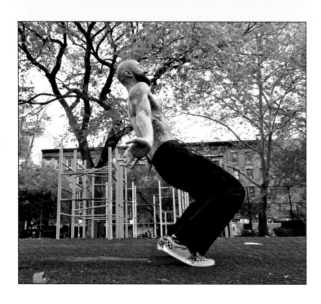
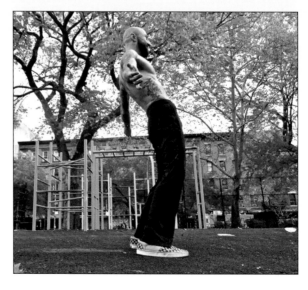

STEP NINE: WUSHU KIP-UP

PERFORMANCE

- Sit on the floor with your knees bent and heels on the ground.

- Roll back and swing your legs up as you place your arms out on the ground, at right-angles from your body.

- Roll onto your upper-back and shoulders and squeeze into a tight ball, with your bent knees close to your head (this will give you a better position to spring out from).

- To gain momentum, "unravel" by exploding your legs in an arc, *up* and then *down* towards the ground as you simultaneously push down through the backs of your arms.

- As your feet touch down, keep your torso and hands forwards.

- Land on the balls of both feet, into a squatting position. Keep pushing the hips and chest forwards until you are stable, and stand upright.

- Squat down, roll back and repeat the exercise.

EXERCISE X-RAY

It's probably natural to assume that the best way to move from regular *kip-ups* (step 7) to *no-hands kip-ups* (Master Step) is to begin using just *one* arm—then moving on to zero arms. In fact this is unlikely to work. Your body is smart, and pretty soon you'll be pushing twice as hard through the single arm. The secret to moving from regular kip-ups to hands-free kip-ups is to learn to use your arms *differently*. The wushu style—with the arms outstretched—will force you to use much less arm power compared to the traditional hands-by-ears pushing position, which is very strong.

REGRESSION

Different arm positions will make this exercise easier. You can begin with the *bridge*-style arm position, but push through the knuckles/backs of the hands instead of the palms. Straighten the arms over time. Holding the arms straight out from the body is the hardest variation.

PROGRESSION

To make the exercise even harder, you can use the straight-leg style described in step 8.

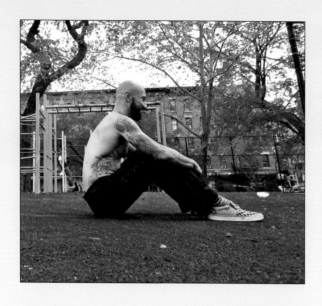 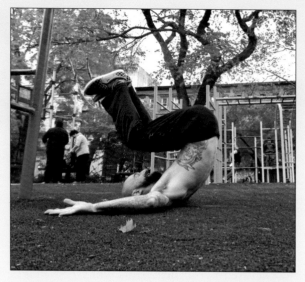

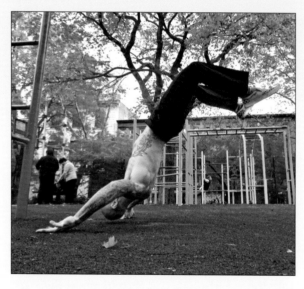 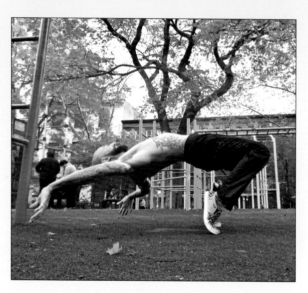

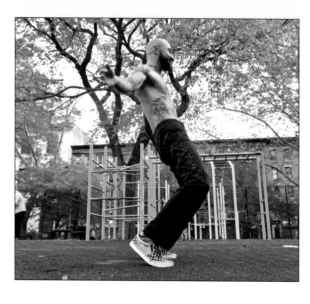 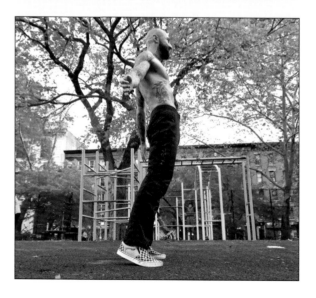

MASTER STEP: NO-HANDS KIP-UP

PERFORMANCE

- Sit on the floor with your knees bent and heels on the ground.

- Roll back and swing your legs up, while keeping your arms to your sides (they must never touch the floor during this move).

- Roll onto your upper-back and shoulders and squeeze into a tight ball, with your bent knees close to your head (this will give you a better position to spring out from).

- To gain momentum, "unravel" by exploding your legs in an arc, *up* and then *down* towards the ground; keep your arms off the floor and to the side of your body.

- As your feet touch down, keep your torso and hands forwards.

- Land on the balls of both feet, into a squatting position. Keep the arms to your side as you stand upright.

- Squat down, roll back and repeat the exercise.

EXERCISE X-RAY

If there is a more impressive—or explosive—way to power up off the floor, then humans haven't invented it yet! Novices who see experts perform this incredible move often assume that the performing athlete must have a neck of steel to get the job done. Although you should avoid this exercise if you have neck problems, it's not true that you need huge neck strength—the neck only acts as a lever for a split-second, if at all. The power here is really generated by the waist and legs. Master this advanced drill, kid, and your total-body speed and agility will start bursting off the charts.

To really make this technique elite, you can apply several of the progressions outlined in this chapter; for example, you can begin the move from a lying position (see page 128), or attempt it with straight legs (as for step 8). Crossing your arms over your chest will also make things brutal.

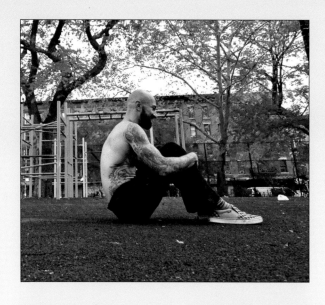
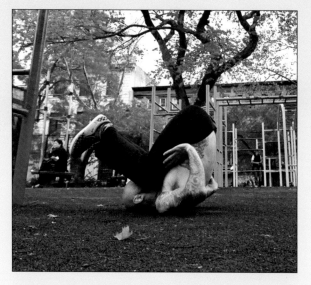
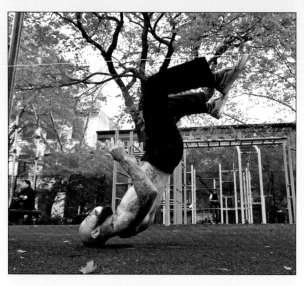
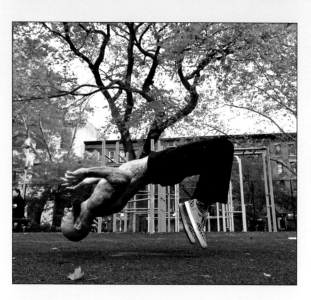
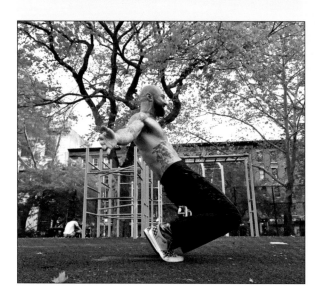
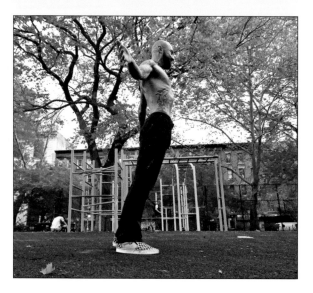

EXPLOSIVE CALISTHENICS

GOING BEYOND

ROLL KIP

An acrobatic variant of the kip-up is the *roll kip*; from standing, perform the beginning stage of a forward roll. When your upper-back contacts the floor, you will be in a position not unlike a roll-up (see page 128)—use the momentum to kick out into a kip-up.

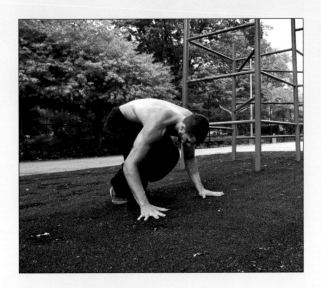
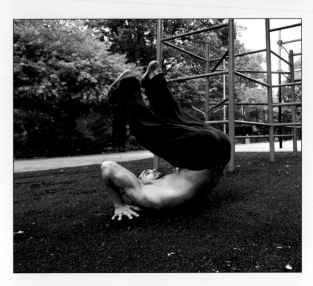
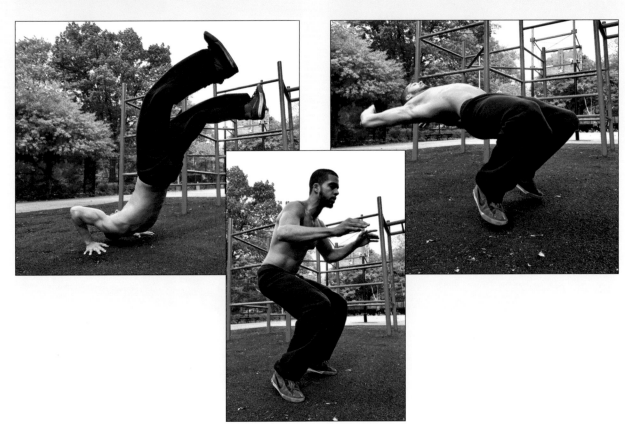

HEAD KIP

A logical extension of the roll kip is the *head kip*. Who says you gotta be on your *upper-back* to kip-up? You can do it from your head with a little practice (although this is obviously much easier if you're comfortable in a *headstand*). I don't necessarily endorse this move—it does little for power, and is flavored more like a *trick* than a sensible training drill. But for those of you with strong necks and a sense of adventure, it's there to explore if you want.

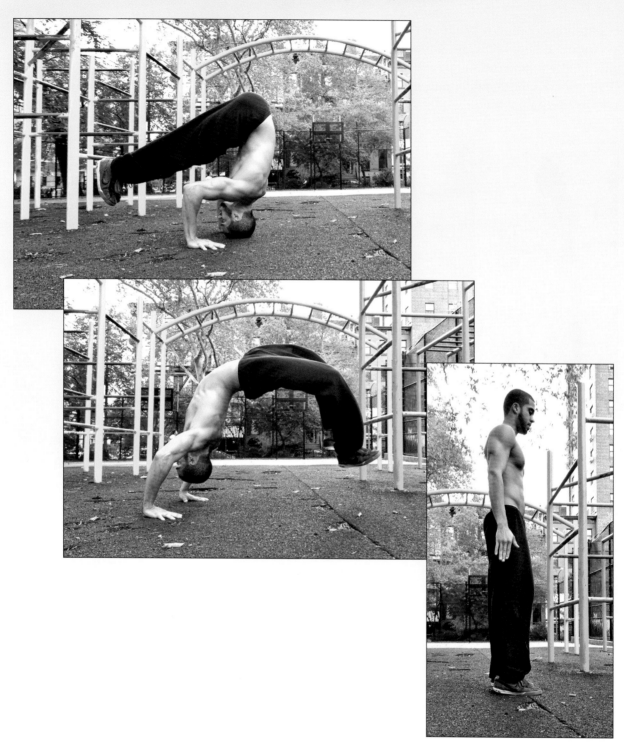

DITANG BREAKFALL

Those of you who want a more vigorous version of the *kip-up* should try the *ditang breakfall*. Developed originally as a martial arts move, you dip and hop back onto your upper-back and shoulders, immediately rebounding via a kip-up using elastic power. It looks cool, but *please* experiment carefully. Start with a soft or cushioned surface and don't attempt it unless you've had a lot of training hours already.

Hip-hop contains a brutal approach to the kip-up known as *rubber banding*. Essentially, you perform a ditang breakfall, kip-up onto your feet, and repeat. The goal is to perform all the reps rhythmically and gracefully. *Easy to say, not easy to do*. Like the head kip and ditang breakfall this is all just for entertainment purposes: I'm not advising you to try 'em. One bad rep could mean one screwed up neck, or worse, clear?

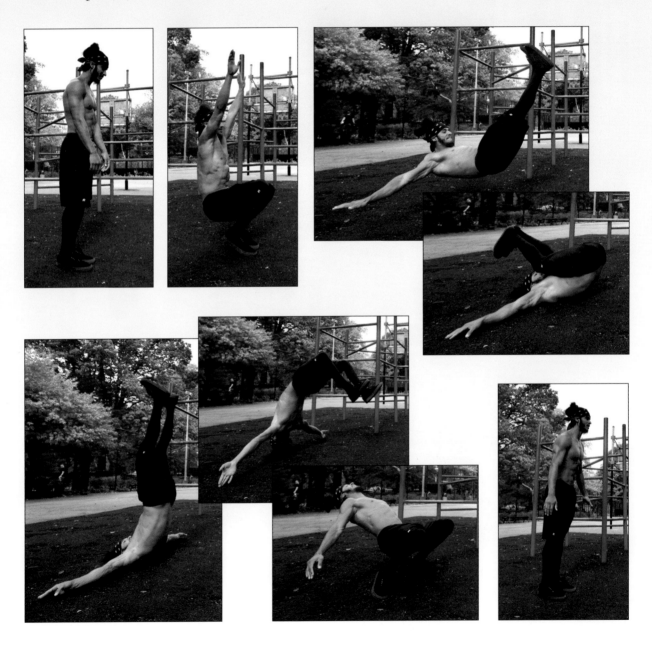

EXPLOSIVE CALISTHENICS

SMALL SPACE DRILLS

Following are three useful speed and power techniques you can utilize in your routine for variety, as ancillary work or to train your muscles from different angles. They are all solo drills, and they require zero equipment. Unlike the progressive exercises in the chains, most of the following drills can be performed rhythmically for higher reps, and can work well when used with any of the chains in this book. In this sense, they can also work as warm-ups or finishing exercises in an explosives session.

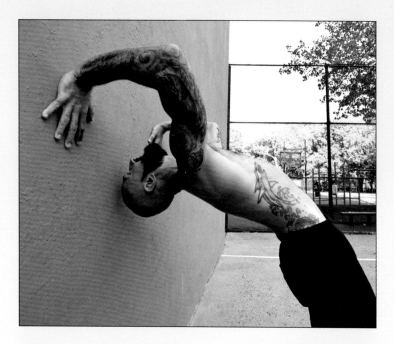

BRIDGE PUSH-OFFS

Stand a short distance from a sturdy wall, facing away from it. Bend back and place your hands on the wall, bending your arms as much as you can. Once your arms are well bent, push away from the wall fast enough to end up standing. This drill is a great one to condition the shoulder and arm muscles for the kip-up hand position. If it's too easy, move further from the wall, or try using just one hand.

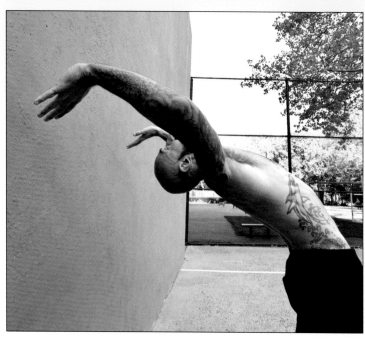

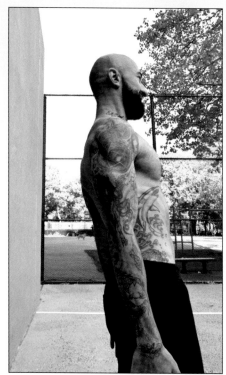

SITTING KIPS

Kneel down on your shins and insteps, Japanese-style (In the photos, Al is performing a slightly easier version on his toes). Throw your arms and torso up with a snap, using the small amount of height you get from this to whip your legs out from under you. Finish in a standing position. The *sitting kip* is a great example of a speed drill, and imparts the kind of hip-snap that's needed in real kips. A few reps of this beauty is a great addition to any routine, especially if you feel like you're slowing down.

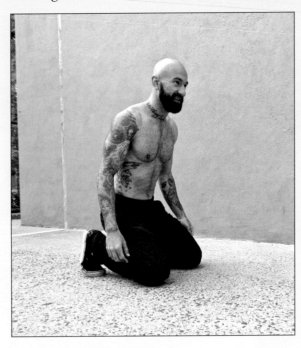
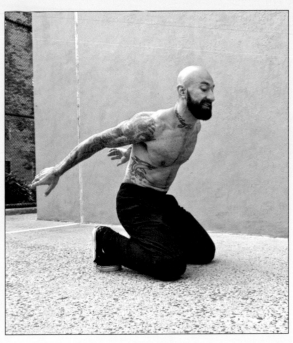
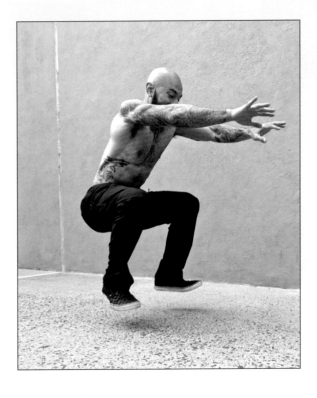
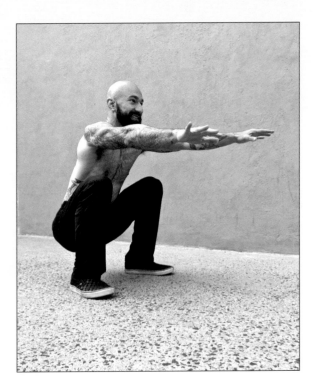

PRONE KIP

This is a fairly rare drill, though it was a favorite of Brett "the Hitman" Hart back in the day. Lay face down with your knees bent and your body and palms supporting you. Push down hard through the hands to gain enough height to whip your legs in underneath you. Finish standing. Can also be done from the palms instead of the fists. Another wonderful variation on the classic *kip-up*.

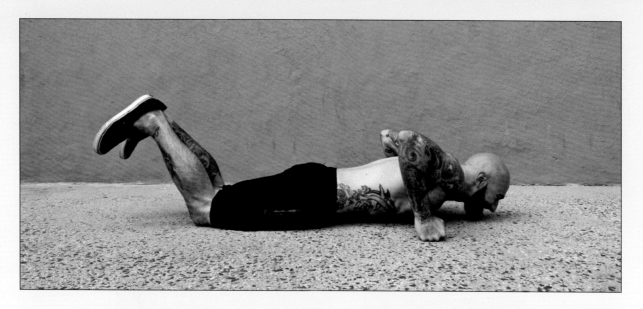

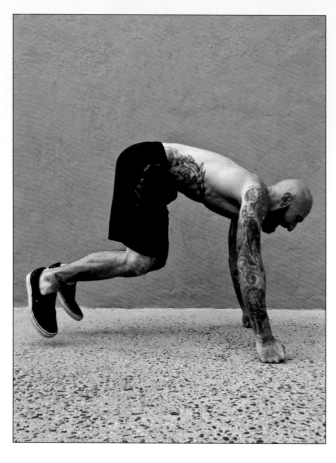

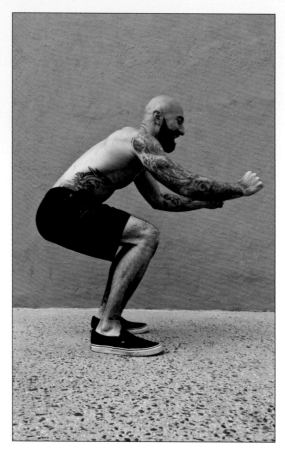

LIGHTS OUT!

At the beginning of this chapter, I mentioned that fact that most kids—most *boys*, anyways—have tried their best to pull off a kip-up. In fact, it's about time more *adult* athletes began exploring this movement as a serious tool in their power armory.

A major part of the reason athletes of all ages avoid kip-ups is that they see them as a binary movement—all or nothing. Some people (the light, lucky ones) can bang out kip-ups the first time of trying. Others know they can't, so they avoid the motion. If this is you, I'm asking ya for a *mindset change*. Stop thinking of kip-ups as a *single movement*, and rather as a *family of techniques*. Some versions are elite-level Shaolin tough; others are more family friendly and can be performed by almost anyone. If you begin at the beginning, you too can progress up through these movements, and be whipping onto your feet with pride.

Trust me, nobody's looking, and nobody cares but you and me. To paraphrase the Godfather of Soul, "*Get down on the floor, then get up offa that thing!*"

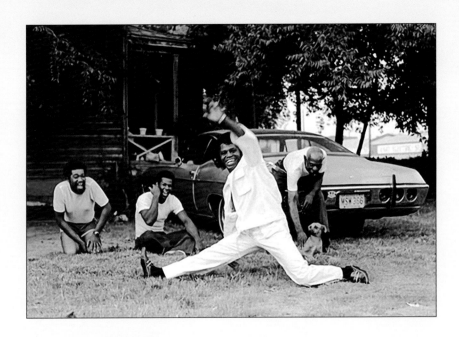

7

THE FRONT FLIP
LIGHTNING MOVEMENT SKILLS

Tthink you're *powerful, explosive, fast?* Would you count yourself as *agile?* Reckon you've got *strong joints* and excellent *coordination* plus *ideal reflexes?*

Well, there's one real quick test to find out if you really are all these things. It won't take long, we won't need any special equipment, and scientific measuring instruments are not required. Just jump up, complete a full 360 degree forward revolution in mid-air, and land on your feet again in the same place you started. Ta-daa! It's a pretty black-and-white test—if you can do it, you're one hell of an explosive athlete. If not, you still have a way to go, right? If so, I want to help.

The movement I described is the *front flip*—known as the *standing front tuck* in gymnastics. If there's an iconic test of power and agility, it's this—trust me, your entire body, from your *toes* to your *neck* needs to be whip-like explosive in order to make this one work. It's simple, ancient, hardcore, and requires no equipment to perform. But God *damn*, it's one hell of a technique, and only the explosive need apply. The good news is that you can *become* explosive, and you can train yourself to perform this iconic stunt, starting anywhere, even if you are out-of-shape. All you need are the progressions and knowledge in this chapter. Get ready to impress the neighbors.

DECONSTRUCTING FRONT FLIPS

Let's examine one of the advanced techniques in the front flip chain: step 9, the *running front flip*. (This awesome move contains many of the components of the other steps.) There are *five* basic stages to look at when analyzing this flip:

RUN-UP

You only need a few steps for this—less than ten feet is optimal for most athletes. A huge long run-up might help with a *long jump* in track and field, but it won't add to your front flip. There is only so much horizontal momentum that you can transform into vertical momentum by blocking anyway. (You should have already mastered the technique of *blocking* via the power jump chain; see pages 41-42). You don't need to sprint, either—a few steps at a fast jog are enough. Approaching the block too rapidly can make it difficult.

TAKE-OFF

The take-off is misunderstood. Jumping—and vertical power—are essential for getting a front flip. But it's a mistake to think that you *jump straight upwards* on take-off. You don't. You *dive* up *and* forwards; a good visualization is to imagine diving head-first over the highest wall you could manage. As you dive, the arms swing downwards from your head, followed shortly afterwards by the explosive forwards sit-up motion of the torso. In explosive forward rotation, the trunk, torso and arms must all play their part in building circular momentum. One of the best drills for developing this momentum is already in this book—the *kip-up*. Yep, the kip-up rotation is partial (only 90 degrees) and the front flip rotation is fuller (the big 360); but the *muscles* are the same. Athletes who have already progressed with—or mastered—the classic kip-up, inevitably find the front flip *much* easier to approach.

TUCK

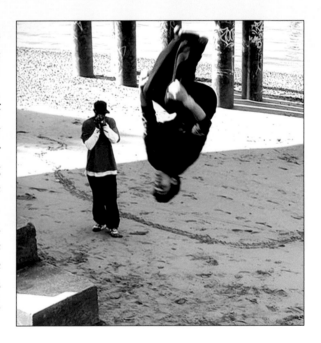

After the take-off—but pretty simultaneous with throwing the torso forward—comes the *tuck*. Have you ever seen an ice skater spinning? Sometimes they pull their leg and arms in close, and this makes the spin accelerate much faster. If you have ever seen this, you have witnessed how drawing the limbs in tight increases *angular momentum*. This is why we tuck tightly during flips—the tucking action makes the body revolve quicker, allowing us to land on our feet in time. Most of the tuck is due to hip and midsection power; if you have worked your way through the power jump drills, you will have an adequate tuck by now—and trust me, you'll need one: this element is so important that gymnasts still call the front *flip* the front *tuck*.

UNFURL

Once the tuck has done its job and got you over—i.e., your legs have revolved past the point of your head, and your body is heading towards horizontal—your next job is to *unfurl* your legs, to start to straighten them for landing. This requires some speed, but no real power. The real difficulty here is *timing*. Most neophytes assume the back flip is harder than the front (because you are going backwards), but I'm convinced that the front flip is harder, and one reason has to do with *vision*. In a back flip, you can actually *see* the floor as you rotate, and your body and brain can work out when to unfurl. With the front flip, you are pretty much flying blind, and will have to rely on instinctive kinesthetic timing: your body will have to *remember* where the floor is. A good (but not perfect) rule of thumb is to unfurl the moment your tuck is deep (i.e., when the knees come as close to the chest as you can manage).

LANDING

The landing is the end point, and the sum of the previous four actions. Remember, these actions aren't discrete units—they all *flow*. They must. In terms of conditioning, lots of jump drills should have prepared your landing reflexes, and fortified the bones and tissues of your feet, ankles and knees. Beyond this, the only advice I can give you is *drill*. Yep, you'll land on your ass a lot. Then eventually you may start to over-rotate and land on your knees and hands. The ideal landing is not easy: the writer G. K. Chesterton once noted that: *there are an infinite number of angles at which one can fall, but only one in which we can stand.* (He was right: where do gymnasts always seem to go wrong? The landing!) But—with time—you'll perfect your rotation.

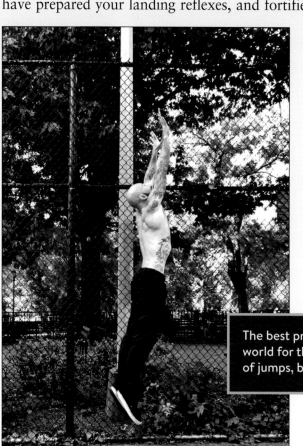

The best pre-conditioning in the world for the front flip? A heavy diet of jumps, baby!

THE FRONT FLIP CHAIN

What's the easiest way to rotate forwards? To roll. So that's what we start with, the *shoulder roll* (step 1), the simplest way of rolling over forwards. The *press roll* (step 2) requires you to direct your roll using your *hands*—which allows some gentle forces to run through the arms and shoulders. These forces ramp up in the *jump roll* (step 3), where your hands contact the floor and briefly take some of your body's weight before you roll through. The *handstand roll* (step 4) is the final roll in the chain, and continues the athletes' conditioning by forcing them to hold *all* their body's weight on their hands—if only for a fraction of a second—before rolling through. Once you've completed a course of all these rolls, your arms, shoulders and back will be conditioned to holding your weight as part of a rotation, and revolving forwards quickly will no longer make you dizzy or nauseous.

When you can do a handstand roll well, you're ready to attempt a *back-drop handspring* (step 5). This involves running and jumping forward into a handspring and pushing off—just like a regular handspring—except you land on your feet and butt. This, essentially, is what it looks like when most people try a handspring for the first time—they get lift off, but can't quite achieve the full rotation, enough to land on their feet. With time and practice—a lot of drilling—you will automatically begin to achieve that. When you land on your feet and stay upright, you're at the *front handspring* stage (step 6). After the front handspring is properly *mastered*—not just performed once—the athlete moves on to tackle the perfect version of the exercise, the *flyspring* (step 7). A flyspring is, essentially a symmetrical front handspring; in the regular version, it's easier to push off one leg more than the other, but in the flyspring you push off both equally.

Once you've got the flyspring right, you'll be able to approach the proper front flip, where the hands don't touch the floor. Like for the front handspring, you'll initially need to drill a stage where you can't rotate fully, and after a run-up and attempt, you land on your feet and butt rather than standing. This is the *back-drop front flip* (step 8). When the rotation becomes complete, you have the *running front flip* (step 9). This is a major milestone—all it takes is to gradually remove the steps in the run-up, and the athlete becomes the proud possessor of the *standing front flip* (step 10). I say "all it takes"—of course—this is a huge leap to make. But it can be done over time, if the athlete is lean enough, and if they continue to work diligently and progressively on the basic power moves (*jumps* and *power pushups*).

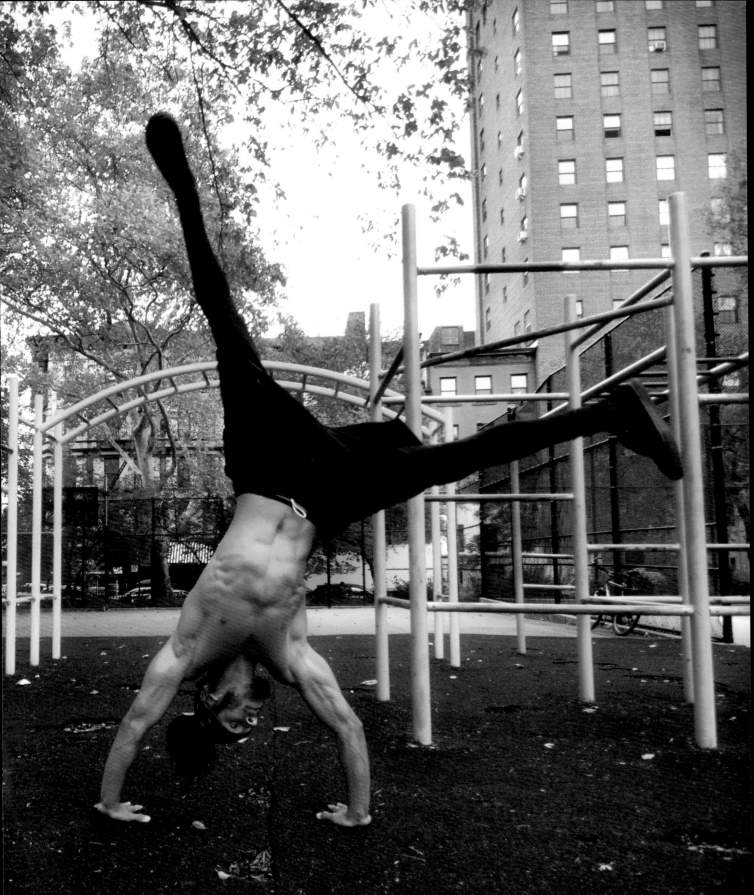

STEP ONE: SHOULDER ROLL

PERFORMANCE

- Squat towards the ground. (Placing the foot of your strongest side forward slightly may feel more comfortable.)

- Place the edge of your palm heel on the ground as you dip down—again, using your strongest side. You can place your free hand on the ground, if it helps.

- Continue lowering slowly down and forwards, until you overbalance. Brace your arm to take most of your weight. As your legs swing, simultaneously bring your hands up and towards your head.

- Let your braced arm and shoulder guide your movement as you roll over—keep your head tucked in and out of the way.

- Roll over your back, trying not to veer to either side.

- Finish the roll naturally, in a seated position.

EXERCISE X-RAY

This type of roll is the easiest on the body and joints; it's the kind of breakfall/front roll (*ukemi*) you will see in many Japanese martial arts, such as jujutsu and aikido. Because the leading upper arm directs the weight of the body straight onto the upper-back, the wrists, elbows and shoulders feel no strain during the exercise. This drill should be performed gently.

REGRESSION

Rolling can make athletes nauseous, if they aren't accustomed to it. To make the spin seem easier at first, carefully lower the head down close to the floor before initiating the rolling motion.

PROGRESSION

Once you can execute this drill slowly with good form, safely pick up speed. Keep the movement smooth—it should be impact-free. When you can perform it quickly, you can use the momentum to stand up at the end (*see photos*). Some martial artists *spin* during the roll, so that they are facing in the opposite direction when they stand—to face their attacker.

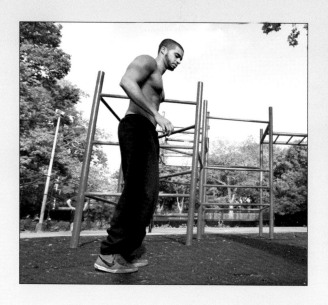 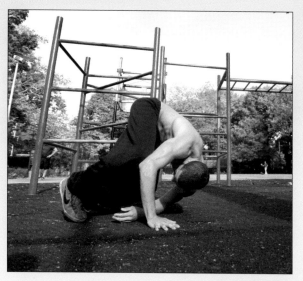

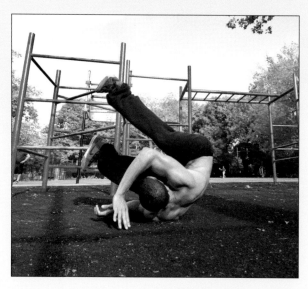 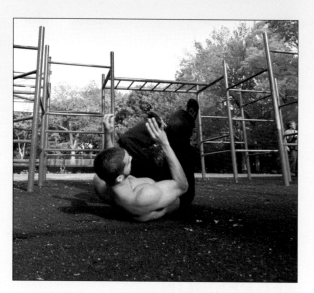

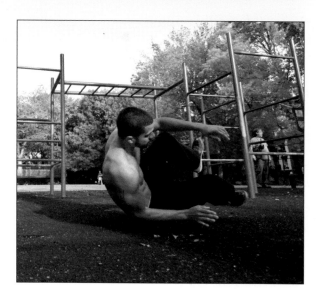 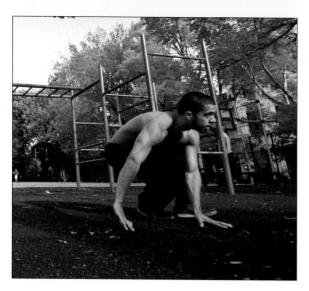

EXPLOSIVE CALISTHENICS

STEP TWO: PRESS ROLL

PERFORMANCE

- With your feet symmetrical, squat towards the ground.

- Place both palms on the floor in front of you as you dip down.

- Continue lowering slowly down and forwards, by squatting and bringing your torso down. Straighten your legs until you overbalance forward. Brace your arms to take most of your weight.

- Let your braced arms guide your movement as you roll over—keep your head tucked in and out of the way. Your head should take virtually no weight.

- Roll over your back, trying not to veer to either side.

- Finish the roll naturally, in a seated position.

EXERCISE X-RAY

During handsprings, your arms have to take the pressure of your spinning body. This form of roll begins to make use of the hands as levers to control the body, albeit in a very gentle way. More advanced rolling drills will progressively increase the forces passing through the upper limbs.

REGRESSION

Rolling can seem intimidating to newbies. A controlled descent of the head, a bracing of the curled trunk (*abdominal tension*) and the use of soft surfaces (grass, carpeting) are all tricks that can be used to make rolls seem easier.

PROGRESSION

In the easiest type of *press roll*, the hands and upper-back take the body's weight at the beginning of the technique, with the head tucked in tightly for protection. To make the drill harder, take more force through the hands, so that the upper-back only takes on force at the last moment.

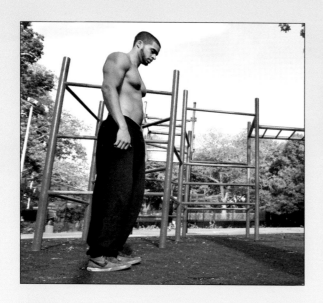
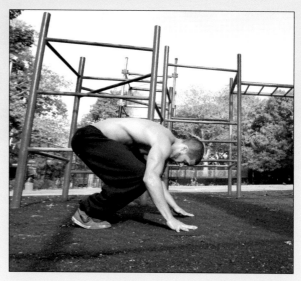
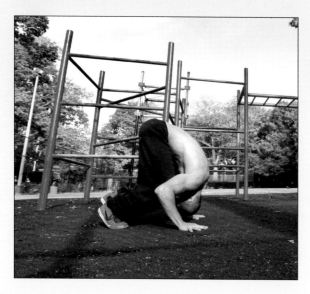
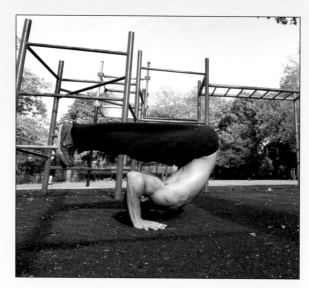
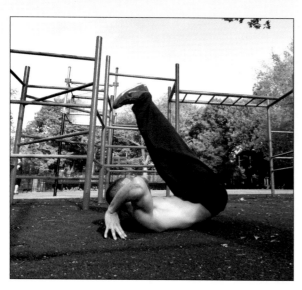
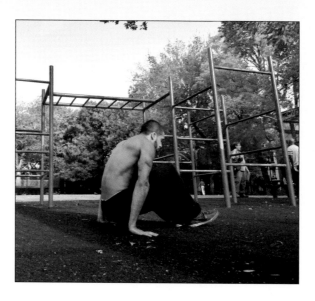

EXPLOSIVE CALISTHENICS

STEP THREE: JUMP ROLL

PERFORMANCE

- With your feet symmetrical, bend forward aiming your palms towards the floor.

- Jump up as you descend, allowing your torso to fall as you drop your hands to the floor.

- Land on your palms, arms fairly straight, just as your feet leave the floor. You are basically catching yourself with your palms.

- Let your braced arms bend to guide your movement as you roll over—keep your head tucked in and out of the way. Your head should take virtually no weight.

- Roll over your back, trying not to veer to either side.

- Finish the roll naturally. By now you should have advanced enough to roll all the way to the standing position.

EXERCISE X-RAY

These roll-drills might not look much like a handstand, but they are a great way for non-tumblers to teach their brains to get used to the *turning* motion before exploring tougher techniques. Gymnasts often learn this roll by diving up and *forwards*—this is called a *dive roll*. In the *jump roll*, however, you build power and explosive strength by jumping *up* more than *forwards*.

REGRESSION

To reduce demands on upper-body power, begin the jump up with the palms already braced on the floor.

PROGRESSION

The higher your hands are from the floor when your feet leave the ground, the more plyometric this drill becomes. (See page 315)

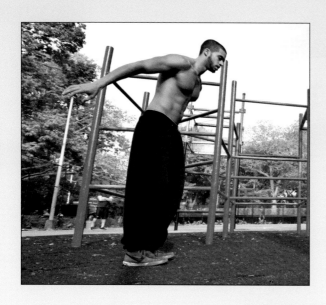 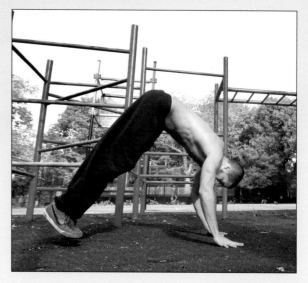

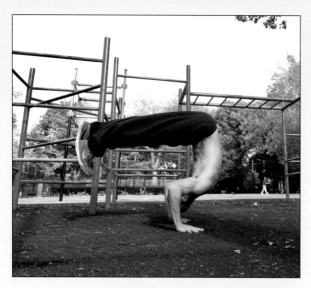 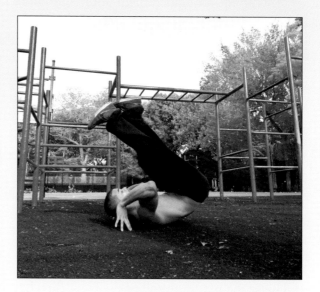

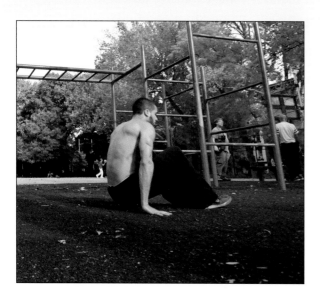 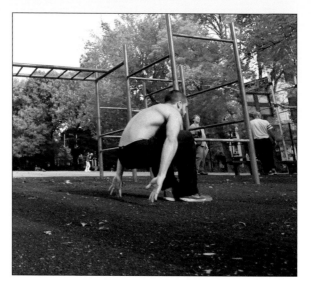

EXPLOSIVE CALISTHENICS

STEP FOUR: HANDSTAND ROLL

PERFORMANCE

- In a split stance with your strongest foot forward, place your palms on the floor and raise your other leg behind you.

- Push yourself up through your strongest foot, swinging back and up with your other foot. Allow your torso to become more vertical as you go.

- Let the momentum from your leg push/swing to carry your legs above your torso; as they whip up, straighten them until your entire body is aligned in a handstand.

- You don't need to hold the handstand. Allow your arms to bend and your trunk to curl up beneath you as soon as you begin to fall forward.

- Let your braced arms guide your movement as you roll over—keep your head tucked in and out of the way. Your head should take virtually no weight.

- Roll over your back, trying not to veer to either side.

- Finish the roll naturally. By now you should have advanced enough to roll all the way to the standing position.

EXERCISE X-RAY

This is the final true roll of the front flip chain. It requires some explosive power to kick the legs up above you, and begins developing the solid arm strength required for *front handsprings*.

REGRESSION

To make this movement easier, keep the arms bent throughout: this avoids the need to attain a handstand position.

PROGRESSION

Begin with your hands off the floor, and kick up with the legs a split-second before your palms make contact with the ground.

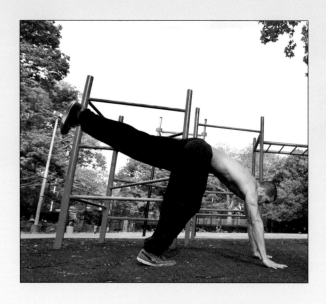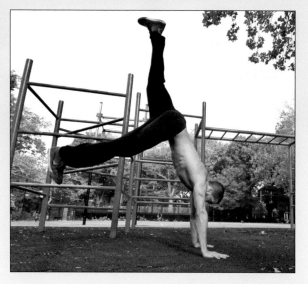
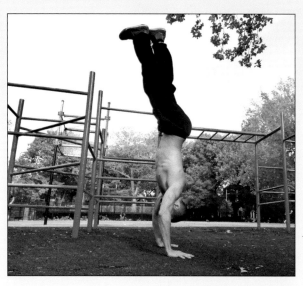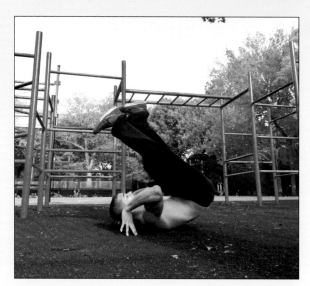
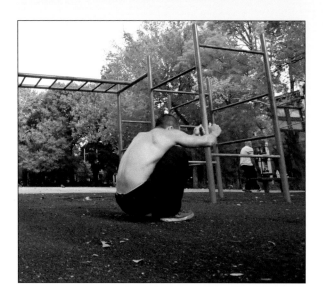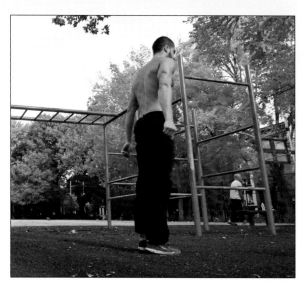

STEP FIVE: BACK-DROP HANDSPRING

PERFORMANCE

- Take a step to build momentum, and with your hands up above you, kick off with your strongest leg.

- Allow your torso to fall as you drop your hands to the floor. As your hands approach the ground, jump up hard, swinging with your highest leg.

- Keep your arms fairly straight, just as your feet leave the floor. You are basically catching yourself with your palms.

- Let the momentum from your jump to carry your legs above your torso.

- Allow your forward momentum to turn you over. As you spin, tuck in your head, curl your trunk, and whip your hands up off the floor.

- The bottoms of your feet should be the first part of your body to touch the ground after your hands lift off.

- Your feet should quickly act as shock absorbers, before your glutes, arms and back also contact the ground.

EXERCISE X-RAY

You are now very, very close to the *front handspring*—a pivotal exercise to learn if you wish to master the *front flip*. This drill looks like a partial handspring, teaching athletes the first portion of the spin out of the handstand. Very little upper-body explosiveness is required to master this, however. Even fairly weak athletes can practice this drill.

REGRESSION

At first you may begin by landing on your glutes or back before your feet can act as shock absorbers. If this is you, you can still practice this drill until you improve, but definitely use padding on the floor. (Use your imagination: how about pillows: cushions: parts of a couch, even a mattress?)

PROGRESSION

As you improve, you will begin to generate enough momentum so that you fall back onto your butt after landing on your feet. That's fine—think of the "fall-back handspring" as a hidden step between the *back-drop handspring* and the running *front handspring*, and drill it until you transcend it.

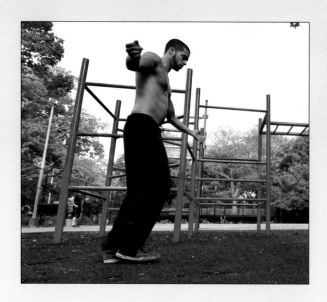
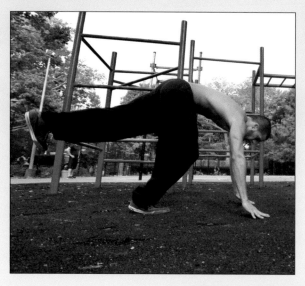
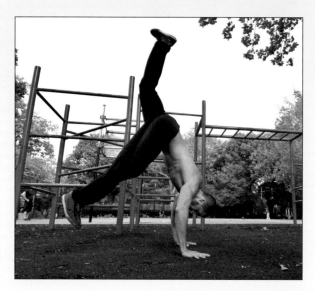
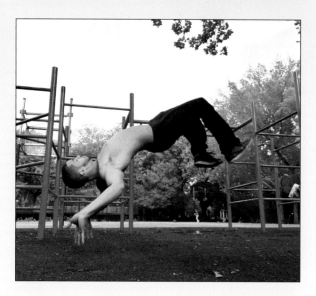
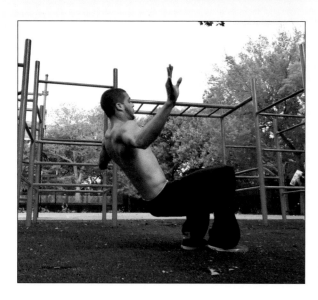
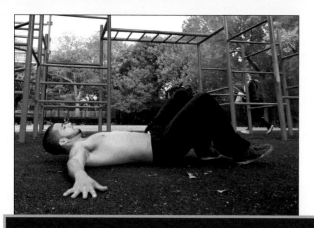

WARNING! Vertical is a master acrobat and can perform this exercise safely, even on a hard surface. Beginners should *definitely* use whatever padding they can find to protect themselves! "

STEP SIX: FRONT HANDSPRING

PERFORMANCE

- Take a run-up to build momentum.

- *Block* (see page 50) by punching down on the floor with your strongest foot. (This will be easier than using both feet, because you can simultaneously swing your rear leg up, as you did for the previous two steps.)

- Kick up hard through your strongest leg, pushing your foot off the ground but allowing your torso to fall as you drop your hands to the floor. Your other foot should swing up behind you, assisting the rotation.

- Land on your palms, arms slightly bent, just as your feet leave the floor. You are basically catching yourself with your palms.

- Allow the momentum from your jump to carry your legs above your torso, into a bent-leg handstand position.

- Don't hold the handstand, but allow your forward momentum to turn you over.

- Extend through your arms and hands to gain extra height.

- Continue pulling your torso forward as you land on both feet. If you need to, step forward to dissipate extra momentum.

EXERCISE X-RAY

Many calisthenics experts consider the *front handspring* a key stage in the development of the *front flip*—it is, but it is also a phenomenal explosive drill in its own right. The athlete who can perform this correctly has reached an excellent level in fundamental skills such as: running, blocking, jumping, explosive pressing (with the upper-body), rotational tolerance and landing.

REGRESSION

Landing in a low squat position will be easier because it requires less rotation; you may also fall back onto your glutes at first.

PROGRESSION

To progress, improve your rotation: a good measure of this is the ability to land with a more *extended* body, instead of in a deep squat position. Avoid over/under-rotation and learn to land without taking any adjustment steps.

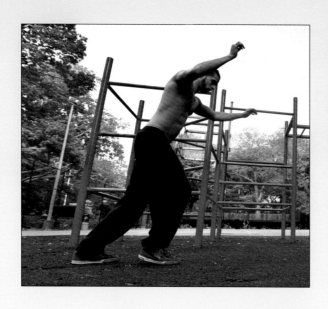
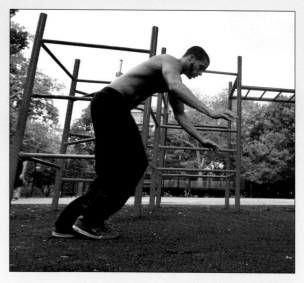
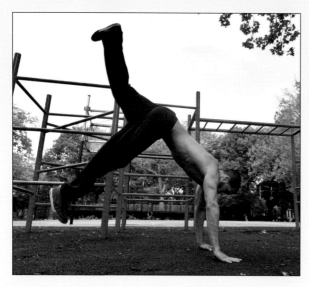
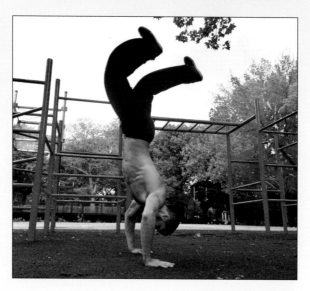
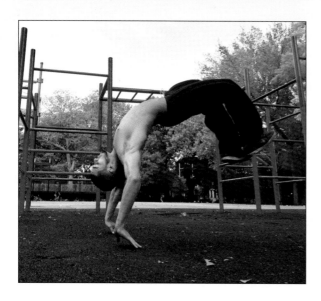
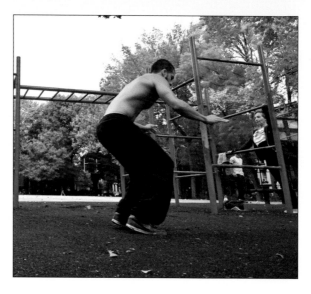

STEP SEVEN: FLYSPRING

PERFORMANCE

- Take a run-up to build momentum.

- Perform a *block jump* (see page 50) with both feet, as you throw your hands down.

- Kick up hard through the legs, pushing your feet off the ground but allowing your torso to fall as you drop your hands to the floor.

- Land on your palms, arms nearly straight, as your feet leave the floor. You are basically catching yourself with your palms.

- Let the momentum from your jump to carry your legs above your torso.

- Allow your forward momentum to turn you over. Extend through your arms and hands to gain extra height.

- Continue pulling your torso forward as you land on both feet. If you need to, step forward to dissipate extra momentum.

EXERCISE X-RAY

Once an athlete has mastered the *front handspring* with a run-up, the next step is to explore the *flyspring*. Whereas the front handspring is performed by kicking off the stronger leg, sometimes landing with the feet apart (or unsymmetrical), in the flyspring you block (jump) off both feet together, and also land on both feet symmetrically. This requires much more total body power. The flyspring has several names—it's sometimes called a *bounder*.

REGRESSION

If moving from front handsprings (step 6) to flysprings is too difficult, try back-drop flysprings at first—lay out some padding and perform the set-up with feet together, but finish in the *back-drop position* (see step 5).

PROGRESSION

To increase difficulty, gradually perform fewer steps in the run-up; ultimately the perfect version can be performed from *standing*—you can also learn the *front handspring* (step 6) from standing. However this requires huge power, and is not necessary to be able to approach the front flip.

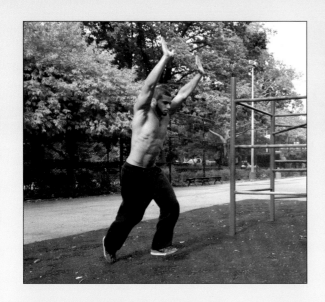
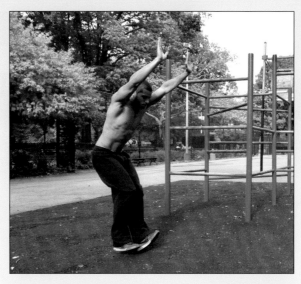
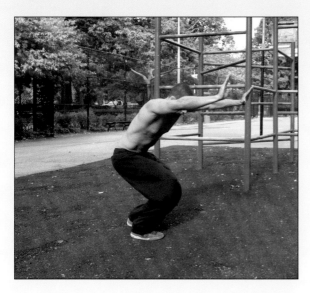
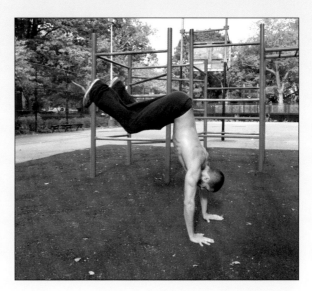
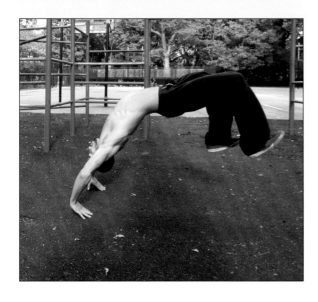
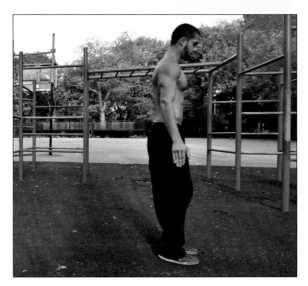

STEP EIGHT: BACK-DROP FLIP

PERFORMANCE

- Take a run up of several steps to build momentum.

- Perform a *block jump* (see page 50) with both feet, as you throw your hands down.

- Jump up hard, simultaneously throwing your hands down and pulling your curled upper body down at the hips.

- Immediately begin to pull your knees up to your chest. This is the *tuck* and will help you rotate.

- As you rotate over, begin to extend the legs. (This extension will help your feet contact the floor before your back, protecting your spine. Never land flat on your back if you can avoid it, even with a padded floor.)

- The bottoms of your feet should be the first part of your body to touch the ground. The feet should quickly act as shock absorbers, before your glutes and back also contact the ground. You can also spread the force by touching down with the hands.

EXERCISE X-RAY

For most athletes—no matter how disciplined you are in applying intelligent progressions—there is gonna come a time when, in the process of mastering the *front flip*, you land on your ass. This, in fact, is a big part of the process. It takes time to gain the power to carry the rotation forwards into a standing or semi-standing position. Embrace *back-drop flips* as the "missing link".

REGRESSION

I know I promote drills with minimal equipment, but this sucker is definitely an exception. *Always* begin this technique with maximum padding to protect your spine. Dragging a thick mattress onto the floor is a good option.

PROGRESSION

At first, you'll land on your glutes more, and less on your feet. In time, you'll land with your weight *over* your feet, until you land in a semi-squat, typically falling back from that position. Once you can land in a semi-squat consistently, it's time to take the padding away and move to step 9.

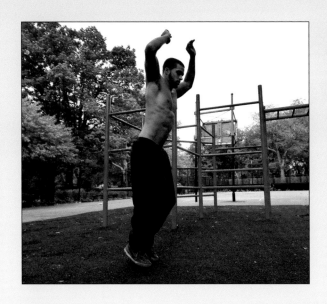

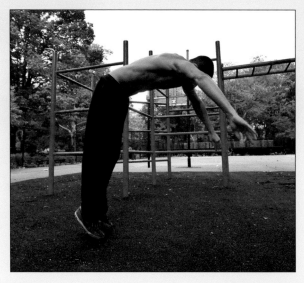

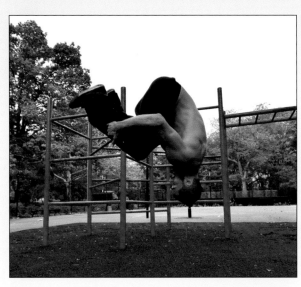

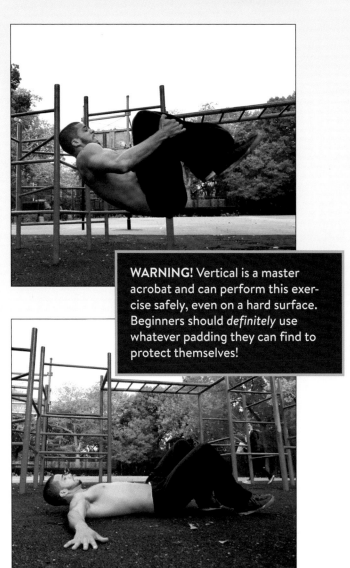

WARNING! Vertical is a master acrobat and can perform this exercise safely, even on a hard surface. Beginners should *definitely* use whatever padding they can find to protect themselves!

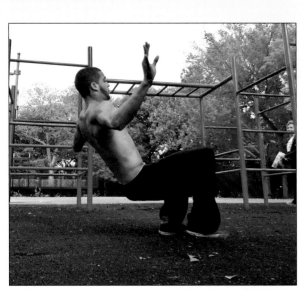

STEP NINE: RUNNING FRONT FLIP

PERFORMANCE

- Take a run up of several steps to build momentum.

- Perform a *block jump* (see page 50) on the floor with both feet.

- Jump up hard, simultaneously throwing your hands down and pulling your curled upper body down at the hips.

- Simultaneously snap your knees up to your chest. The tighter your tuck, the better you will rotate.

- As your rotate over, quickly whip your legs out beneath you.

- Land on the balls of your feet with slightly bent knees to absorb the shock; continue taking a few steps forwards (or even backwards, if you under-rotated) to steady yourself, if you need to.

EXERCISE X-RAY

The Master Step of this chain, the *front flip*—the hardest variation of this exercise—is performed from *standing*. This preliminary step, the *running front flip*, is significantly easier, because taking a run-up—even a few steps—adds forwards momentum to the rotation, as well as vertical momentum (through *blocking*: see page 41). This drill is used in calisthenics disciplines as diverse as parkour and martial arts "tricking", and any athlete who reaches this stage should be proud as hell of his or her achievement.

REGRESSION

As with the *back-drop flip*, a simple way of overcoming fear is to use padding beneath you—a mattress at first, later cushions, pillows and similar lighter padding. This is partly for safety reasons, but is mostly psychological, to help counter the primal fear of crashing. Eventually you must remove all padding—when you do, try the drill on grass if you can.

PROGRESSION

Progress by taking fewer steps in the run-up—this will force your own body to produce the explosive power required to complete the rotation.

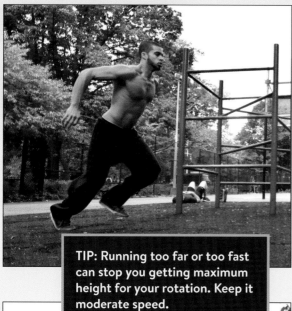

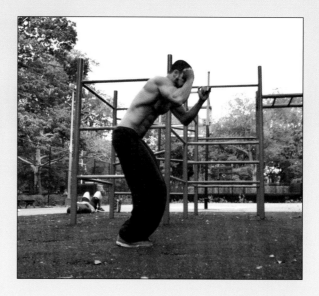

TIP: Running too far or too fast can stop you getting maximum height for your rotation. Keep it moderate speed.

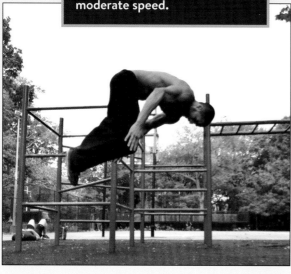

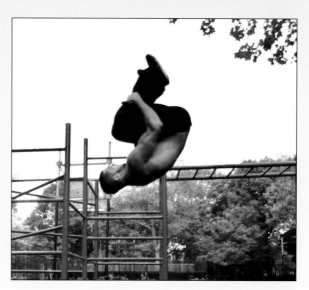

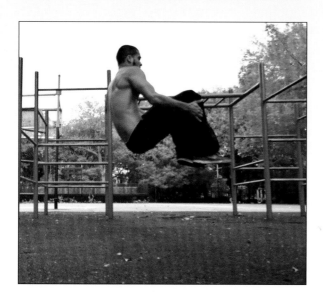

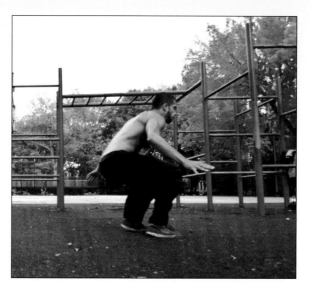

MASTER STEP: FRONT FLIP

PERFORMANCE

- Stand with your feet less than shoulder-width apart, and your arms above your head.

- Begin by rising onto your toes to generate a little extra "bounce".

- Dip down at the knees and hips, and explode your legs upwards as you simultaneously snap your torso and arms downwards.

- The *upwards* leg push combined with the *downwards* torso/arm thrust will cause mid-air rotation.

- As soon as the feet leave the floor, tuck the knees into the chest. The tighter you tuck, the quicker you'll rotate. Speed is of the essence in a standing front flip. On their downwards path, your hands may meet your shins—some athletes even grip their shins or knees to enhance the tuck. (See also the *catch tuck jump*, page 58.)

- As your rotate over, quickly whip your legs out beneath you.

- Land on the balls of your feet with bent knees to absorb the shock; extend the arms out in front for balance if you need to.

EXERCISE X-RAY

Make no mistake—the *front flip* is THE explosive exercise *par excellence*. It is the "super-drill" for any athlete wanting speed, agility and explosive power. All the components of supreme human speed and agility are tested to the max in the front flip: jump velocity, hip and waist explosiveness (in tucking), arm speed, and plyometric force absorption (in landing). Yes, it is easiest to learn *front handsprings* before exploring *back flip* work, simply because these the reverse overhead rotation drills are more *intimidating*—but the front flip is actually the more demanding explosive exercise, both technically and in terms of raw power. There is also a big gap in difficulty between the run-up front flip (step 9) and the standing version, where incredible speed is required—don't be embarrassed about training using floor padding to drill a standing *back-drop front flip* variation where you land on your feet then glutes (see step 8). Ultimately, there is only one way to attain the front flip...and that's by drilling easier steps over, and over, and over again, until the components are like lightning. So get moving!

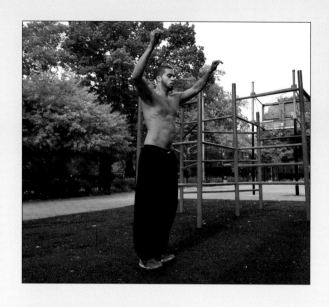
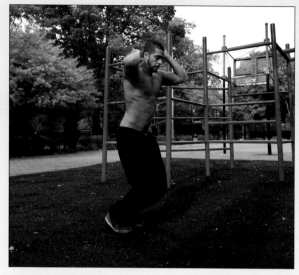
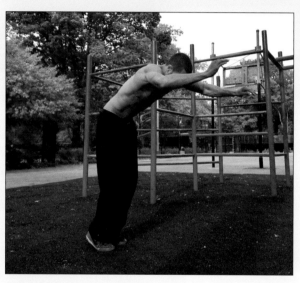
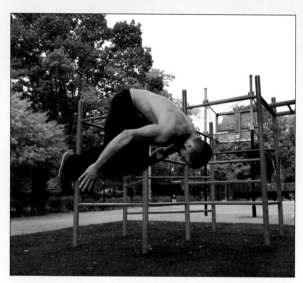
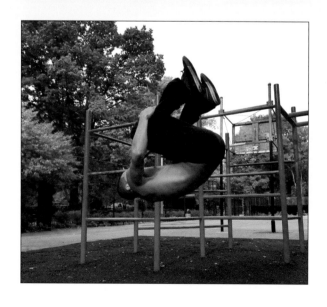
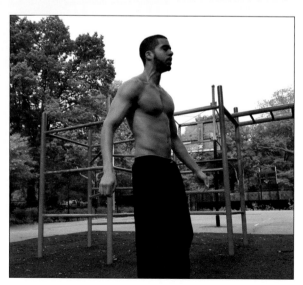

GOING BEYOND

Many athletes who graduate to at least step 9 of the front flip chain (the *running front flip*) can consider *combining* acrobatic movements at this stage, depending how far advanced they are with the back flip chain. None of this is necessary for increased power—it's a skill feat, really—but some athletes will be interested in expanding their acrobatic repertoire. If you wish to explore combinations, it's a good idea to add an extra rotational movement to your arsenal: the *round-off*. The round-off is a lot like a *cartwheel*. Whereas a cartwheel rotates an athlete sideways, the round-off finishes with a slight turn, leaving you facing the way you came.

THE ROUND OFF

The importance of the round-off for combining acrobatic movements is simple; as the name suggests, it turns you around. You start the movement facing front, and can finish facing 180 degrees the other way. This turns your *forward* momentum into *backwards* momentum, for *back flips* or *back handsprings*.

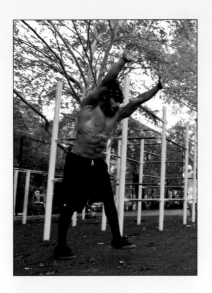 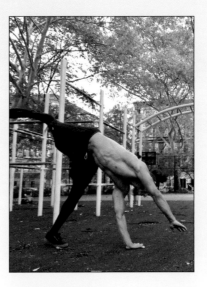 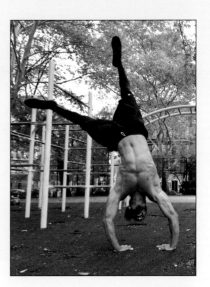

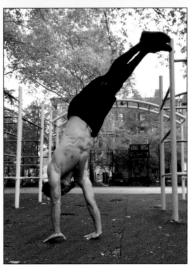 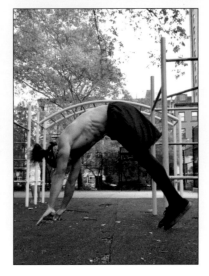 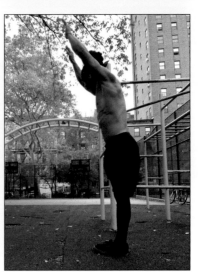

EXPLOSIVE CALISTHENICS

Once you have the round-off in your box of tricks, potential combination sequences include:

- Round-off to back handspring
- Round-off to back flip
- Round-off to back handspring to back flip

...etc. Another interesting combination coming from a slightly different idea, is to combine a *handstand* with a *roll* into a *front flip* (see page 168). The movement feels totally different but will perhaps appeal to hand-balancing aficionados: there are very few ways cooler than this for finishing up a handstand, provided you have the space to do it.

THE CARTWHEEL

The cartwheel can be viewed as a basic progression leading to the round-off. Both cartwheels and round-offs are excellent additions to any athlete's power training regime, in that they add basic *lateral* rotational power to the body, just as the flips add *front*-and-*back* rotational power.

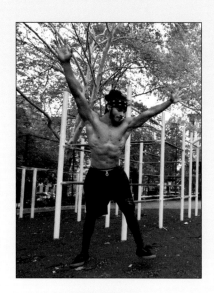
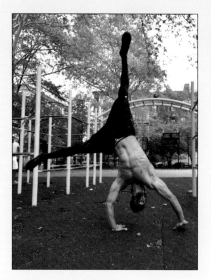
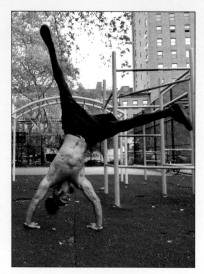

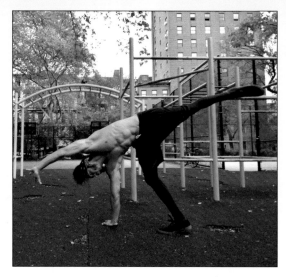
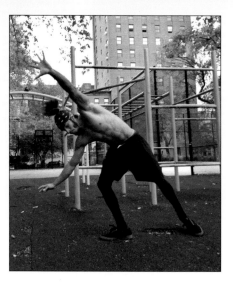

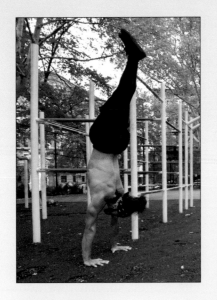
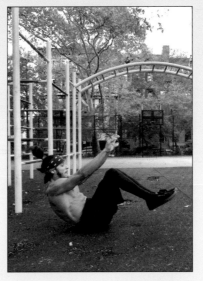
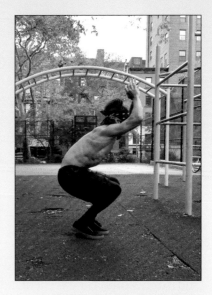
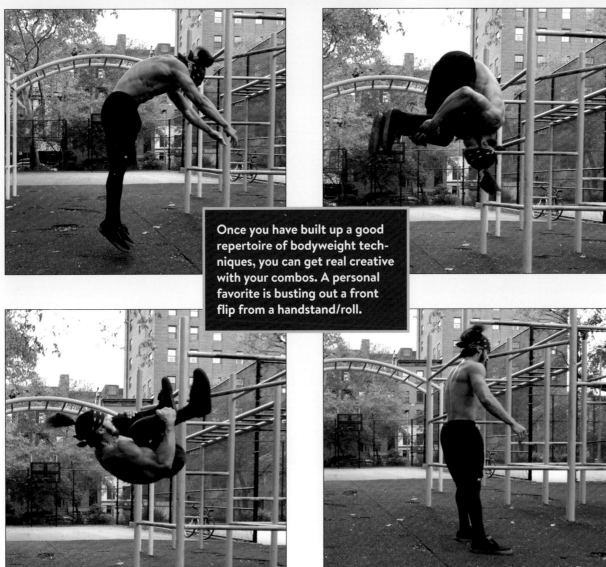

Once you have built up a good repertoire of bodyweight techniques, you can get real creative with your combos. A personal favorite is busting out a front flip from a handstand/roll.

As far as individual techniques go, progressing beyond the front flip is a big task, but it can most certainly be done—such a journey will take you into the sophisticated, asymmetrical-type flipping movements performed in acrobatics, "tricking" and some forms of martial arts.

Bear in mind that these advanced flip forms require incredible skill levels. For sure, many of the athletes who perform them are exceptionally explosive and perhaps even powerful, but it doesn't follow that progressing from front flips to these movements will add very much more explosiveness to your body. It's mostly coordination. Explore them if it interests you, but if it's *power* and *explosiveness* you want, you don't really need to move beyond the standing front flip—you're better off just improving your form and speed on that exercise, while simultaneously increasing linear progression on your basic jumps and power pushups.

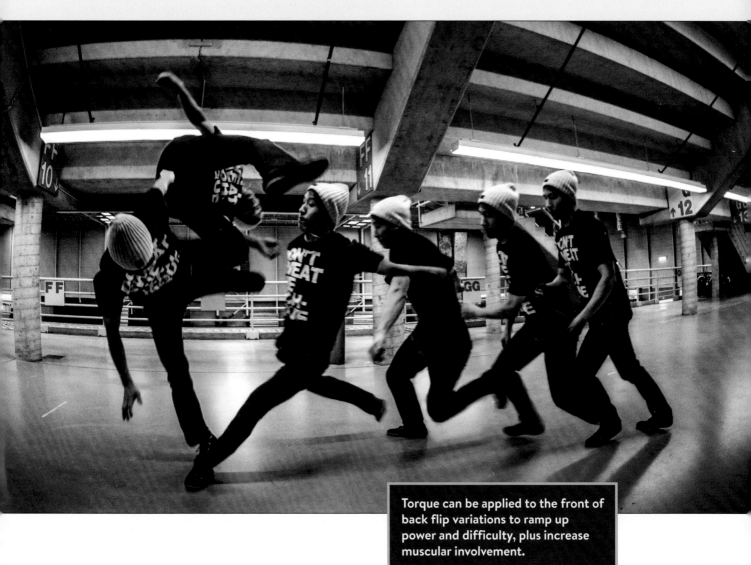

Torque can be applied to the front of back flip variations to ramp up power and difficulty, plus increase muscular involvement.

SMALL SPACE DRILLS

Following are three useful speed and power techniques you can utilize in your routine for variety, as ancillary work or to train your muscles from different angles. They are all solo drills, and they require zero equipment. Unlike the progressive exercises in the chains, most of the following drills can be performed rhythmically for higher reps, and can work well when used with any of the chains in this book. In this sense, they can also work as warm-ups or finishing exercises in an explosives session.

KOJAKS

Bend over and place your palms on the floor, as if you were going to perform a *pike pushup*. Bend the arms until your skull kisses the floor, then straighten them explosively, enough to push yourself off the ground some way. When your hands leave the floor, quickly slap the top of your head with them, before you fall and have to "catch" yourself again. This is a great preliminary to build the kind of explosive pressing power needed in the *front handspring*.

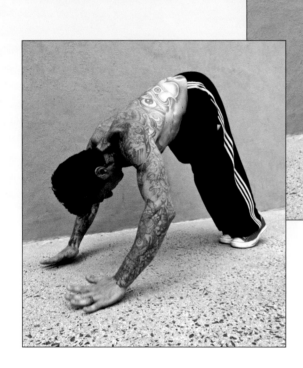

THRUSTERS

These are sometimes called "burpees", depending where you are. In the pushup position explode your knees up into your chest, then immediately thrust them back straight, into the starting position. Essentially this is a kind of prone tucking exercise and is a great example of how some small space drills can be performed for high repetitions for a cardio benefit.

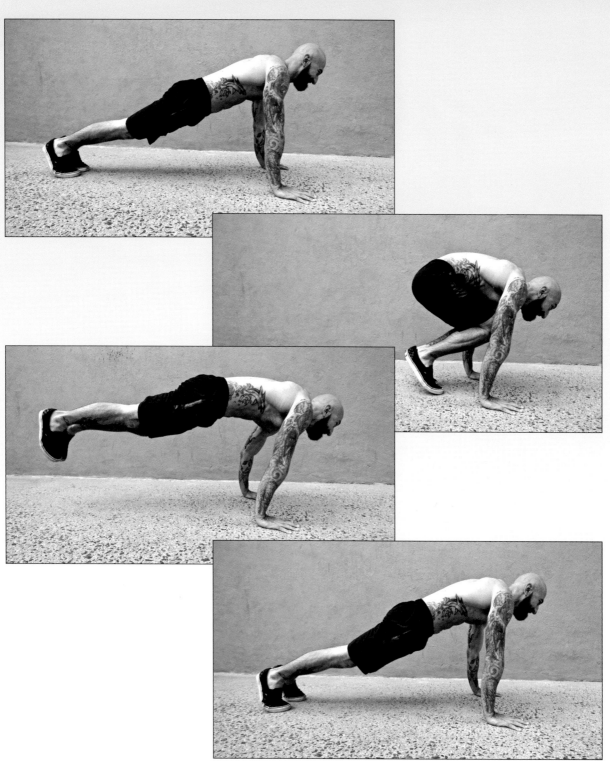

UNILATERAL JUMP

This one's ideal for the strong brothers and sisters who have mastered the one-leg squat. With one leg chambered, squat down on the loaded leg, and spring back up. You can go all the way down into a "pistol", but if you do, ensure you pause at the bottom. Plenty of benefits for this move, ranging from increased coordination, landing balance, stronger ankles, etc.

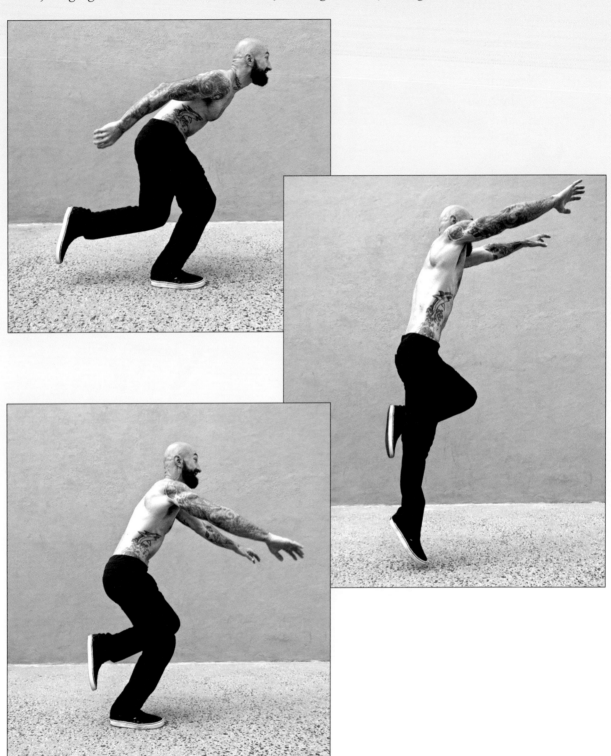

LIGHTS OUT!

I can take a stab at how many folks can do a proper *pullup* but I can't predict what percentage of athletes can perform a *standing front flip*. The number is vanishingly small, even amongst super-athletes like MMA fighters, pro footballers or basketball players. The combination of power, *total body speed*, agility and skill it takes is *tremendous*.

If you want to become one of the very few masters of this exercise—*you can*. It may take years for you to get there or you may achieve it relatively quickly. I can't know without training you myself. I can promise you this much though—when you get there, you WILL be the most explosive athlete in the room, no matter what else you can or can't do. In pretty much any room. But it will take time, and it will take dedication.

So many would-be athletes—potential super-men and women—waste their time thinking about training, reading about training, and cruising the internet looking for training info. Can you imagine if you took all that wasted time and channeled it into front flip chain drills, instead? You woulda had this under your belt, years ago!

So, what are you waiting for now?

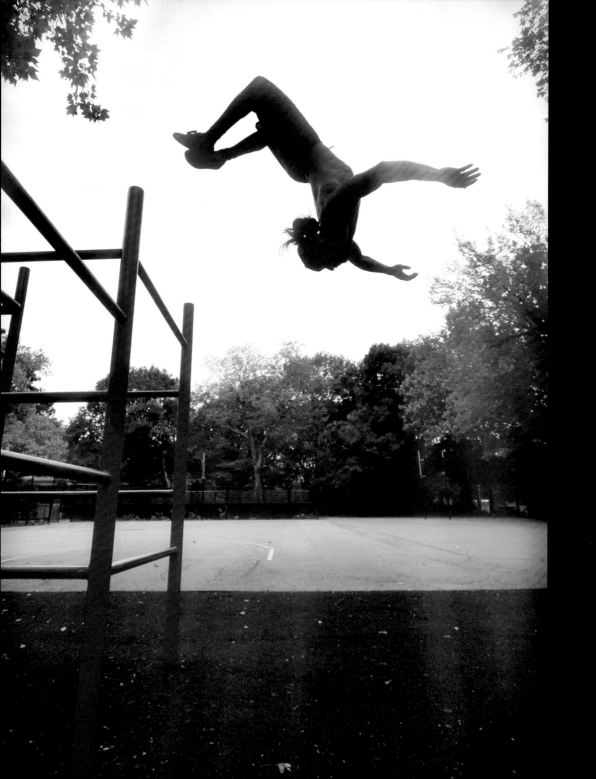

8

THE BACK FLIP
ULTIMATE AGILITY

When the average human being pictures true *agility*, only one exercise comes to mind—the *back flip*. Check out Hollywood—any time a character is meant to possess physical dexterity, the first thing you see them do is a back flip, or some kind of *back handspring*. These are always the moves that mesmerize kids the most, when they see them on TV—and during any gymnastics class, the back flip is always the movement students will ask about first. You wanna be a contender for the power crown? You've gotta own that back flip, baby!

Why is this? The *front flip* is actually the more difficult exercise, and requires more power. I think the feature that gives the back flip almost mystical status is the fact that the athlete jumps *backwards*, leaping into a space unseen. As a species, we have the stereoscopic vision of our predator ancestors: we are only truly comfortable proceeding in this direction. We *walk forwards*, we *run ahead*, we *press on. Jump as hard as you can and spin backwards? Are you nuts?!*

The good news is: you don't have to be crazy to attempt this movement, let alone master it. You just need to take it step-by-step, and let your body feel its way slowly. I'll give you all the tools you need in this chapter.

The back flip *can* be yours!

DECONSTRUCTING BACK FLIPS

The technical chain leading to the back flip is varied; the only commonality is the backward rotation. It has to be this way—there are a number of skills to pick up. So rather than just focusing on the techniques at the very end of the chain, I'll pump out a few general tips for moving through the steps efficiently. Most of it—as ever—is about work on the basics, and if you've been working on the stuff in the opening of the front flip chapter (page 142 onwards) that all applies equally to the back flip. They are acrobatic siblings.

GET HIGH

The higher you can jump, the easier it is to fully rotate. The simple message is—lots of power training. Jump drills aiming at verticality are the best approach.

STRENGTHEN YOUR SPINE

The *back handspring* is a key component in the back flip chain, and in many ways it can be seen as an explosive version of the classic *bridge* exercise. Your spine arches backwards at high velocity to allow your hands to impact the floor. This requires strength and robustness in the spine and its deep tissues. The best way to get this is by lots of conditioning with bridges. *Bridge holds* and *bridge pushups* are the way to go. Bridges will also condition your spine and shoulders for the *monkey flip (macaco)* steps, too—especially one-arm bridge variants, like the *gecko bridge*. Working with these movement patterns will really bulletproof those joints prior to the unusual angles they'll encounter in the macaco.

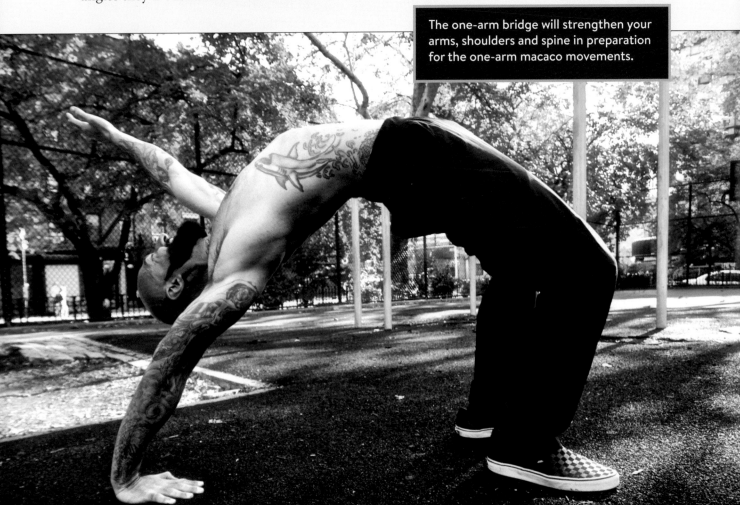

The one-arm bridge will strengthen your arms, shoulders and spine in preparation for the one-arm macaco movements.

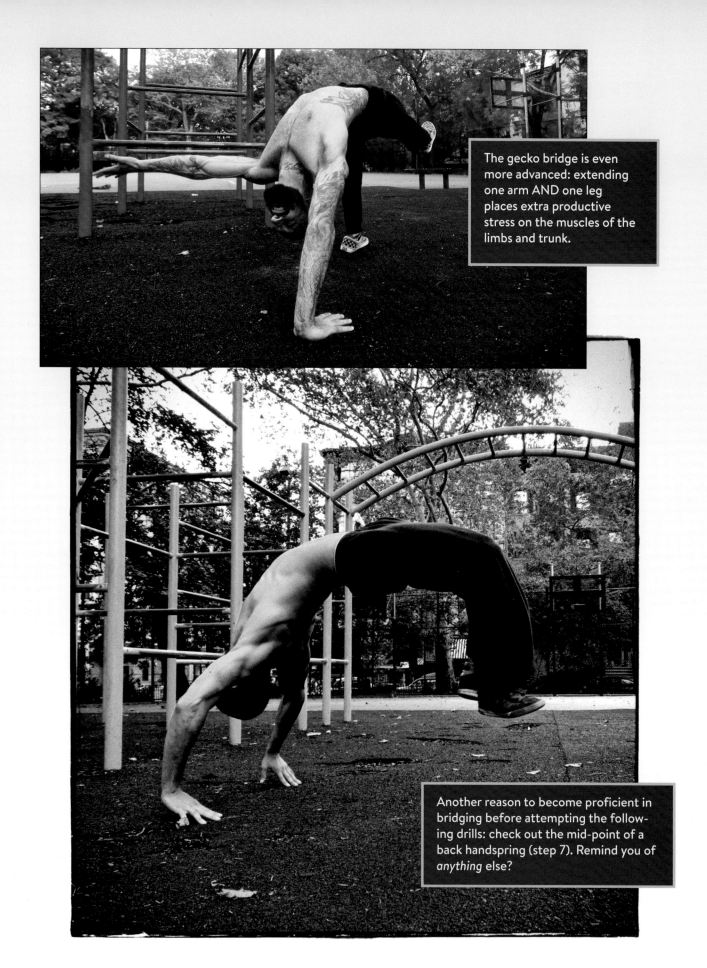

The gecko bridge is even more advanced: extending one arm AND one leg places extra productive stress on the muscles of the limbs and trunk.

Another reason to become proficient in bridging before attempting the following drills: check out the mid-point of a back handspring (step 7). Remind you of *anything* else?

STRENGTHEN YOUR ARMS AND SHOULDERS

Before they master the *back flip*, most athletes need to become expert in the *back handspring*. This really exposes the hands and shoulders to high forces. Athletes should condition themselves over time using:

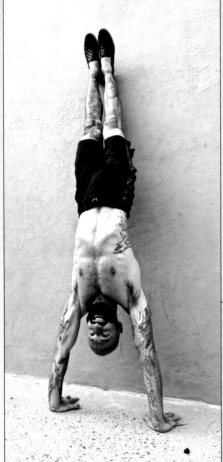

- Basic pushups
- Power pushups
- Free handstands
- Wall handstands
- Handstand pushups

The *monkey flip* (step 6) requires that you hold your body on one arm, for a split second. If you are crumbling under the weight—or if your joints are hurting—a course of *handstands*, building to *one-arm handstands*, is the way to go. As with all these preliminary drills, just achieving the correct position once or twice isn't enough. It takes *time* for the muscles, joints, soft-tissues and even bones to adapt to stresses. Give them the time and consistent training they need to get the job done.

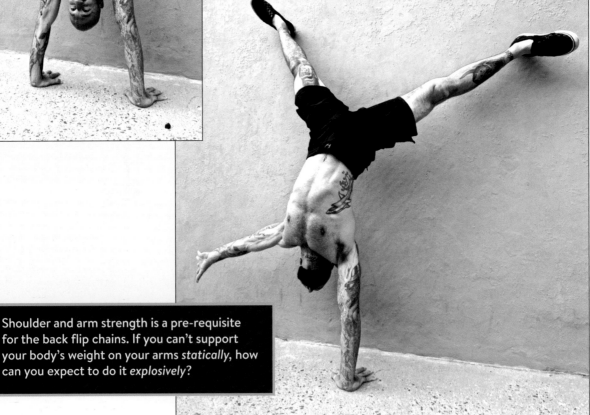

Shoulder and arm strength is a pre-requisite for the back flip chains. If you can't support your body's weight on your arms *statically*, how can you expect to do it *explosively*?

BUILD A POWERFUL TUCK

The back flip is called a back *tuck* in gymnastics for a reason. It's the upwards tuck position of the knees that enhances the angular rotation you need to land on your feet. The best way to master the tuck? Work through the *power jump* chain and you'll have it.

LEARN TO LAND

The impact on the feet, knees and hips from a back flip can be considerable. Before you attempt the harder steps, your lower body *must* be conditioned to the impact—again, this can best be achieved via jumps—lots of 'em. An even more specific technique to drill, if you're having trouble with your landing, is the *depth jump*. Instead of starting a box jump on the floor, start on the box. Then jump down (either backwards or forwards) before immediately shooting back up. A great way to condition your joints and nervous system to landing.

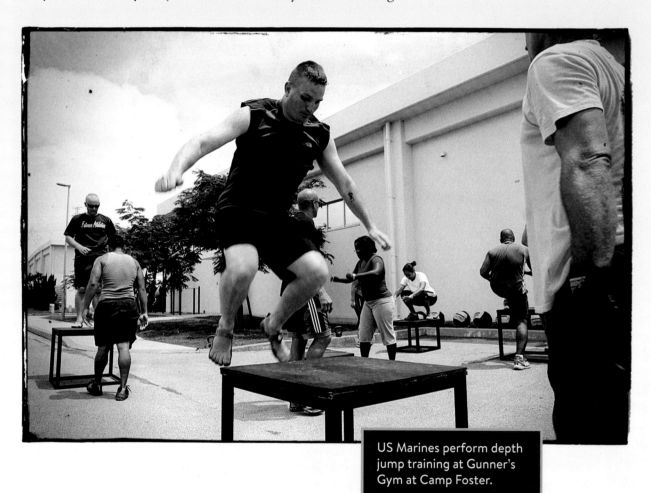

US Marines perform depth jump training at Gunner's Gym at Camp Foster.

THE BACK FLIP CHAIN

The most important aspect in finally achieving the *back flip*—or even the *back handspring*—is starting with very easy exercises. It's important that the athlete is as confident and successful as possible from day one, and then builds up ability organically and gradually. The chain begins with backwards rolls. These get the athlete's brain and vestibular system used to rear rotation, and they're easy and relatively safe. The athlete starts with *rear shoulder rolls* (step 1) which (obviously) involve rolling backwards over a shoulder. In the next step, *rear press rolls* (step 2), the hands become involved, which transfers some load to the arms and shoulders.

Once the athlete is used to rear rotation, they make things more difficult by kicking over from a bridge (step 3) using a wall or similar solid object. This involves the arms even further, and in many ways is like a *back handspring*, which we're moving towards.

At this stage, most athletes will be happy in rotating backwards, but will lack the confidence to jump up and back onto the hands, as for a handspring. The next three steps are gradual variations on the *monkey flip* (a.k.a. the *macaco*), and are designed to gradually teach the ability to perform back handsprings. First you perform an easy monkey flip from a *side* angle, the *side macaco* (step 4), then you perform a *monkey flip* where you kick up and *backwards* over your head, the *back macaco* (step 5), then finally, you perform the back macaco but beginning with your hands off the floor: the full *monkey flip* (step 6).

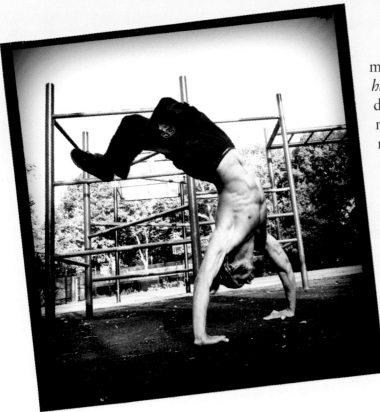

The full monkey flip only requires a little modification of angle to become a *back handspring* (step 7). This is a crucial level of development in the chain, and a real achievement—it's an incredible exercise in its own right, but it's also a general rule that without a good back handspring, a back flip will be impossible. Before moving forward, the athlete should have an excellent back handspring—high, powerful and confident. One option to ensure this is to build to a *one-arm back handspring* (step 8) although this step isn't absolutely necessary to progress.

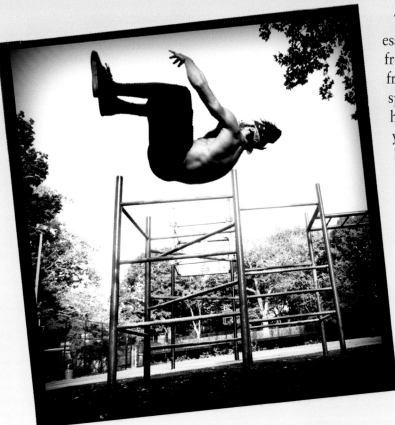

The *four-point back flip* (step 9) is an essential transitional tool to take athletes from the back handspring to the (hands-free) back flip. In the classic *back hand-spring*, after the initial jump, your hands touch the ground, followed by your feet. To progress, the athlete must build a faster rotation—and this includes beginning to tuck the knees in—as well as trying to "delay" placing the hands down as long as possible. Eventually, as improvement occurs, the feet will begin to touch down just a *fraction* after the hands, and then eventually at the *same time* (hence the term *four-point*, as the hands and feet land simultaneously.)

As the athlete gets the hang of the four-point back flip, there will come a time when the feet touch down 5—before the hands. This is usually only possible if the knees are tucked in well to increase angular momentum. (Have you ever seen a skater spinning around? When they bring their arms and leg in, they seem speed up. The principle is the same—if you tuck your knees in while rotating, you'll rotate faster, which is one reason I emphasized the skill of *tucking* so much in the power jumps chapter.) As soon as the feet are touching down first, you have in principle, reached the Master Step: the *back flip*. With consistent drilling, you'll be able to finish these without touching the floor with your hands at all.

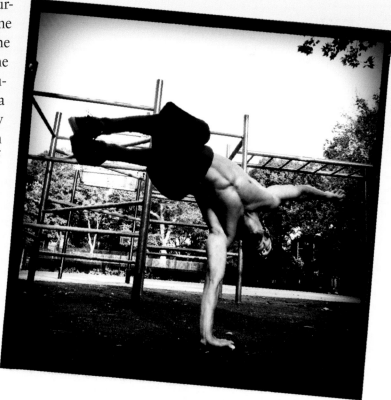

STEP ONE: REAR SHOULDER ROLL

PERFORMANCE

- With one foot out front, squat towards the ground.

- With your spine curled forwards, gently drop back onto your glutes. You can slip your rear leg behind you if this feels right.

- Continue your momentum by pushing through your strongest leg, encouraging your body to roll backwards.

- Swing your legs over your head as you roll over your strongest shoulder. Keep your head tucked in.

- As you roll over your shoulder and your legs approach the floor behind you, allow the braced arm of that shoulder to guide you back up.

- As your feet touch down, try to use your momentum to finish the roll naturally, in a standing position. Push up with your hands if you need to.

EXERCISE X-RAY

This kind of rear roll is the best for beginners because it is low impact and protects the neck and skull. It is similar to the rear rolls (*ushiro ukemi*) found in some Japanese martial arts. When performed correctly, it should look like the front *shoulder roll* (page 146), but performed in reverse.

REGRESSION

There are many ways to perform basic, easy rear rolls, and this is just a common one. You can alter the form as it suits you. The keys to easy rolls are keeping the head tucked in and safe, and rolling over the arm and shoulder, rather than the neck, to protect the joints.

PROGRESSION

Once you can perform this drill slowly—having mastered the key points mentioned above—feel free to pick up the speed. Don't worry about being "explosive" at this stage. This is just a preliminary technique.

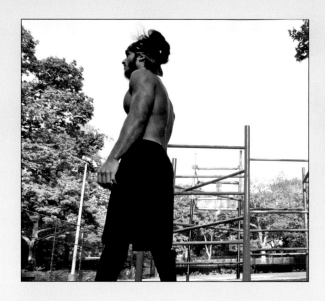

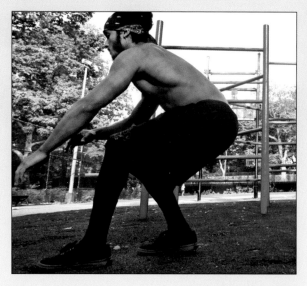

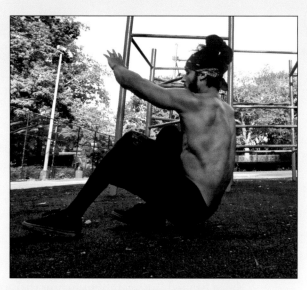

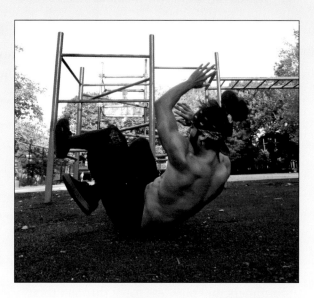

TIP: Do *not* roll directly back, over your head and neck—use your shoulder.

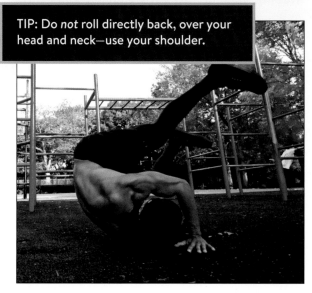

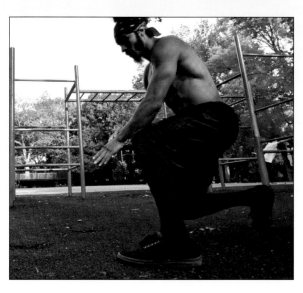

STEP TWO: REAR PRESS ROLL

PERFORMANCE

- With your feet symmetrical, squat towards the ground.

- With your spine curled forwards, gently drop back onto your glutes.

- Roll back, bringing your legs over your head. Simultaneously slip your palms either side of your head, and push through your arms.

- Let your braced arms guide your movement as you roll over—keep your head tucked in and out of the way. Your head should take virtually no weight.

- Roll over your back, trying not to veer to either side.

- Finish the roll naturally, in a seated position. As your feet touch down, push up with your hands into a crouching or standing position.

EXERCISE X-RAY

Just as with the frontal roll progressions, backwards rolls exist primarily to get the athlete's brain and nervous system used to spinning 360 degrees in a short space of time. Also like the frontal roll progressions, once you have mastered the most basic gentle rolling motion, the next step is to begin controlling the body with the upper limbs via the palms.

REGRESSION

Beginners will take less force through their arms, keeping them braced but well bent, using them for control and to protect the neck only, relying on momentum to carry them over.

PROGRESSION

Progression is about taking more and more force through the arms during the roll; eventually you will be pushing up to standing in a semi-press motion, handling much more of the body's weight than you did at first. More confident rollers can perform see-saw drills: a *rear press roll* immediately followed by a front *press roll* (see page 148), repeated for reps. This also works for *shoulder rolls/rear shoulder rolls*, and many other roll and flip drill combinations. You can mix and match, too (*shoulder roll/rear press roll*, etc).

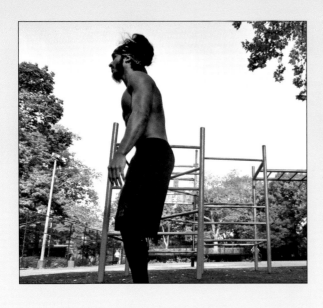
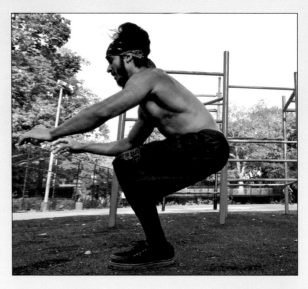
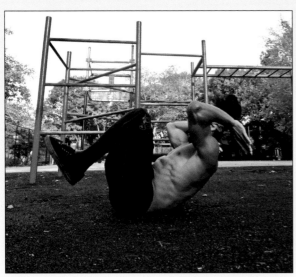
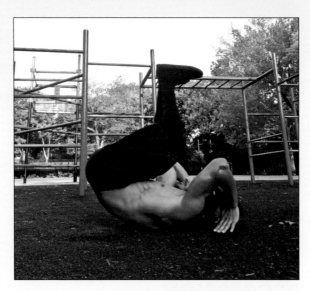
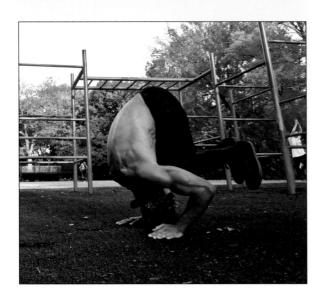
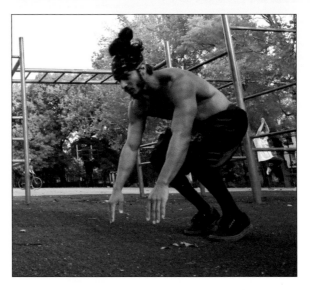

STEP THREE: BRIDGE KICK-OVER

PERFORMANCE

- Lie flat on your back with your toes next to a sturdy vertical object like a wall, column, pole, etc. Your knees should be well bent.

- Place your palms by your ears with your fingers pointing to your toes and your elbows angled to the ceiling.

- Press yourself up into a full *bridge hold*, using the power of your arms and legs.

- Lift one leg and press your foot firmly against the object.

- Under control, press firmly against the wall with your foot, until your second foot leaves the floor. Extend that foot over the hips.

- Keeping your arms braced, continue pressing against the wall until your legs flip over you.

- Land on one foot first, with your hands still in contact with the floor. Be careful not to kick the ground with your toes.

EXERCISE X-RAY

Most athletes are just not prepared to flip back on their hands—their shoulders, elbows and wrists can't take the sudden forces, and their brains and vestibular systems find the 360 degree spin totally alien. This simple drill cures all that. If *back handsprings* scare you, this step is the antidote.

REGRESSION

Make this easier by pushing off the *top* of an object—like a bed instead of the wall. The higher the object, the better. Kicking off stairs is another option, trying to kick off a lower stair every time. When you progress to a vertical wall, you can begin by "walking" up the wall using several steps, if you need to.

PROGRESSION

At some point you will be able to perform this exercise by kicking off the *floor*, rather than a wall—however this variation is advanced, and not necessary if you wish to learn the back handspring.

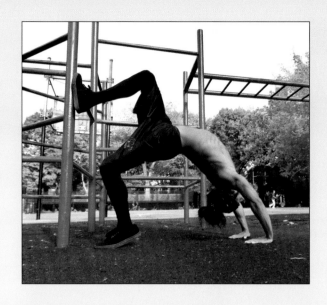

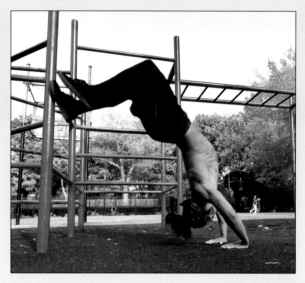

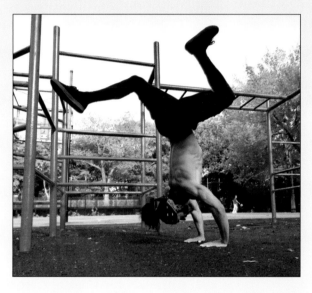

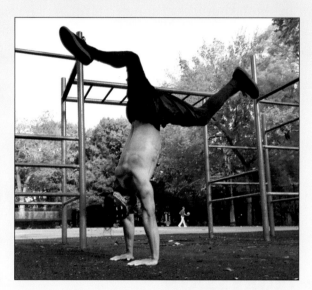

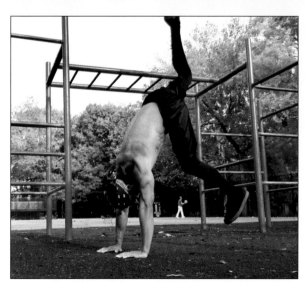

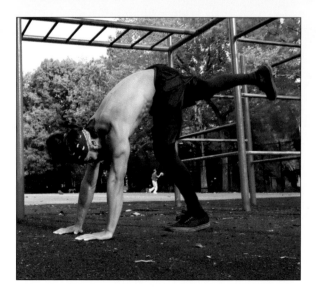

STEP FOUR: SIDE MACACO

PERFORMANCE

- With your feet fairly close together, squat down and lean back. Support yourself by placing your one palm on the floor behind you, thumb pointing away from you and your inner-elbow facing out with a locked arm.

- Thrust up through your hips, swinging your free arm up and over your head.

- Keep the momentum going by pushing off the floor with your legs. (Your main pushing leg should be on the same side as whichever arm you are swinging overhead.)

- With your locked arm as a pivot, swing your furthest leg up and round the side of your head in an arc, with your other leg following beneath it.

- Touch down with your foot behind the level of your hand.

- As your feet touch down, push through your arm and use your momentum to stand up. (Your main swinging foot may touch down first.)

EXERCISE X-RAY

The *macaco* (*monkey*) is a drill often associated with capoeira, and it's a brilliant way to gradually ease into the *back handspring*. It requires strong shoulders—don't try this unless your handstand is solid (see page 178).

REGRESSION

The height of your swinging feet and how far you rotate are the key progression variables for this drill. Begin small, with your feet close to the floor. As you improve, your feet should be as high as your head.

PROGRESSION

To improve, just increase the height of your swinging legs. This drill is a preparation exercise to get your joints and nervous system ready for the *back macaco* (step 5), so your legs should not go above the height of your head yet.

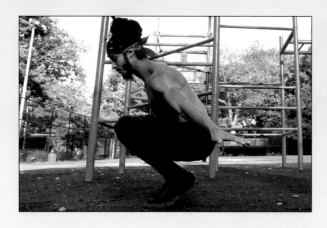
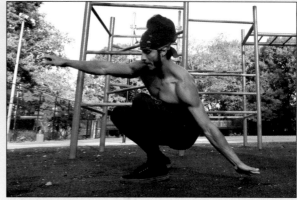

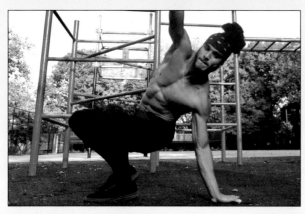
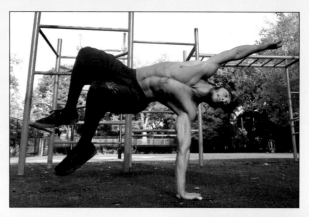

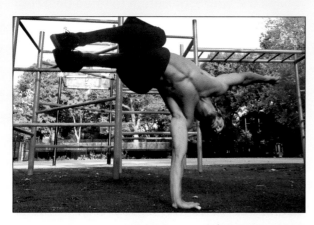
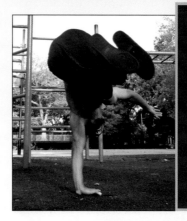

TIP: This is a rotating motion, so you need to make sure your inner-elbow was facing out when you started, so that your arm and shoulder can safely revolve (like an axle).

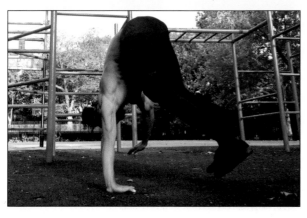
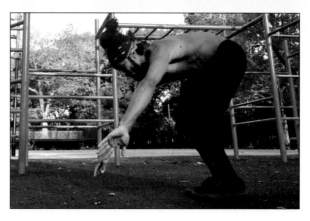

EXPLOSIVE CALISTHENICS

189

STEP FIVE: BACK MACACO

PERFORMANCE

- With your feet fairly close together, squat down and lean back. Support yourself by placing one palm on the floor behind you, thumb pointing away from you and your inner-elbow facing out with a locked arm.

- Thrust up through your hips, swinging your free arm up and over your head.

- Keep the momentum going by pushing off the floor with your legs. (Your main pushing leg should be on the same side as whichever arm you are swinging overhead.)

- Swing your legs up and over your head, leading them with your swinging arm. For a split second your legs will be over your head, with your entire body supported by one arm. As soon as you can, set down the swinging arm to help take the load.

- Flip right over yourself, and touch down with your foot behind where your back used to be. Initially, the leg which is on the same side as your locked arm will land first: in time you'll gain symmetry.

- As your feet touch down, push through your arm and use your momentum to stand up. (Your main swinging foot may touch down first.)

EXERCISE X-RAY

This movement is an evolution of the *side macaco* (step 4). Instead of swinging your legs around your side, you swing them straight up over your head. Don't attempt this until you're comfortable with the side version. By now you'll see that you're getting pretty close to something that looks like a *back handspring*.

REGRESSION

As this drill is an evolution of the side macaco (step 4), veering off towards your loaded arm will make things easier at first.

PROGRESSION

To perfect this motion, the legs must go right over the head—the straighter your legs during this motion, the harder the exercise. Ensuring that the non-loaded arm swings over close to the side of the head will help with this.

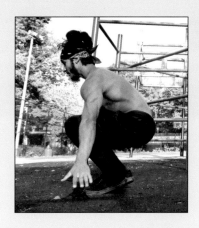 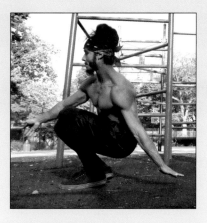 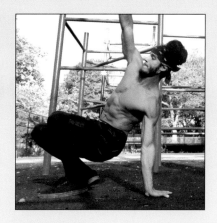

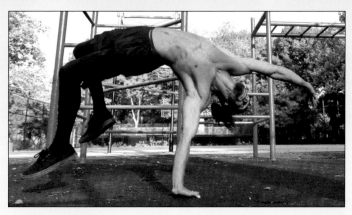

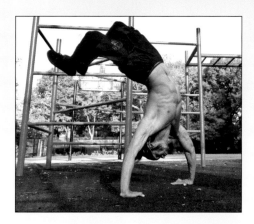 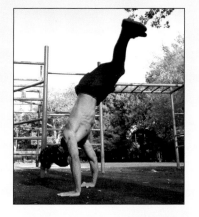

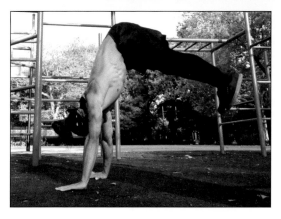 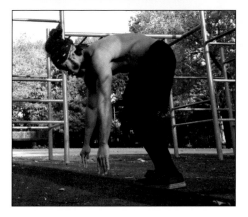

STEP SIX: MONKEY FLIP

PERFORMANCE

- Begin standing, with your feet fairly close together.

- Squat down as you drop your palm to the floor, but begin to explode up even before you touch down; your loaded palm should be about to touch down as your feet leave the floor.

- As you explode up, thrust through the hips and swing your other arm up over your head and next to your ear, twisting to reach the ground.

- Reach for the floor with your non-loaded arm, as you swing your legs up and over your head, leading them with your swinging arm.

- Flip right over yourself, and touch down with your feet behind where your back used to be.

- As your feet touch down, push through your arms and use your momentum to stand up.

EXERCISE X-RAY

The *monkey flip* should look very similar to the *macaco* drills you learned in the previous two steps. In fact, the monkey flip is only a slightly harder version of the macaco—which is exactly what you want in progressive calisthenics training. The difference is that you begin the jump in the *side* and *back macaco* with your hand *on* the floor, while you begin the monkey flip jump standing, with your hand *off* the floor. This is the ultimate version.

REGRESSION

Begin the movement in a semi-squat position with your pivotal hand only a very short distance from the ground—an inch—and build to greater distances over time. You want to get to the point where the backwards fall/jump adds to your swinging momentum.

PROGRESSION

As you improve with this movement, you'll be able to delay swinging your pivot arm onto the floor. You'll also be able to swing it further and further back, away from your body.

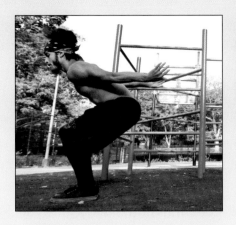
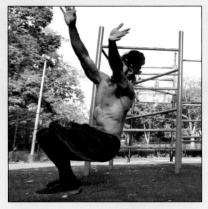
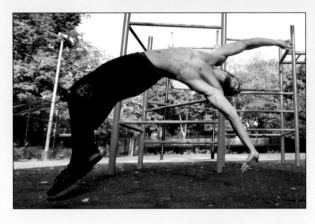
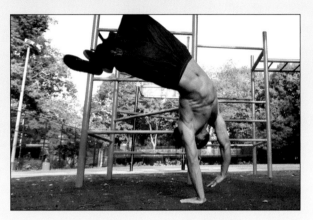
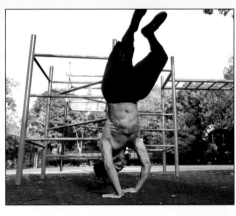
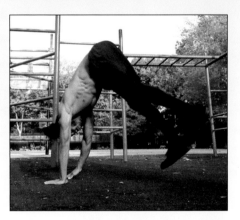
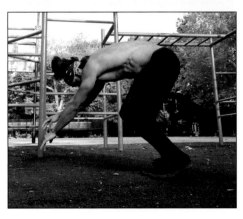
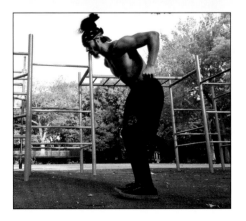

EXPLOSIVE CALISTHENICS

STEP SEVEN: BACK HANDSPRING

PERFORMANCE

- Stand with your feet shoulder-width apart, and your hands out in front of your head, or a little higher.

- Dip down at the knees and hips, as you swing your arms down and behind you. Keep looking forward as you descend.

- Explode up and backwards—approximately diagonally—swinging your hands above you as you go.

- As you jump, look behind you. Arching the back a little will help you rotate. Your hands should follow your line of vision.

- Make contact with the floor with your arms locked if you can, and at about shoulder-width.

- Once your legs reach a vertical point, whip your feet down to the ground rapidly.

- When your feet are planted, step (or hop) to catch your balance if you need to, and extend your body again.

EXERCISE X-RAY

The true block towards a good *back handspring* is *fear*—your body's fear of explosively flipping back over your head. Athletes who have mastered the *monkey flip* will have deprogrammed this fear by approaching flipping side-on, and will not find true back handsprings all that challenging.

REGRESSION

If you can do a solid monkey flip, you can do a back handspring. What holds athletes back is that last bit of anxiety. To help with the psychology, practice on soft surfaces, like grass, or pad the ground with pillows and cushions.

PROGRESSION

Improve your form by landing with an extended body—overcome the "crouch" style of landing. For added difficulty, bring your feet close together.

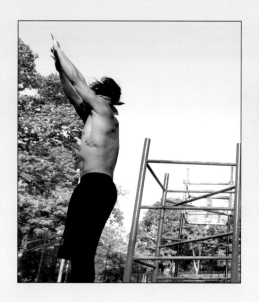

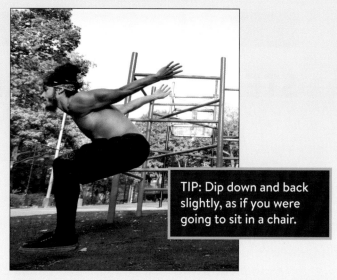

TIP: Dip down and back slightly, as if you were going to sit in a chair.

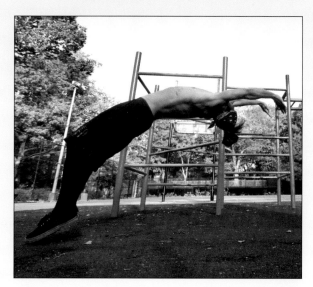

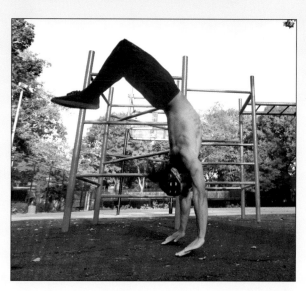

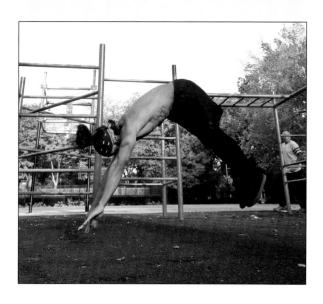

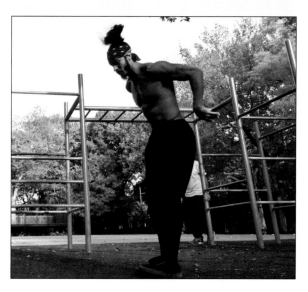

STEP EIGHT: ONE-ARM
BACK HANDSPRING

PERFORMANCE

- Stand with your feet shoulder-width apart, and your hands held high.

- Dip down at the knees and hips, as you swing your arms down and behind you. Keep looking forward as you descend. Dip down and back slightly, as if you were going to sit in a chair.

- Explode up and backwards—approximately diagonally—swinging your hands above you as you go.

- As you jump, looking behind you and arching the back a little will help you rotate. Your hands should follow your line of vision.

- As you are inverted, reach out with one arm to make contact with the floor directly below your head. If your timing is good, this placement with be the natural end of the backwards arm-swinging motion. Keep your other arm pulled closer to your head.

- Once your legs reach a vertical point, whip your feet down to the ground rapidly.

- When your feet are planted, catch your balance and extend your body again.

EXERCISE X-RAY

You don't necessarily need to be able to perform a back handspring with one-arm in order to learn a *back flip*—in fact, some back-flippers can't do this exercise! But it works as a great training drill because it forces athletes to become less dependent on their arms during the flip, relying on leg power and momentum instead. If your back handspring is good and high, you can probably skip this step.

REGRESSION

You can approach this exercise by utilizing a slightly different two-hand version—try with close hands, asymmetrical hands, etc. until your confidence grows and one-arm is achievable.

PROGRESSION

The loaded arm should really only act as a pivot, for a fraction of a second; over time, touch it down quicker and with less force behind it.

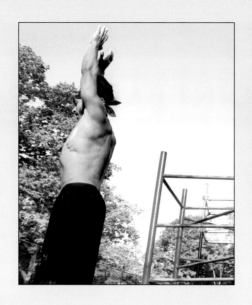
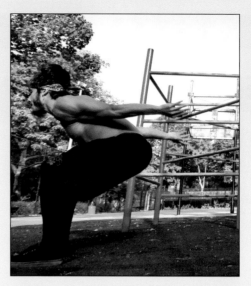
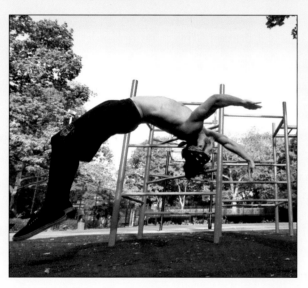
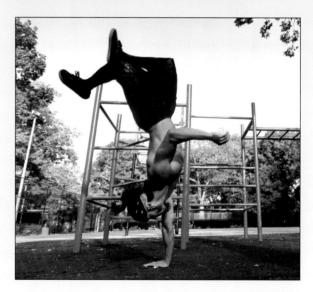
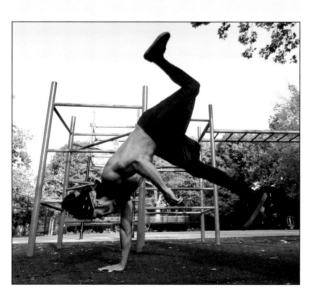
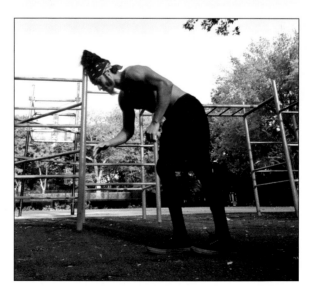

EXPLOSIVE CALISTHENICS

STEP NINE: FOUR-POINT BACK FLIP

PERFORMANCE

- Stand with your feet shoulder-width apart, and your hands held high.

- Dip down at the knees and hips, as you swing your arms down and behind you. Keep looking forward as you descend.

- Explode up and backwards—approximately diagonally—swinging your hands above you as you go. Your goal is to jump higher than for a regular *back handspring*.

- As you jump, looking behind you and arching the back a little will help you rotate. Your hands should follow your line of vision.

- Once your legs reach a vertical point, whip your feet down to the ground rapidly.

- Delay putting your arms down for as long as you can—wait until the very last moment. For this drill, your hands and feet should make contact with the floor at about the same time.

- When your feet and hands are supporting you and the motion is finished, stand up straight.

EXERCISE X-RAY

One-arm back handsprings should have taught you to depend on leg power, instead of your arms, like a two-arm *back handspring*. It should also have given you some *height*. In this stage you are using that height to whip your legs around *earlier* than for back handsprings; at first the difference in speed will be small, but eventually your hands and legs with touch down at the *same time*. Before long your legs will touch down *first*—the *back flip*!

REGRESSION

This is a transitional drill. At first, your hands will land *before* your legs—that's fine. Just keep trying to jump higher and whip down the legs sooner, and you'll be landing four-point style in time.

PROGRESSION

Eventually you will be landing on your feet before your hands—in a deep squat. This, essentially, is a back flip. From here you just need to tighten up your form by adding a tuck. This is where the Master Step comes in.

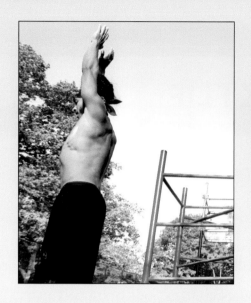
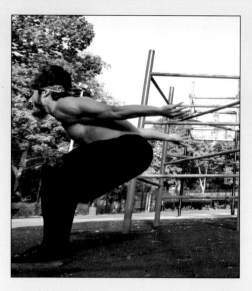
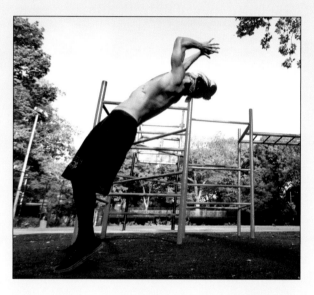
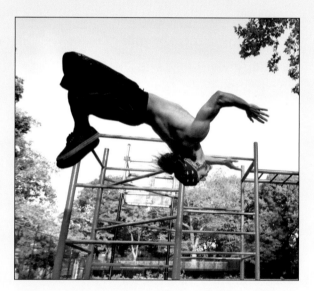
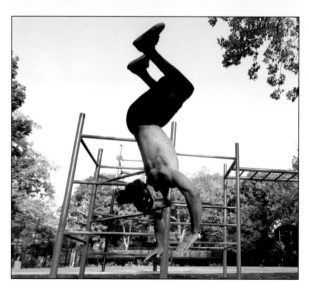
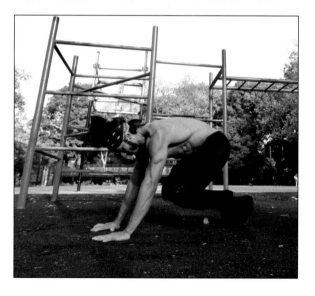

EXPLOSIVE CALISTHENICS

MASTER STEP: BACK FLIP

PERFORMANCE

- Stand with your feet shoulder-width apart, and your hands held high.

- Dip down at the knees and hips, as you swing your arms down by your sides. Keep looking forward as you descend.

- Jump up hard, swinging your hands above you as you go. You can look up as you jump. Too many athletes fail because they begin this drill by jumping back. Don't! Jump vertically!

- When your body is fully extended at maximum height, explode your knees up into your chest as hard as you can. (Gymnasts call this a *tuck*.) The momentum of this tuck helps you rotate.

- Bring your arms to your sides, or your thighs, as you spin over.

- When you begin to see the ground below you, whip your legs out straight to make contact with the floor.

- When your feet are planted, catch your balance and extend your body again.

EXERCISE X-RAY

If you got this far—and everyone can get this far, if they put the time and effort into the previous nine steps—then congratulations! You are the envy of every ninja and b-boy wannabe since 1963! You are the owner of the *back flip*: not the hardest acrobatic feat in the world, but definitely the most archetypal. More important than looking damn cool—and if a back flip doesn't make you look damn cool, then you are already dead—the back flip displays integrated mastery of some of the most fundamental traits required for total explosive strength. I'm talking about a super quick jump, massive hip snap, a powerful, agile waist and spine, and an upper-body that can generate high-levels of responsive force like *lightning*. Once you can pull off the back flip, speed, power and agility will be in your toolbox whenever you need 'em.

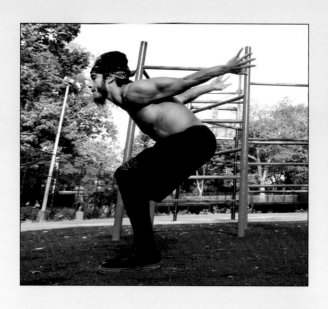
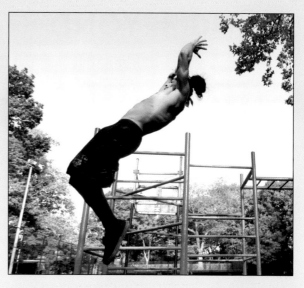
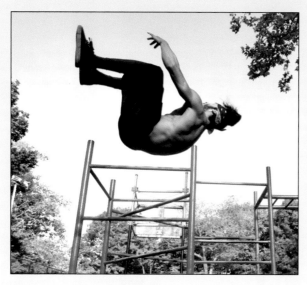
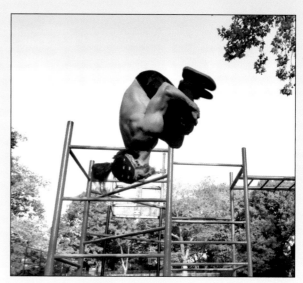
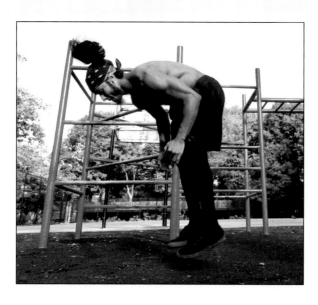
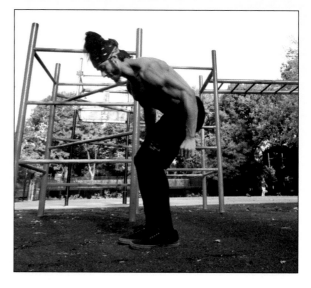

GOING BEYOND

Beaten the sacred back flip? You might consider *combining* acrobatic movements at this stage: and I discuss this option more in the *front flip* chapter (see page 166). Aside from this, there are plenty of interesting solo *back flip* variations to explore. Most folks are familiar with the *partner flip* (where your partner holds your foot and helps with the flip: a.k.a. the *pitch tuck*), but you can replicate this yourself by placing one foot up on something at knee-height. If that floats your boat, you can move forward by raising both feet. Find a low wall, and you have a basic parkour move.

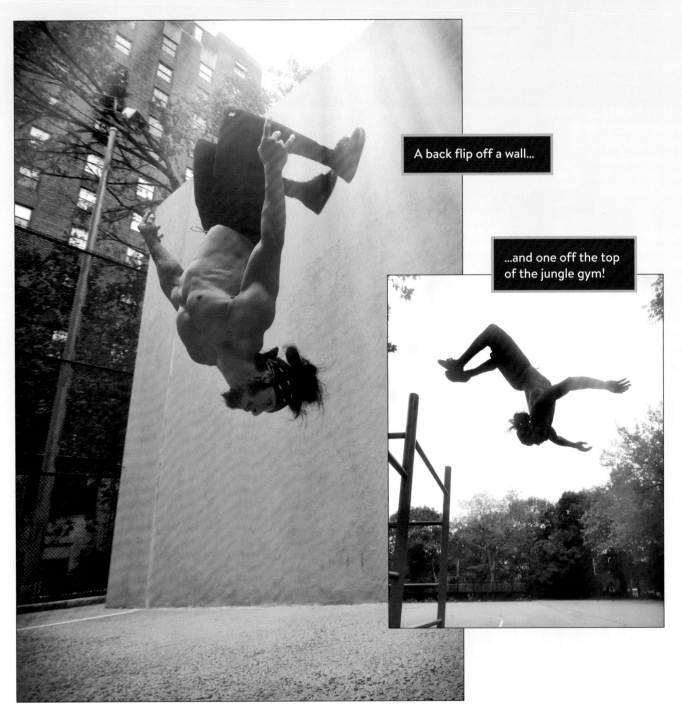

A back flip off a wall...

...and one off the top of the jungle gym!

Another variation of the back flip involves extending one leg and keeping the other tucked. (There are various ways you can approach this.) This is sometimes called a *flashkick*.

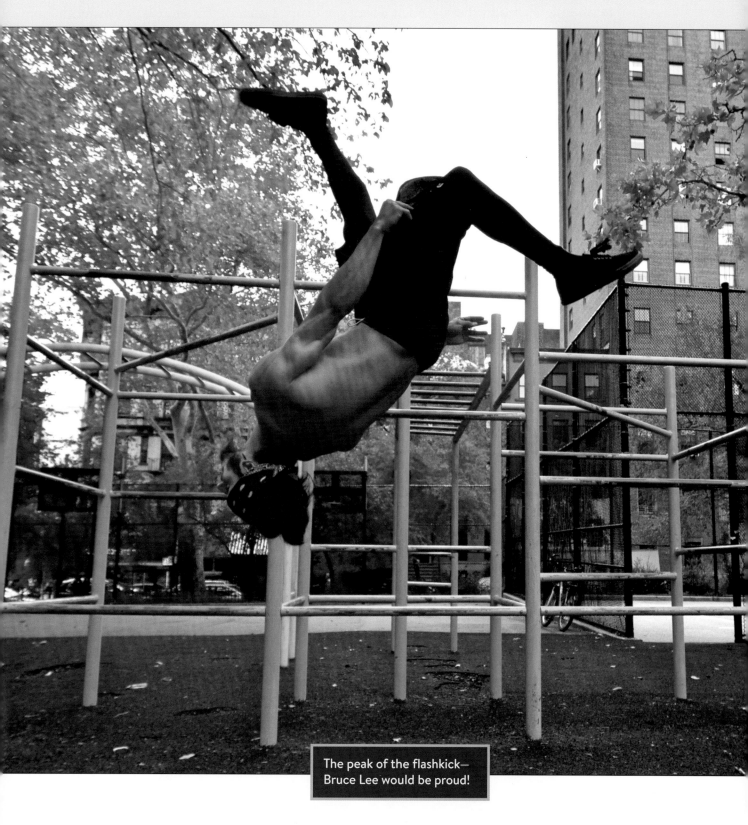

The peak of the flashkick—
Bruce Lee would be proud!

EXPLOSIVE CALISTHENICS

A movement similar to the flashkick is the *gainer*. An athlete typically lands a back flip at approximately the same point they push off. In fact, there are several variations of this theme: you can either land slightly forward of the point where you jump (a *gainer*), or even rear to the launch point (a *loser*). It's also possible to flip off one leg, transitioning to land on the opposite leg. This is called a *switchflip*.

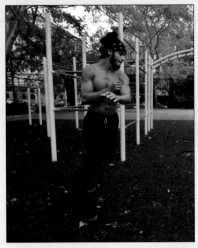
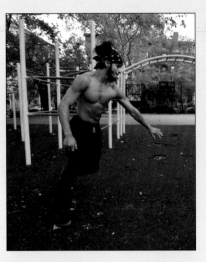
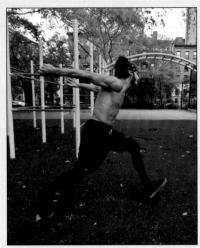
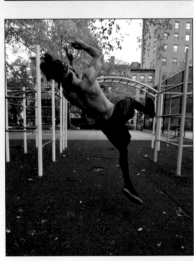
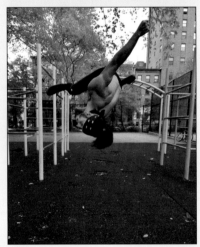
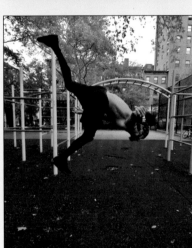
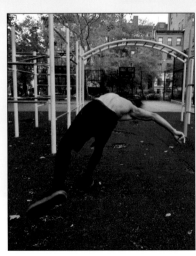
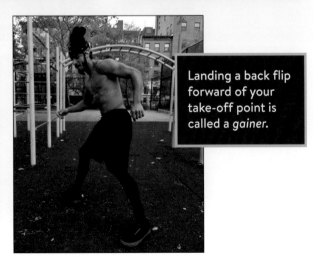

Landing a back flip forward of your take-off point is called a *gainer*.

SMALL SPACE DRILLS

Following are three useful speed and power techniques you can utilize in your routine for variety, as ancillary work or to train your muscles from different angles. They are all solo drills, and they require zero equipment. Unlike the progressive exercises in the chains, most of the following drills can be performed rhythmically for higher reps, and can work well when used with any of the chains in this book. In this sense, they can also work as warm-ups or finishing exercises in an explosives session.

ONE-ARM WALL PUSH-AWAYS

Lean against a wall with one arm; keep your feet well back. Bend the arm as for a *one-arm wall pushup*, then explosively push yourself away from the wall. Finish standing. A great exercise for powerful, bulletproof elbows. To make the exercise progressive, place your feet further back.

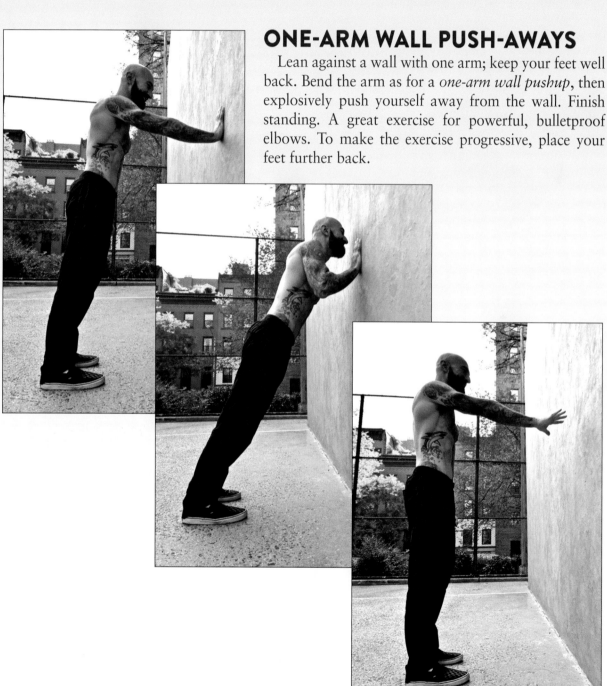

DONKEY KICK

Support yourself on your palms and feet, with locked arms and bent legs. Jump up with the legs, and straighten them out in mid-air, like a donkey kicking. There are many small space drills which force the *waist* or *abdominal* muscles to fire explosively, but the *donkey kick* is useful to know because the *spine* and *posterior chain* does most of the firing. That makes it a useful warm-up or ancillary drill for exercises like *back handsprings*, which require quick, powerful spinal muscles.

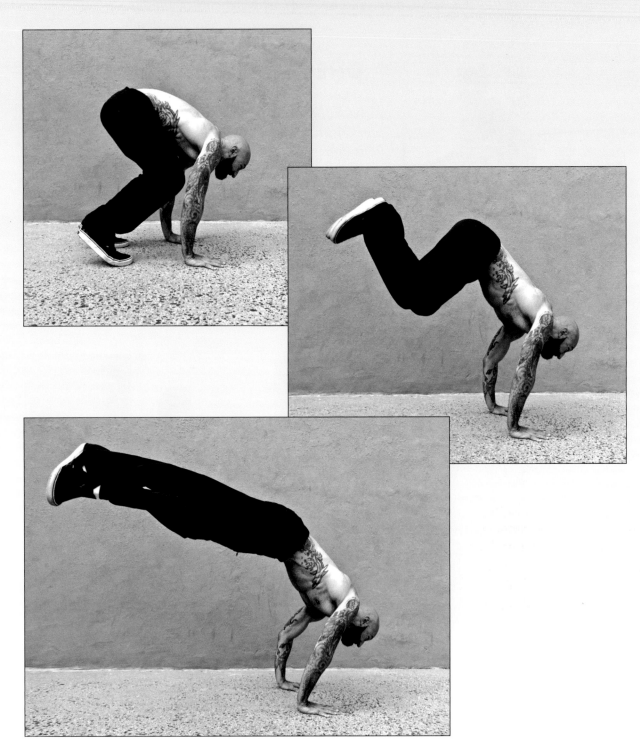

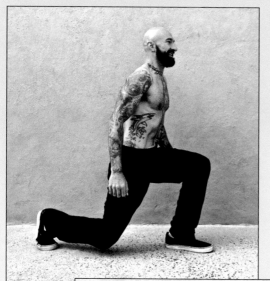

SCISSORS JUMP

From a split position—one leg in front of the other—dip down into a lunge, and explode up. Switch your legs in mid-air to land on the opposite side, then repeat. This drill is great for jumping, but also for super-quick *hip movements*: something essential for any flip. The twist is also a useful ancillary benefit, to keep all your trunk muscles nice and explosive.

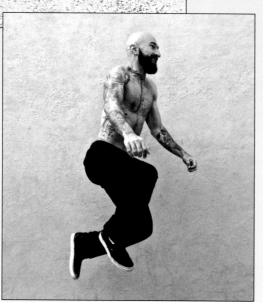

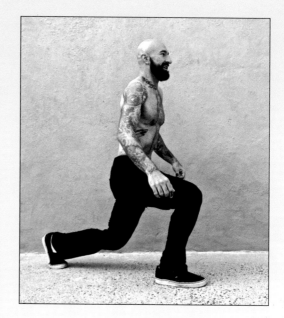

LIGHTS OUT!

For total-body explosiveness, you don't need to be performing box plyometrics or a bunch of ball apparatus exercises. Weight-lifting won't get you to the elite levels either. You need to move your *entire body*: nothing else will get you there. The *back flip* is a legendary physical movement and is arguably the greatest test of explosive power, true speed, and agility found in nature. It requires a powerful jump, a strong hip-midsection tuck, fast arms, excellent coordination, lightning reflexes and superior kinesthetic skills.

In the past, this bodyweight feat has been considered something that can only be approached by the super-athletic elite. Not anymore. In this chapter I've given you all the drills you need to *become* the elite.

I'm here for ya, champ. We can ace this thing together.

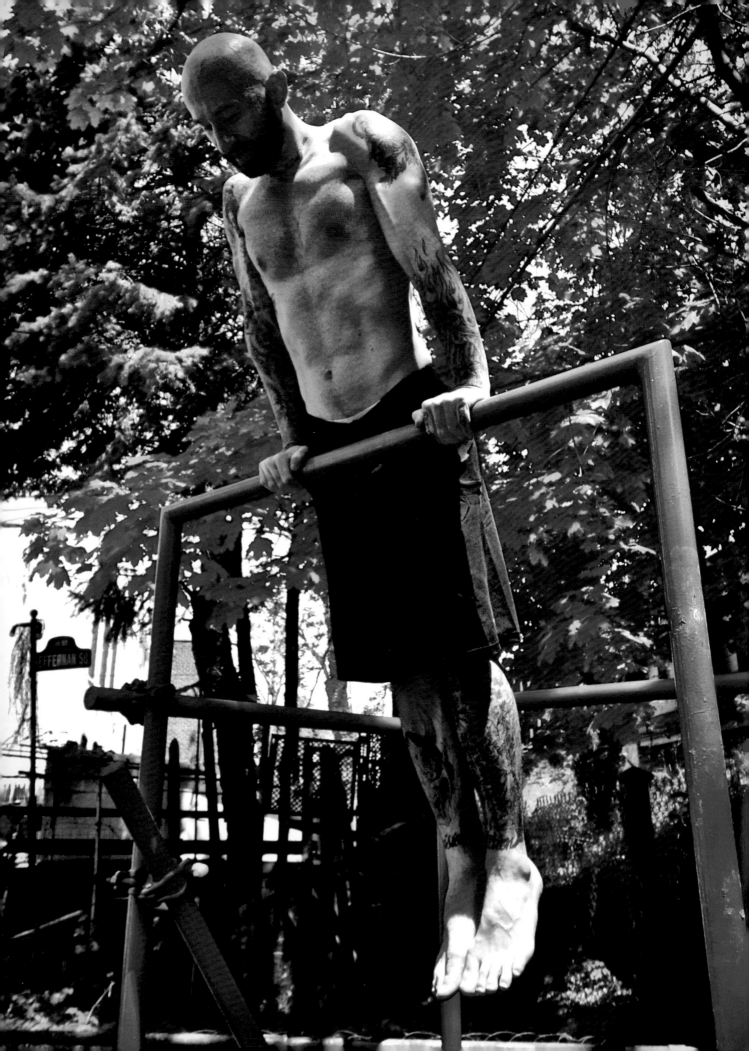

9

THE MUSCLE-UP
OPTIMAL EXPLOSIVE STRENGTH

I f I had to write a "top ten" list of the planet's hottest bodyweight moves, the *muscle-up* would definitely rocket straight to number one—with virtually no competition! Thanks to the growing popularity of street calisthenics, and its adoption by a new generation of bodyweight masters like Al Kavadlo, everyone interested in bar work has seen this exercise on *YouTube*. And, better still, everybody wants to achieve it! Very few enthusiasts will be able to manage this exercise of course...unless they approach it *progressively*. In this chapter, you'll learn all the secrets and tactics you need to totally *own* this exercise. In no time, it will be *you* powering yourself over that bar, to envious glances from lesser mortals. Just stick with me, kid.

What is this super exercise? Putting it simply—too damn simply—a muscle-up involves hanging from an overhead bar, and pulling your torso over the bar, before pressing yourself upwards to arm's length.

Younger readers might find this surprising, but ten years ago, if you spoke to calisthenics athletes about "muscle-ups", 99% of 'em wouldn't have had a clue what you were talking about. Even the name is pretty new; I have trained in bodyweight strength methods for over four decades, and I only heard the term "muscle-up" for the first time in 2006. In jail we used to call this exercise the *sentry pullup*—"sentry", I guess, because it looks like you are pulling yourself over something to take a look in the distance. Of course, gymnasts know all about this technique—it's the Movement One of all hanging gymnastics work; it's how gymnasts pull themselves up on the horizontal bars or rings, to initiate a routine!

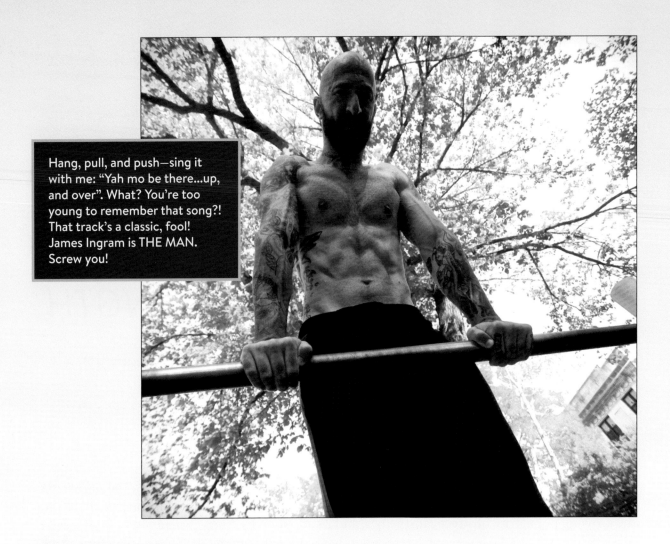

Hang, pull, and push—sing it with me: "Yah mo be there...up, and over". What? You're too young to remember that song?! That track's a classic, fool! James Ingram is THE MAN. Screw you!

BENEFITS OF THE MUSCLE-UP

Although the crazy popularity of the muscle-up is a fairly modern phenomenon, the muscle-up movement itself is *not* new—hell no. The exercise is an ancient one, which stretches all the way back to our primate ancestors. To this day, if you go to a zoo you may be lucky enough to watch a chimp or a monkey climbing up and over a branch—and you'll get to see an animal muscle-up! Species which evolved using *arboreal locomotion* as a survival tool (that's tree-climbing, to schlubs like me) had to be able to pull themselves up and over horizontal branches, and they did it, pretty much, with the muscle-up...or something that looked a lot like it. We humans were one such species.

Fast-forward to the modern era, and this up-and-over movement is still an essential survival tool. I remember being chased around as a kid, back in the Bay, and having to scramble over walls on more than one occasion. Too fat, too outta shape to make that wall? You got your ass caught—or worse. Military calisthenics courses all have short walls for just this reason—and they are often the toughest part of the course, for some trainees (unless they can perform a muscle-up already, that is). Cops and firefighters all need to be able to scale short walls, using the "up-and-over" technique. It's an essential survival movement, in the way a barbell curl or bench press just...*isn't*.

Since physical development systems began, muscle-up movements have garnered an important and honored place in their training curriculums. This was as true for the Greeks and Romans as for the early modern pioneers, like Georges Hébert and Francisco Amoros. Of course, it all died out in recent times, when bodybuilding became king, and guys were only worried about the size of their arms...as opposed to what they could *do* with those arms. (Let's not fall into that mistake, eh?)

If old-school guys with handlebar moustaches took muscle-ups seriously, so should you, dude.

Okay, so the muscle-up is useful. It's "functional". *So what? So's a spatula. I want speed and power, son.* Well, the muscle-up can give you that, too. It really is a unique exercise when it comes to strength and conditioning. Unlike the vast majority of strength techniques, the muscle-up requires a very explosive *pull*—to get you up on the bar—plus a *push*, to get you over it. So it pretty much works the entire upper-body; the back and biceps pull, the chest, triceps and shoulders push. The grip needs to be insanely strong, and you need a stomach of steel and a very athletic posterior chain to initiate the kip and hip-thrust needed to get you up there. On top of that, without coordination, timing and total-body tendon strength, you can forget it—the muscle-up just won't happen. This isn't just blowing smoke; I've met very strong, very fit men who can do pushups and pullups all day, who got their asses handed to them by the muscle-up because they lacked that elusive total-body-sync X-factor which this exercise can teach you. It's this X-factor that's the secret to building insane explosive power in a highly compressed timeframe.

So swallow that coffee and read on, Jack. I'm gonna show you how to own this sucker.

DECONSTRUCTING MUSCLE-UPS

Many newbies look at the muscle-up (or try it) and assume: *superhuman strength and power is necessary to make that movement happen.* Don't get me wrong, strength and power are important—no *weakling* could perform this exercise—but you might be surprised the role *skill* plays; I've trained with plenty of guys who were easily jacked enough to perform the muscle-up, but were miles away from ever pulling it off, because they just never had the know-how. Although you can train muscle-ups like a power exercise—using sets and reps—there's a good argument for training it as a skill technique, because the technical components of this exercise are so crucial. I could write a book about the different elements involved here, but let's break 'em down into four basics: the *kip*, the *pull*, the *pull-over*, and the *press*.

THE KIP

To begin the muscle-up, you don't just perform a very fast pullup—you need to perform a *kipping* pullup. This means that you are not yanking yourself up *vertically*, but swinging *backwards*, and pulling yourself up and *in* to the bar. Think about it for a second—if you want to perform a muscle-up, you need to get your hips to the bar, so you can lean over it (this is called a *pull-over*) before you press yourself up. Pulling yourself straight up vertically—like a regular pullup—and getting your *chin* over the bar is an accomplishment for most people, let alone getting your *hips* all the way up to the bar! So forget the idea of the muscle-up being an extension of a regular pullup. It really isn't. The art of kipping in this respect involves the ability to swing the body back, and slightly up in an arc (you will always swing back and up in an arc if you keep your arms fairly straight—think of a rope swing, or a pendulum in motion). One of the goals of this chain is to get higher and higher on the backswing of the *swing kip*: eventually, your head will be level with the bar on the backswing, and this is what makes a true, *power-based* muscle-up possible.

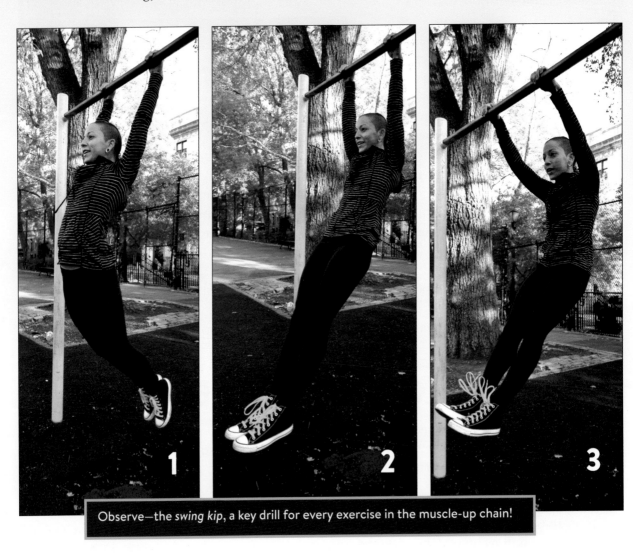

Observe—the *swing kip*, a key drill for every exercise in the muscle-up chain!

1. In the first photo, Grace swings forward as she pushes her hips/chest forwards and shoulders back. She simultaneously flexes her spine, and it goes into a concave position (not unlike a *bridge*, but gentler).

2. In the second image, Grace begins to rebound, straightening her trunk as the backswing begins.

3. Finally, the backswing: Grace harnesses the backward momentum, by pulling down with her hands and arms—the elbows don't bend at this point—and "curling" her abs (like a *crunch*), rendering her entire body convex, or "hollow".

All these changes happen very rapidly, but the end result sees Grace heading *behind* the bar with some momentum assisting her: this is a very powerful position from which to explode *upwards* and *inwards*, pulling your chin, chest, or even abs to the bar, by thrusting your hips up and snapping back with the arms. It's not a pullup!

THE PULL

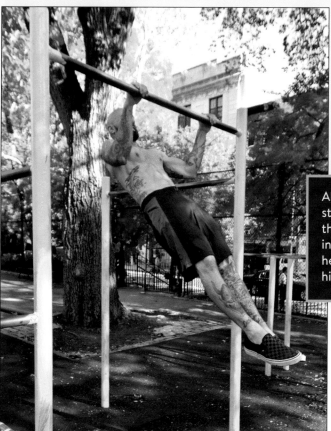

Because of the kip, the pull in a muscle-up is different from the *pull* in a regular pullup. Instead of slowly pulling yourself *up*, the arms quickly snap *back* to the waist—combined with a hip thrust, this punches the lower abs into the bar.

Al pulls himself towards the bar, from the third stage of the *swing kip* (see previous page). Note that—since the kip put him *behind* the bar, and arcing upwards—he doesn't pull straight *up*. Instead, he pulls his arms *back* and *down*, while thrusting his hips *diagonally* up and forward.

THE PULL-OVER

A big problem many athletes face—even those who are great at regular pullups—is that they just can't get their torso over the bar. If the kip and pull, described above, are performed correctly, this should be much easier. Another key point to remember is the grip—your forearms will need to *rotate* above the bar, to form struts for pushing with later. This requires a split-second relaxation of your grip, to allow the hands to spin around the bar.

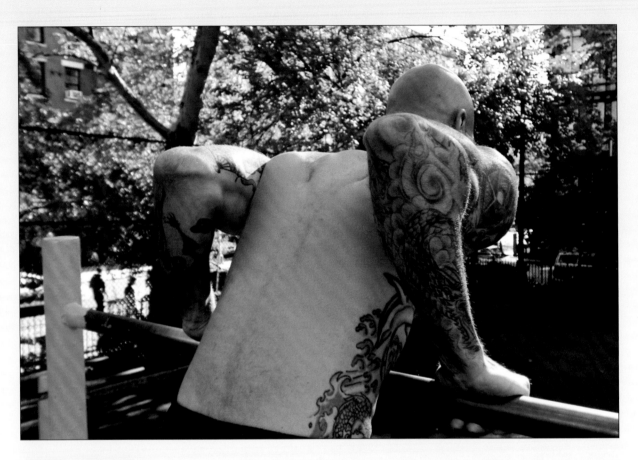

THE PRESS

Once you complete the pull-over, the keys to the *press* are having vertical (or *almost* vertical) forearms to push from, tilting the legs forward for balance, and employing the *false* (thumbless) grip. A thumbless grip—which you need from the start of the exercise—aids the hand rotation in the pull-over, but also provides a wider pressing base. You also need the raw strength—not *power*, just slow *strength*—to perform the push. (If you are still lacking a little, don't worry—starting page 238 I've included enough *dipping* progressions to take any athlete from zero to hero.)

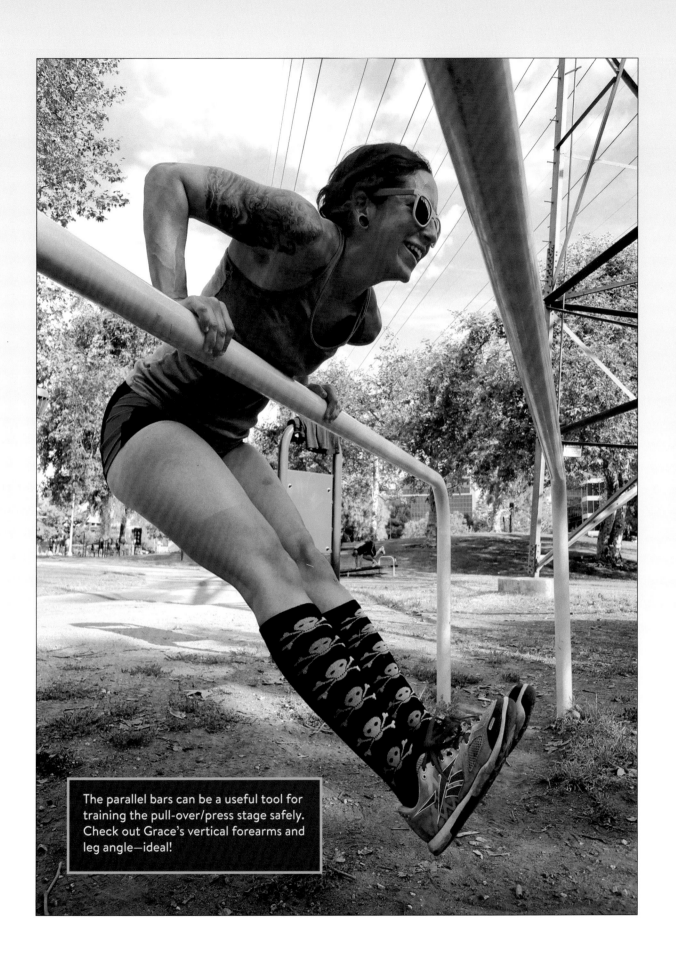

The parallel bars can be a useful tool for training the pull-over/press stage safely. Check out Grace's vertical forearms and leg angle—ideal!

EXPLOSIVE CALISTHENICS

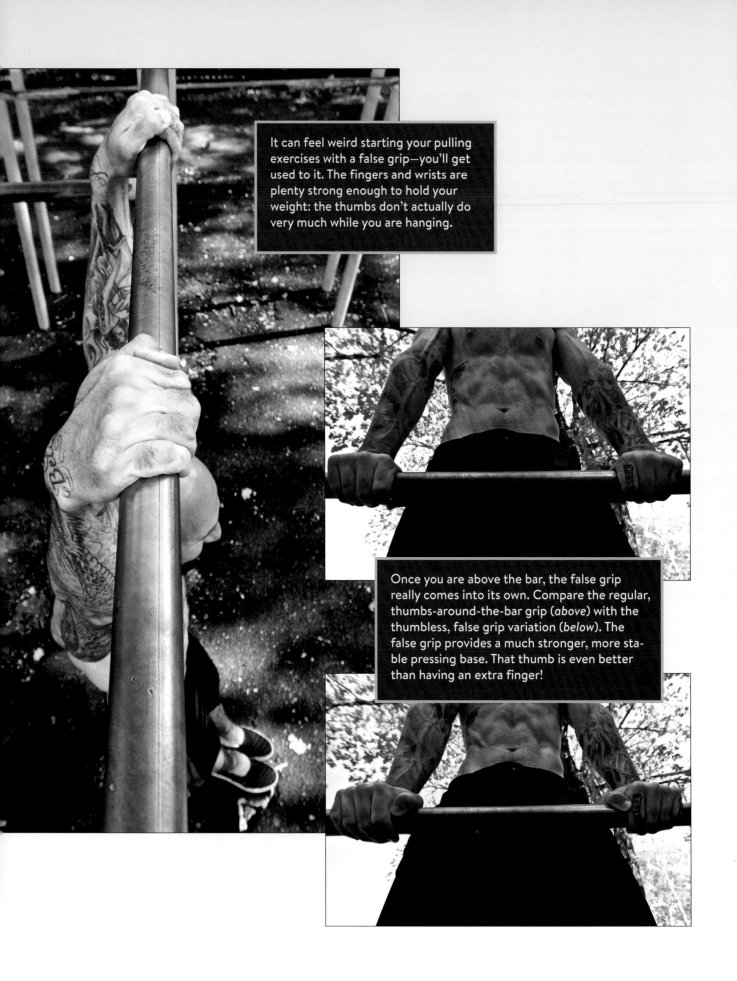

It can feel weird starting your pulling exercises with a false grip—you'll get used to it. The fingers and wrists are plenty strong enough to hold your weight: the thumbs don't actually do very much while you are hanging.

Once you are above the bar, the false grip really comes into its own. Compare the regular, thumbs-around-the-bar grip (*above*) with the thumbless, false grip variation (*below*). The false grip provides a much stronger, more stable pressing base. That thumb is even better than having an extra finger!

EXPLOSIVE CALISTHENICS

THE MUSCLE-UP CHAIN

If the different skill-aspects of the muscle-up I discussed in the previous section seem intimidating at first, don't worry—the muscle-up chain has been designed to teach you those skills, step-by-step. *Swing kips* (step 1) will teach you the basic but subtle movement of building momentum by curving and straightening your body while hanging from an overhead bar. *Jumping pullups* (step 2) teach you the art of pulling *in* to the bar from behind it, but this is made easier since you can push up and backwards off a base. Athletes are encouraged to practice swing kips and jumping pullups *together* until both are fully mastered. When this is the case, you'll be able to combine both these moves into a *kipping pullup* (step 3). These beauties might look like regular pullups, but they are much more explosive, requiring you to swing *back* behind the bar, and pull yourself *in*, until you finish with your chin over the bar.

Once you can pull your chin over the bar, kip-style, it's time to increase your power even more. This starts with *pullup hops* (step 4) where you release your hands briefly from the bar at the top of the movement. When you can release your hands well, the next stage is to clap them—and we have a version of the classic *clap pullup* (step 5). By now, you should really be mastering the kip-pull groove with power to spare, so we'll try to pull the chest into the bar (step 6), and then the hips (step 7).

Once you can kiss your hips to the bar, the pull stage is essentially mastered. The next trick to learn is to throw the head and trunk over the bar, in the pull-over position (see page 214). A surprising number of athletes have difficulty with this, so I like to teach it utilizing a jump to make the power element easier, to allow the athlete to focus on the technique of pulling over. This is the *jumping pullover* (step 8). Once the movement is better understood, the athlete moves to regular *bar pullovers* (step 9) performed from a dead hang under the bar.

Once you can pull your torso over the bar, the "only" thing left is to press yourself up—this stage is the Master Step, the complete *muscle-up* (step 10). Now, pressing yourself up is the element of the exercise which is more about raw strength than power or skill, and this might be where a few athletes need some help. If you do need a bit of work pressing your entire bodyweight over a horizontal bar, I've included a complete series of *dip progressions* to help you on your way, starting on page 238. Don't say I don't love you guys.

STEP ONE: SWING KIP

PERFORMANCE

- Hang from an overhead horizontal bar, with a shoulder-width grip. Keep your shoulders pulled down tight, and your body braced.

- Thrust your hips and chest forwards, while pushing your arms back and bringing your feet behind you. Your body should be curved and flexed. Your knees can bend slightly.

- Don't hold the back-curve, but allow your body to spring out of it, assisting with a contraction of your abs.

- As your glutes and hips shoot back, pull down with your hands and lats (keeping the arms straight).

- At the peak of the rebound, allow your body to curl slightly (the *hollow body position*). You should look like a letter "C", with your feet raised a little, and your trunk *curved* (not just bent at the hips). This is the *backswing*.

- Continue this back-and-forth, building a little momentum, and trying to get as high as you can on the backswing.

EXERCISE X-RAY

This drill might look like a simple swing, but in reality the *swing kip* is the key to unlocking the *muscle-up*—in fact, it's the cornerstone of virtually all explosive bar work. It's also a fantastic conditioning exercise: swing kips condition the deep tissues of the shoulders, spine and hips, as well as the grip, and forearm/elbow complex. These are all "power" areas.

REGRESSION

Any explosive hanging work—even this first step—can be hard on an untrained body. I would advise that an athlete is very comfortable with *pullups* before even approaching this series. That said, if swing kips prove too tough, begin by just hanging from the bar. Start swinging slowly, exploring *pendulum swings* without worrying about "kipping" too much. When swinging backwards and forwards is easy, begin building kipping form.

PROGRESSION

Build a stronger kip by generating more height in the *backswing*. Eventually athletes can perform a modified swing all the way up to the bar; this is a more advanced movement known as a *full kip* (see page 252).

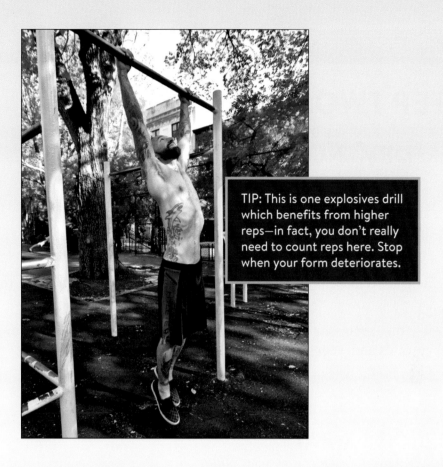

TIP: This is one explosives drill which benefits from higher reps—in fact, you don't really need to count reps here. Stop when your form deteriorates.

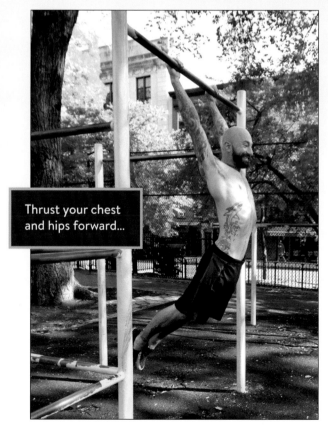

Thrust your chest and hips forward...

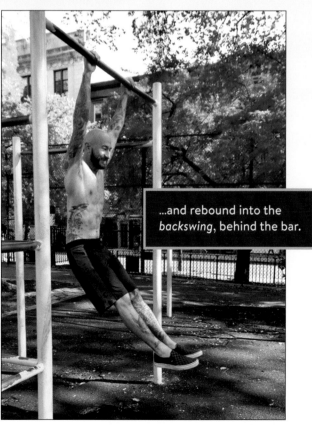

...and rebound into the *backswing*, behind the bar.

STEP TWO: JUMPING PULLUP

PERFORMANCE

- Grab an overhead bar with a shoulder-width grip.

- You should be standing in a semi-squat rather than hanging, so you can use a low bar or stand on a sturdy object.

- Holding the bar, leap up and back, to emulate the *backswing* of the *swing kip* (step 1).

- As you explode up, pull down and in with the arms. You will have to pull yourself *in* to the bar, since you jumped up *and* back.

- Use the combination of the momentum of the jump, plus the arm pull, to carry yourself upwards until your jaw is higher than the bar.

- Lower yourself quickly, but under control.

EXERCISE X-RAY

Have you been doing your regular *pullups* in a slow, strict, controlled fashion? Congratulations kid—that's the best possible way to build muscle and strength! But for *explosive* pulling power—the kind that's absolutely essential if you want to get the *muscle-up*—you need to change gears, neurologically and kinesiologically. *Jumping pullups* are the key. You *can* do jumping pullups by jumping (and pulling) straight *up*, but if you want to use jumping pullups to build to muscle-ups, you should remember to jump up and *back*, so you will have to pull up *and* in—an elliptical motion which mimics the arc of a proper *kipping pullup* (step 3).

REGRESSION

Using more leg involvement will make this easier. This can be done by using a lower bar, or pushing off a higher base. Alternatively, you can just focus on jumping higher.

PROGRESSION

The converse principle holds for progression: the higher you have to jump to grab the bar, the harder the exercise; the less distance you have to jump, the easier the exercise. If you can't raise the height of your horizontal bar, you can make the exercise a little tougher by jumping up off one leg. Remember to alternate legs each rep. At some point you can begin the exercise without gripping the bar—you'll have to jump up and grab the bar and pull up/in.

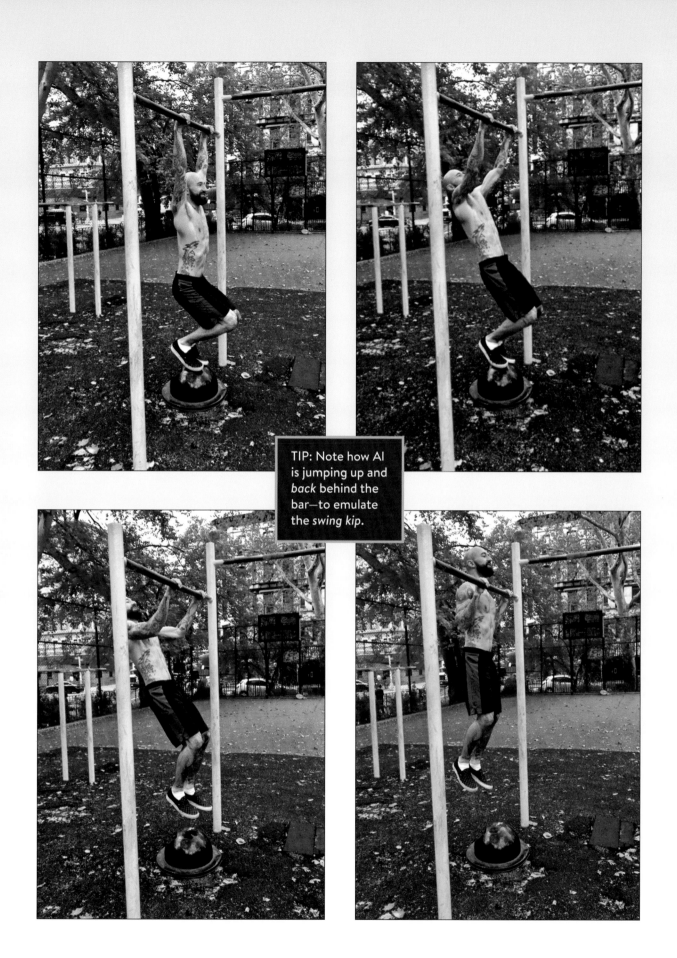

TIP: Note how Al is jumping up and *back* behind the bar—to emulate the *swing kip*.

STEP THREE: KIPPING PULLUP

PERFORMANCE

- Grab and hang from an overhead horizontal bar.

- Your grip should be approximately shoulder width, with your shoulders pulled down tight into the armpits. (This protects the shoulder socket.)

- Use the *swing kip* (step 1) to build some momentum prior to the pull.

- As you reach the peak of the *backswing*, thrust your hips forwards as you simultaneously pull down on the bar by bending the arms and shoulders.

- Use the combination of the backswing, plus the arm pull, to carry yourself upwards until your jaw is higher than the bar.

- Lower yourself quickly, in a reverse path. This will see you swinging forwards slightly. As you reach the bottom position, use this momentum to thrust your chest forwards again into a *swing kip*.

EXERCISE X-RAY

Once you have spent enough time really mastering *swing kips* (step 1) and *jumping pullups* (step 2), the next step is to combine these movements into the *kipping pullup*. The kipping pullup is the cornerstone of all power training on the bar—take the time to master it!.

REGRESSION

If starting the movement with just *one* swing kip is too difficult, utilize a chain of them, to build as much momentum/backswing as you can.

PROGRESSION

At first, you will only be expected to get your jaw over the bar. As this gets easy, instead of making the exercise stricter (which would strip it of power/momentum) keep trying to get your head/shoulders even higher over the bar at the top of the movement.

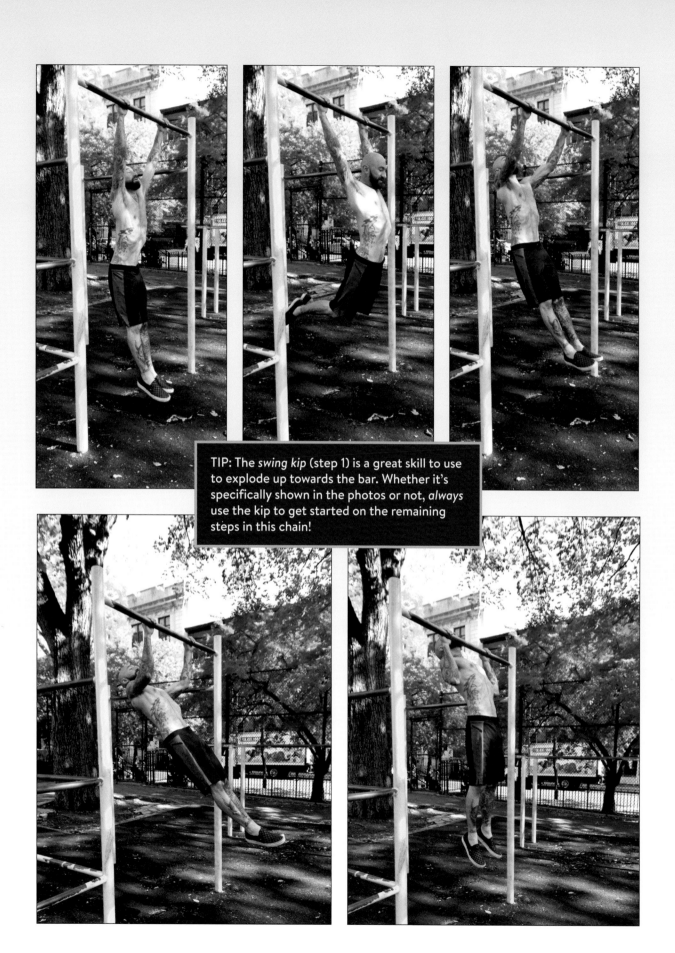

TIP: The *swing kip* (step 1) is a great skill to use to explode up towards the bar. Whether it's specifically shown in the photos or not, *always* use the kip to get started on the remaining steps in this chain!

STEP FOUR: PULLUP HOP

PERFORMANCE

- Grab and hang from an overhead horizontal bar.

- Your grip should be approximately shoulder width, with your shoulders pulled down tight into the armpits. (This protects the shoulder socket.)

- Use the *swing kip* (step 1) to build some momentum prior to the pull.

- As you reach the peak of the backwards swing, thrust your hips forwards as you simultaneously pull down on the bar by bending the arms and shoulders.

- Use the combination of the backswing, the momentum of the knees, plus the arm pull, to carry yourself upwards.

- At the very peak of the movement, quickly lift your hands off the bar for a fraction of a second.

- Re-grip the bar and lower yourself back into the swing kip.

EXERCISE X-RAY

Once you have mastered the *kipping pullup*, you will be beginning to build some good levels of explosive power. But before you can progress to the coveted *clap pullup*, it's a good idea to work with this preliminary drill. *Pullup hops* are, for clap pullups, what *pop-ups* are for *clap pushups*. With either exercise, before you can clap, your body needs to learn the skill of creating "airtime"—it needs to leave its comfy base. The only difference is that for pullups the base is a bar; for pushups, it's the floor.

REGRESSION

At first, just work on building speed. It can help to begin by just alternately lifting one hand off the bar at the top of the movement, to get the feel of the exercise.

PROGRESSION

Initially, athletes exploring this exercise will be lucky to just loosen their grip and recapture the bar. As you get stronger, begin building some height—a master of this exercise should be able to lift their palms six inches or more from the bar at the top of the movement.

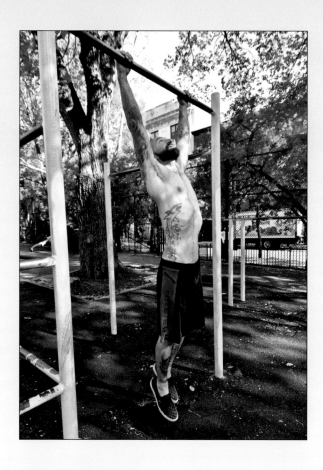
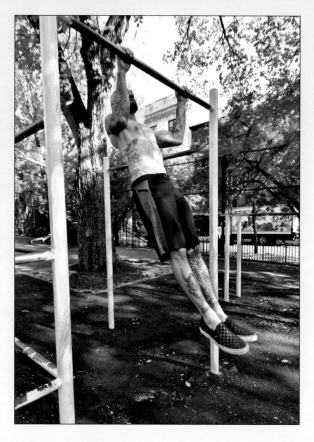
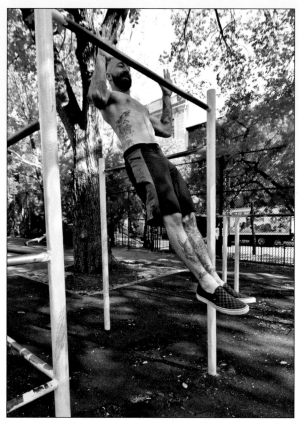
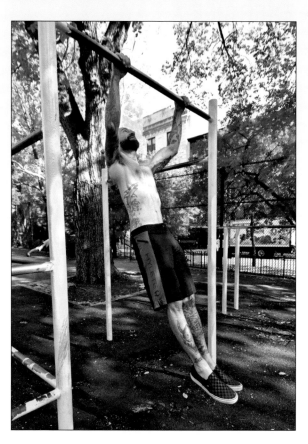

STEP FIVE: CLAP PULLUP

PERFORMANCE

- Grab and hang from an overhead horizontal bar.

- Your grip should be approximately shoulder width, with your shoulders pulled down tight into the armpits. (This protects the shoulder socket.)

- Use the *swing kip* (step 1) to build some momentum prior to the pull.

- As you reach the peak of the *backswing*, thrust your hips forwards as you simultaneously pull down on the bar by bending the arms and shoulders.

- Use the combination of the backswing, plus the arm pull, to carry yourself upwards.

- At the very peak of the movement, quickly lift your hands off the bar and audibly clap them together.

- Re-grip the bar and lower yourself quickly, into the swing kip.

EXERCISE X-RAY

Some folks might think that *vertical* momentum might be better for getting the height needed to pull off your first *clap pullup*. Not so. The most efficient way to learn the clap is through swinging up in a *curve*, like you learned in *kipping pullups* (step 3). When you *swing kip* yourself up *behind* the bar—instead of trying to get *above* it—you'll find there's plenty of room for your forearms and hands to clap *behind* the bar. You don't need to pull yourself a mile *over* it. Don't overdo it and try to push yourself away from the bar, either—just follow the natural curve you worked on earlier in the chain.

REGRESSION

An easier progression involves just removing one hand at the top of the movement, and slapping your opposite forearm.

PROGRESSION

You guessed it—if this is too easy (!), work on those *double* and *triple claps*.

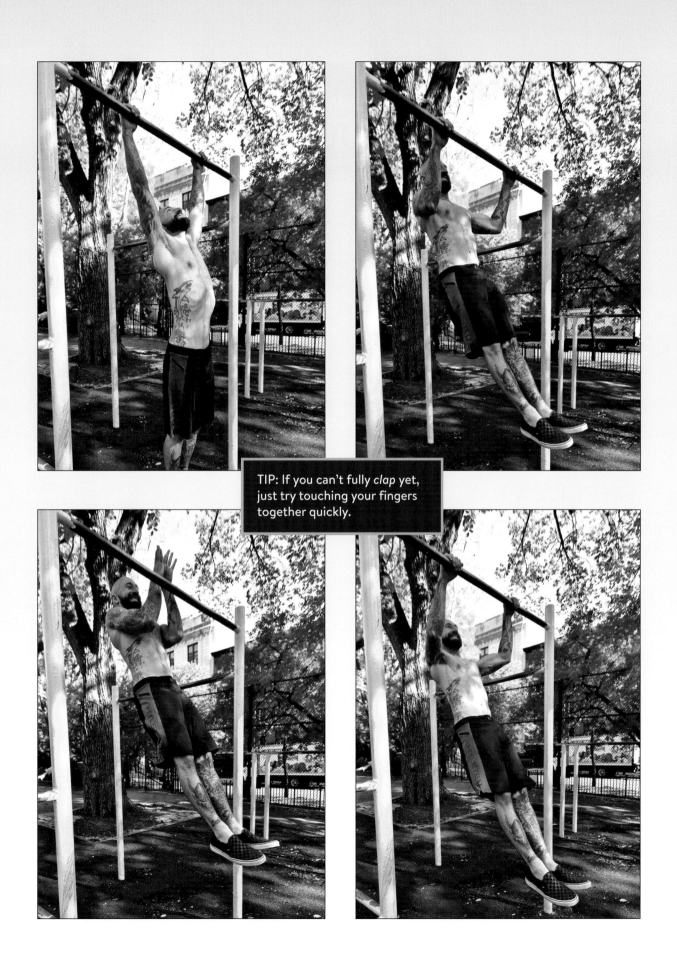

TIP: If you can't fully *clap* yet, just try touching your fingers together quickly.

STEP SIX: CHEST PULLUP

PERFORMANCE

- Grab and hang from an overhead horizontal bar.

- Your grip should be approximately shoulder width, with your shoulders pulled down tight into the armpits. (This protects the shoulder socket.)

- Use the *swing kip* (step 1) to build some momentum prior to the pull. By this stage, your swing kip should be more powerful, to the point where your backswing takes you higher than in the first few steps.

- As soon as you are close to the peak of the backswing—when your head is nearing the level of the bar—begin pulling your elbows *back* as hard as you can.

- Keeping pulling back until your elbows are behind your body, and your chest kisses the bar.

- Lower yourself down quickly, into the swing kip

EXERCISE X-RAY

Up to this point in the chain you have been pulling your torso more or less upwards, in the backwards swing caused by the swing kip. Now the pattern changes. At the height of your backswing, you change direction, and pull your elbows *back*—until they are *behind* you. This is what draws your chest into the bar, and if you do it right then at the peak of the movement your forearms will be *diagonal*; not vertical, as for regular pullups.

REGRESSION

If touching the bar with the sternum (*breastbone*) is too difficult, begin by kissing the bar with your upper chest. Experiment carefully, however—if you miscalculate your ability early on, it's possible to hit your face against the bar.

PROGRESSION

As your swing kip gets you higher and higher, keep trying to touch the bar lower and lower against your torso. Eventually you will be pulling the bar into your stomach, then your lower abs—and this leads us neatly to the next step.

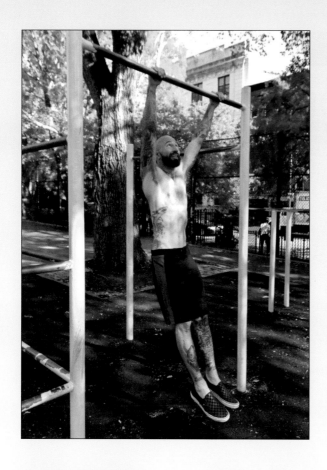
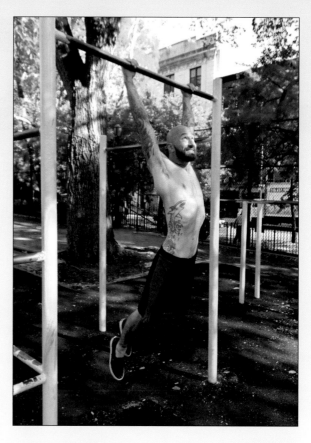
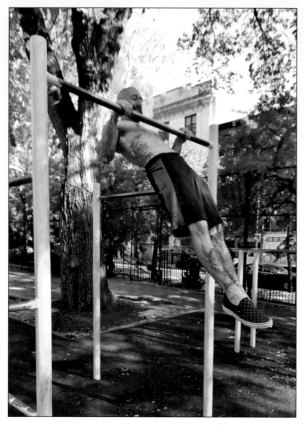
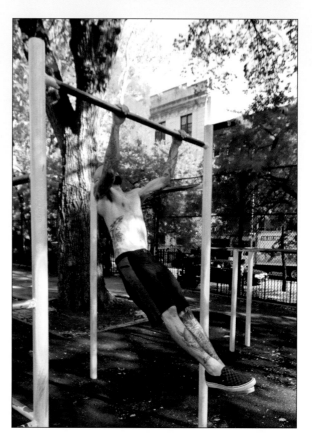

STEP SEVEN: HIP PULLUP

PERFORMANCE

- Grab and hang from an overhead horizontal bar.

- Your grip should be approximately shoulder width, with your shoulders pulled down tight into the armpits. (This protects the shoulder socket.)

- Use the *swing kip* (step 1) to build some momentum prior to the pull. By this stage, your swing kip should be more powerful, to the point where your backswing takes you higher than in the first few steps.

- As soon as you are close to the peak of the backswing, snap backwards with your arms; this is a short tug backwards to change direction, not the full range pull you used for *chest pullups*.

- Simultaneously clench your glutes and posterior chain to thrust your hips upwards toward the bar. Thrust hard enough so that your lower stomach kisses the bar.

- Re-grip the bar and lower yourself quickly, into the swing kip.

EXERCISE X-RAY

There is an important distinction between *chest pullups* and *hip pullups*; with chest pullups, you pull *in* to the bar with your arms at the peak of the movement. With hip pullups, your arms only bend a little—most of the force at the top is generated by a hip thrust. Believe it or not, once you can achieve the *hip pullup*, you have pretty much achieved the *muscle-up*—the pulling portion, anyways. The next step will teach you how to channel this strength into the *pull-over* position.

REGRESSION

As before, the height at which your body touches the bar is key. If you can't pull your lower abs into the bar, try your upper abs.

PROGRESSION

At this point, you have achieved pretty much the height you need to start working on the middle portion of the muscle-up—the pull-over. If you want to, you can keep building height—it's possible to explode the upper thighs into the bar.

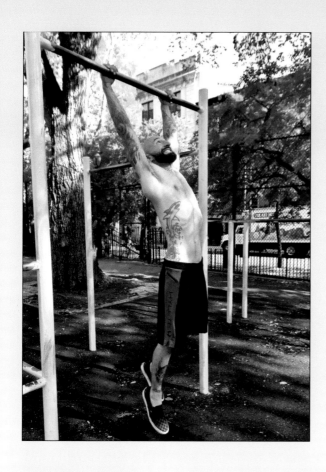
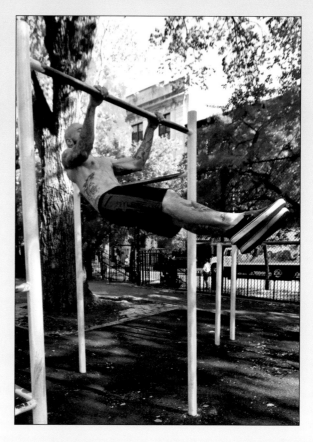
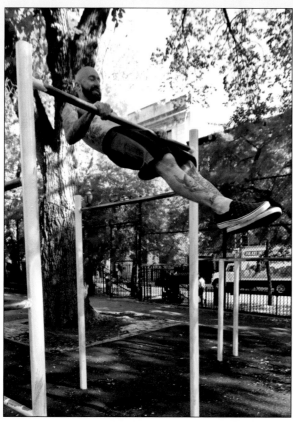
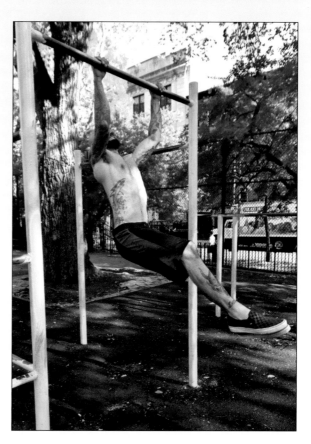

STEP EIGHT: JUMPING PULLOVER

PERFORMANCE

- Grab an overhead horizontal bar. Your grip should be approximately shoulder width, with your shoulders pulled down tight.

- Utilize a "false grip"—i.e., thumbs over the bar. (See pages 214-216 for more information on the correct grip.)

- You can either use a low bar (*shown*) or place one (or both) feet on a stable box or base beneath you; something that will allow you to push with your legs.

- Bend the loaded leg/s, and jump *up* and *back*, in the direction of the *swing kip* (step 1).

- As soon as you are close to the peak of the jump-assisted backswing, snap backwards with your arms, pulling yourself towards the bar.

- Simultaneously clench your glutes and posterior chain to thrust your upper abs into the bar.

- Keep pulling back hard with the elbows, as you hurl your torso forward over the bar.

- Rotate your wrists as you reach the final pull-over position (see page 214). You should finish up with the bar under your upper abs, with your head and chest over the bar, legs tilted forward slightly. Your forearms should be vertical struts. Pause in this position.

EXERCISE X-RAY

If you can attain *hip pullups* (step 7), then you have the power to perform the pull section on a *muscle-up*. You just need to learn the correct technique for pulling your torso over the bar. This is where *jumping pullovers* come in—the extra power from the legs allows you to work on pulling your trunk over the bar, before you do it for real (step 9). Train this exercise alongside hip pullups, to retain the power you've already built.

REGRESSION

The higher the base/lower the bar, the easier it is to self-assist.

PROGRESSION

Make the self-assist harder by jumping off a lower object, or using just one leg to push from.

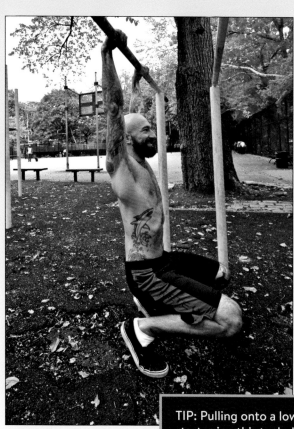

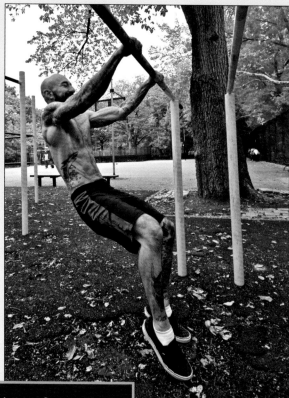

TIP: Pulling onto a low bar is a perfect way to start using this technique. As you gain in confidence, move to the higher horizontal bar and push (jump) off a base, like a box or a chair, etc.

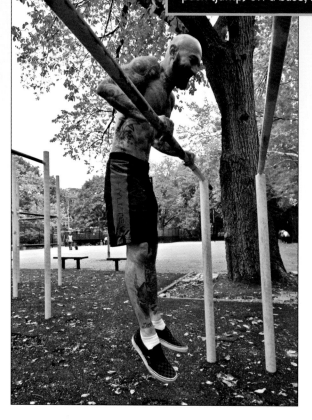

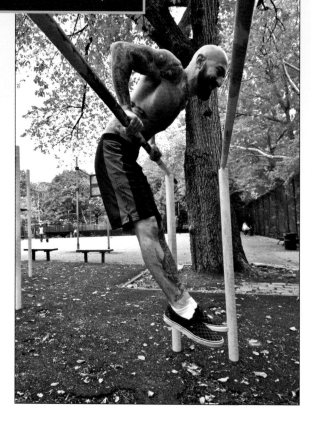

STEP NINE: BAR PULLOVER

PERFORMANCE

- Grab an overhead horizontal bar. Your grip should be approximately shoulder width, with your shoulders pulled down tight.

- Utilize a "false grip"—i.e., thumbs over the bar. (See pages 214 to 216 for more information on the correct grip.)

- Use the *swing kip* (step 1) to build some momentum prior to the pull. By this stage, your swing kip should be more powerful, to the point where your backswing takes you higher than in the first few steps.

- As soon as you are close to the peak of the backswing, snap backwards with your arms.

- Simultaneously clench your glutes and posterior chain to thrust your upper abs into the bar.

- Keep pulling back hard with the elbows, as you hurl your torso forward over the bar. Keeping your legs tilted will help with this.

- Rotate your wrists as you reach the final pull-over position (see page 214). You should finish up with the bar under your upper abs, with your head and chest over the bar, legs raised. Your forearms should be vertical struts. Pause in this position.

EXERCISE X-RAY

Calisthenic pullovers are not only an incredible exercise for harnessing nuclear-level explosive strength, they are also *functional* as hell—you are learning to pull your bodyweight *up and over*. Whether it's a tree, a fence, or a wall, having this technique under your belt may even save your life in an emergency. Almost as cool, master the *bar pullover*, and you are just one set of straight arms away from one of the most admired bar moves on the planet—the *muscle-up*!

REGRESSION

Initially you may not be able to pause over the bar—if you can't get your trunk forwards far enough. At first, just be satisfied with completing the movement: the pause will come in time.

PROGRESSION

Finish the repetition by rolling forwards over the bar.

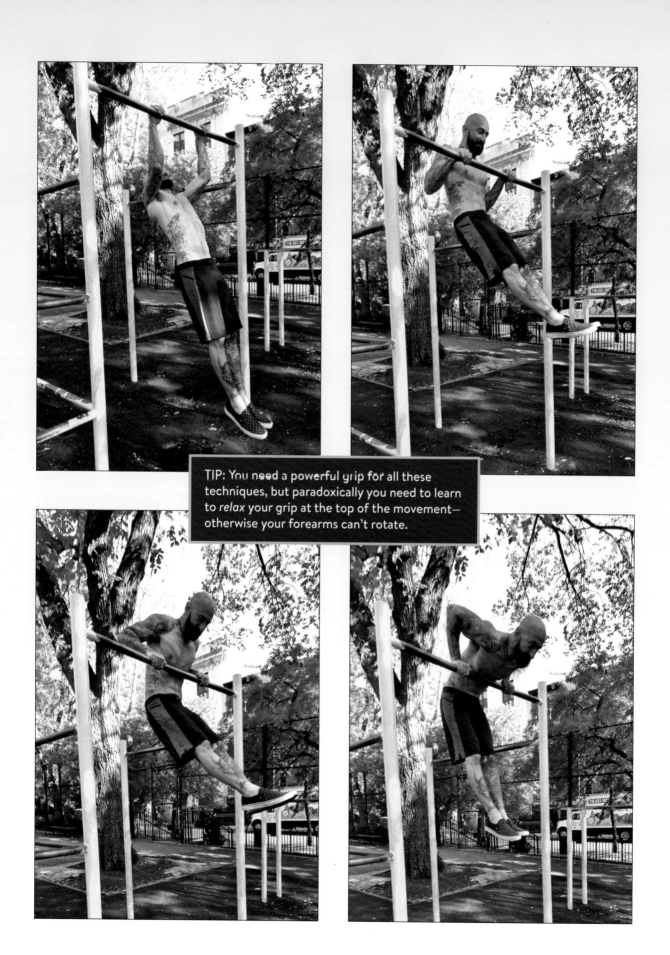

TIP: You need a powerful grip for all these techniques, but paradoxically you need to learn to *relax* your grip at the top of the movement—otherwise your forearms can't rotate.

MASTER STEP: THE MUSCLE-UP

PERFORMANCE

- Grab an overhead horizontal bar. Your grip should be approximately shoulder width, with your shoulders pulled down tight.

- Utilize a "false grip"—i.e., thumbs over the bar. (See pages 214 to 216 for more information on the correct grip.)

- Use the *swing kip* (step 1) to build some momentum prior to the pull. By this stage, your swing kip should be more powerful, to the point where your backswing takes you higher than in the first few steps.

- As soon as you are close to the peak of the backswing, snap backwards with your arms.

- Simultaneously clench your glutes and posterior chain to thrust your upper abs into the bar.

- Keep pulling back hard with the elbows, as you hurl your torso forward over the bar. Keeping your legs raised will help with this.

- Rotate your wrists as you reach the pullover position (see page 214). The bar should be under your upper abs, with your head and chest over the bar, legs raised. Your forearms should be vertical struts.

- Press yourself up by straightening your arms. It will help to look forwards with the head up as you dip up. Pause at the top.

EXERCISE X-RAY

If one popular strength exercise ever qualified as a "complete" feat of ability, it would probably be the mighty *muscle-up*. Unlike the vast majority of strength exercises it features a strong *pull* component, plus a strong *push*—add to these the need for speed, power, balance, timing, total-body coordination and a midsection of steel, and is it any wonder the muscle-up is one of the most jealously admired skills in all bodyweight training?

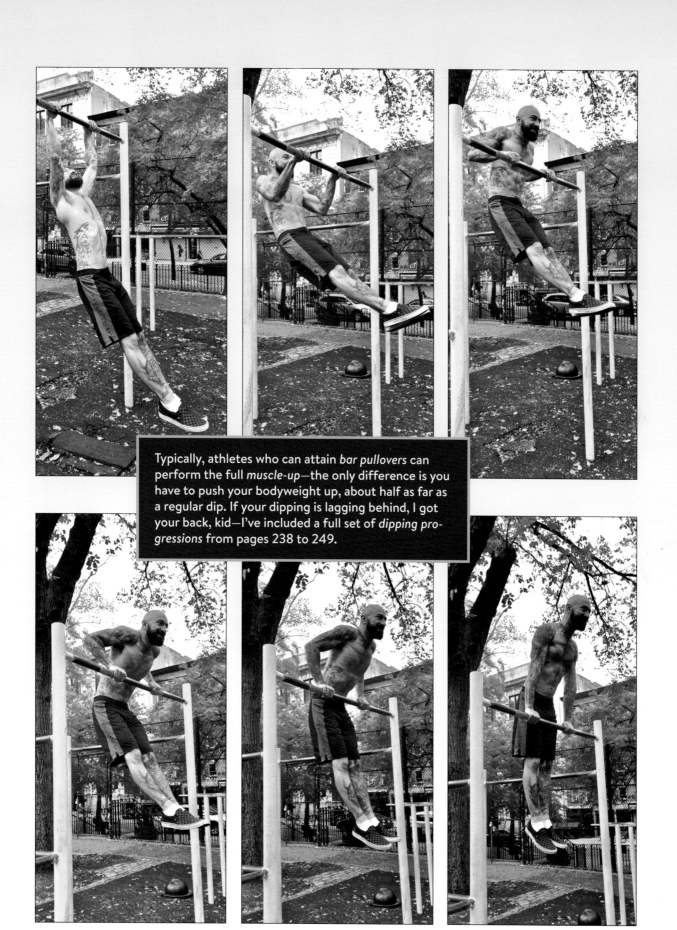

Typically, athletes who can attain *bar pullovers* can perform the full *muscle-up*—the only difference is you have to push your bodyweight up, about half as far as a regular dip. If your dipping is lagging behind, I got your back, kid—I've included a full set of *dipping progressions* from pages 238 to 249.

BONUS PROGRESSIONS: DIPS

The dip-press from the bar is the final concentric aspect of the muscle-up: without being able to depend on speed or momentum, most athletes are forced to push up with raw *strength*. Yep, there's technique involved—there always is—but if the basic muscle strength is lacking, forget it.

This is why the dip-press is the part of the muscle-up that so many folks struggle with. The only way to build that strength is through plenty of progressive dipping. If you can comfortably perform a *horizontal bar dip* (a dip on top of the horizontal bar), then your chances of completing a muscle-up have skyrocketed.

Do you really need dips in your routine? As a permanent movement, I'm a bigger fan of *pushups*, for various reasons. But if you want to master the muscle-up, dips as an ancillary drill are a good idea: you need to be able to dip well. In addition, many famous calisthenics masters—notably Al Kavadlo and Matt Schifferle—take dips seriously as a part of their basic training. There are many roads to Mecca, right?

The majority of dips—being *strength*-based—are really not *power* exercises, per se. But since they help so much in the muscle-up, I've included a summary of a ten step chain of dip progressions here for anyone who needs them. There are no progression standards here; just use your intuition and "milk" the exercises until you become expert in them before moving on. Since this manual is about explosive power, I've also included some more explosive dipping variations after the progressions.

1. BENT DIPS

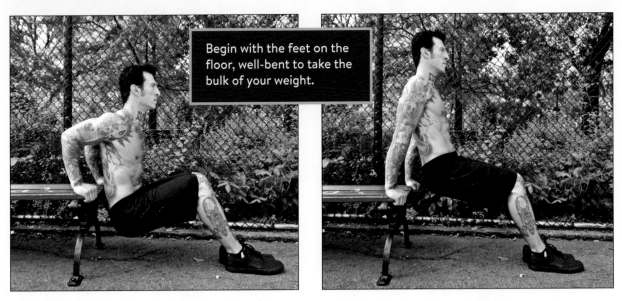

Begin with the feet on the floor, well-bent to take the bulk of your weight.

2. STRAIGHT DIPS

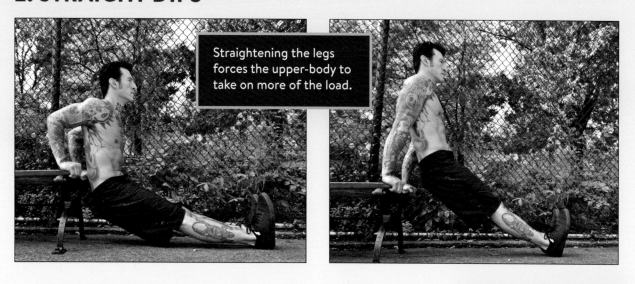

Straightening the legs forces the upper-body to take on more of the load.

3. FEET-ELEVATED DIPS

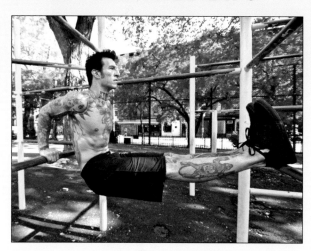
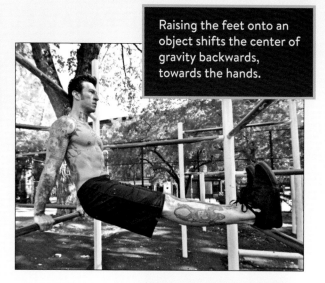

Raising the feet onto an object shifts the center of gravity backwards, towards the hands.

4. FEET-UP PARALLEL BAR DIPS

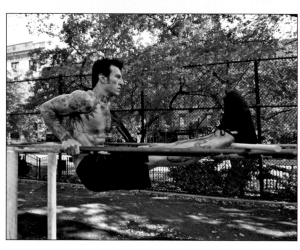
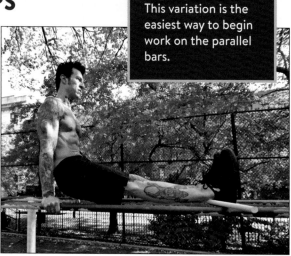

This variation is the easiest way to begin work on the parallel bars.

5. SELF-ASSISTED PARALLEL BAR DIPS 1

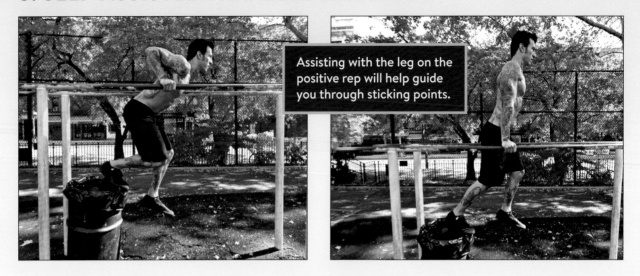

Assisting with the leg on the positive rep will help guide you through sticking points.

6. SELF-ASSISTED PARALLEL BAR DIPS 2

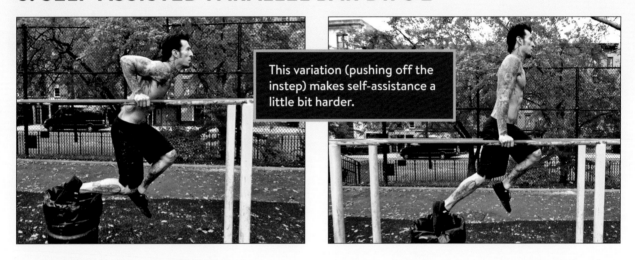

This variation (pushing off the instep) makes self-assistance a little bit harder.

7. PARALLEL BAR DIPS

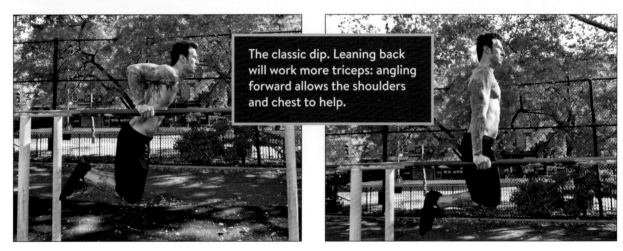

The classic dip. Leaning back will work more triceps: angling forward allows the shoulders and chest to help.

8. LEGS FORWARD PARALLEL BAR DIPS

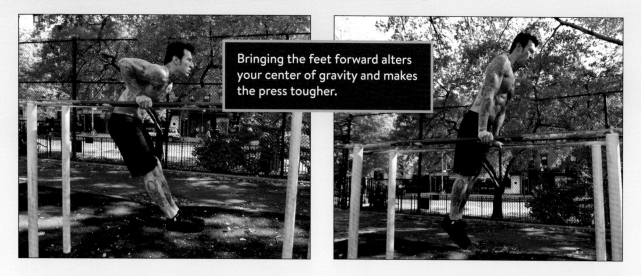

Bringing the feet forward alters your center of gravity and makes the press tougher.

9. PERPENDICULAR DIPS

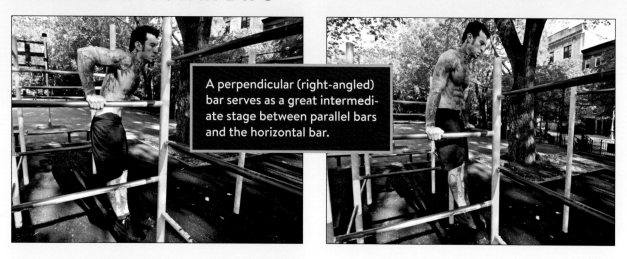

A perpendicular (right-angled) bar serves as a great intermediate stage between parallel bars and the horizontal bar.

10. HORIZONTAL BAR DIPS

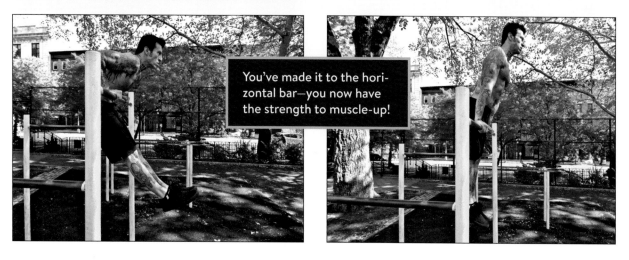

You've made it to the horizontal bar—you now have the strength to muscle-up!

RUSSIAN DIPS

Dips are an incredibly versatile exercise, and once you're advanced, there are various options you can try. *Russian dips* are sometimes used as an ancillary exercise to *muscle-ups*: using the parallel bars, you lower under control down to your elbows, then shift your weight forward and straighten your arms. Some coaches feel that this pattern mimics the pull-over well.

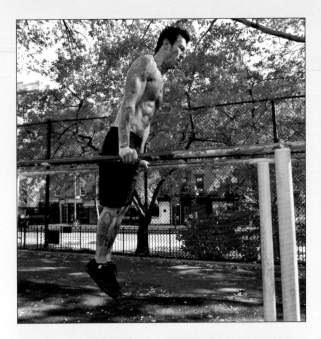
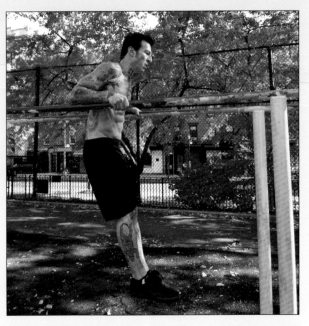
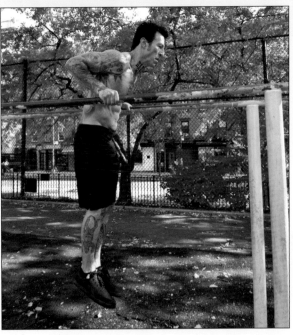
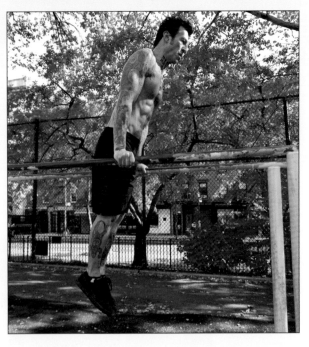

L-HOLD DIPS

Performing parallel bar dips with your legs locked out in front of the hips (called an *L-hold*, or an *L-sit*) is an interesting advanced dipping variation. As well as training the midsection, the position shifts your center of gravity forward, making the exercise much tougher.

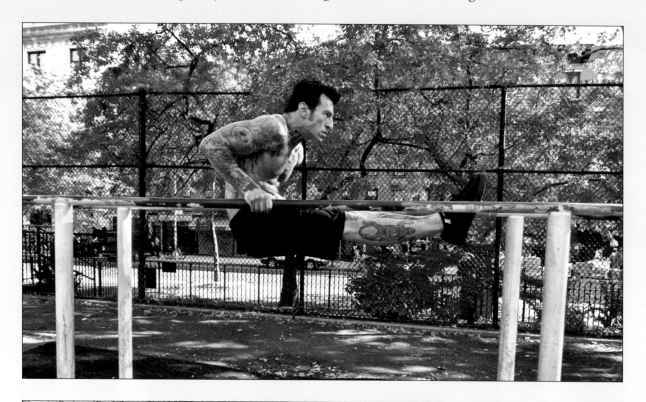

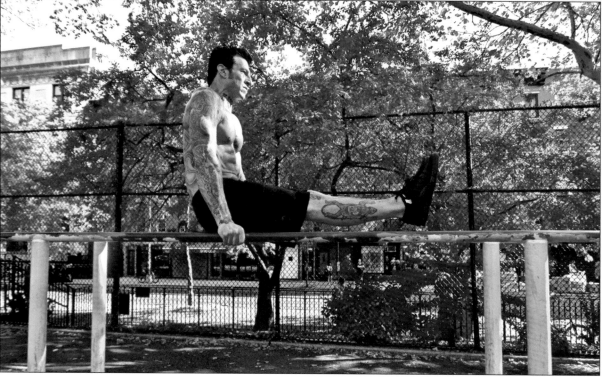

KOREAN DIPS

For those of you wanting to take your dipping to superhuman levels, how about *one-arm dips*? Believe it or not, they are possible, if you push up off the top of a wall. For information on this (and lots more) check out Steve Low's superlative volume of progressive gymnastics, ***Overcoming Gravity.*** While you're in a book-buying mood, you need to check out the greatest resource on dips (amongst other things) ever written: Al Kavadlo's ***Raising the Bar.***

Korean dips are a crazy variation of the straight-bar dip, where the bar is behind you. Gorilla shoulders only!

DOUBLE DIPS: EXPLOSIVE VARIATIONS

The dipping chain I've just presented is designed for building slow strength, the kind of strength that's useful in the very top portion of the muscle-up. But this book is about *explosive power*, right? So it'd be remiss of me not to show you a few ways to work the dipping movement for speed-strength. Get ready to amp up that upper-body...I'm talking power dips, gorgeous!

WALKING DIPS

Once you have progressed in dips to the point where you can perform a few strict parallel bar dips, you can begin experimenting with explosive variations. The basis of all these variations is the *walking dip*. This forces your joints and muscles to accommodate a little shock as you "step" along the bars. A perfect start.

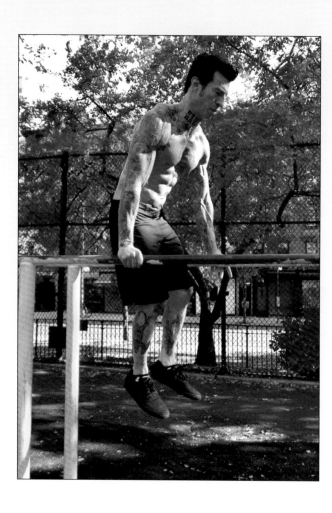
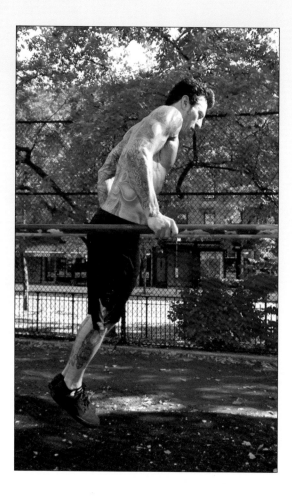

HOPPING DIPS

Once walking is a breeze, you can step up the shock factor by hopping up and down in the dip position. The *hopping dip* requires a powerful enough press to lift your hands off the bars. As you gain power, you can elevate yourself further. The hands and forearms also get a power workout by "catching" the bars again.

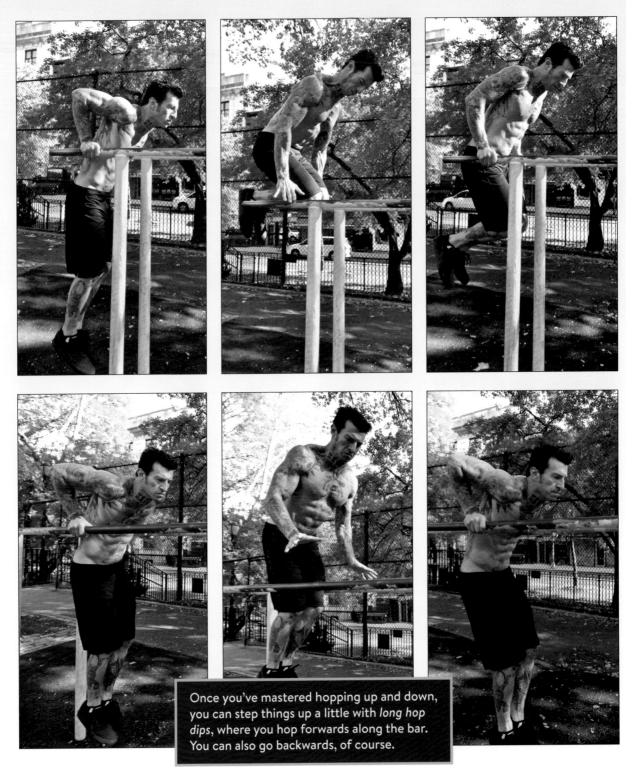

Once you've mastered hopping up and down, you can step things up a little with *long hop dips*, where you hop forwards along the bar. You can also go backwards, of course.

246

EXPLOSIVE CALISTHENICS

CLAP DIPS

Once your hopping is powerful enough, you will be able to perform *clap dips*. If you think *clap pushups* are tough, try this number, where your arms have to move your *entire* bodyweight explosively! Make sure you build up to this kind of brutal power exercise, or it's an injury waiting to happen.

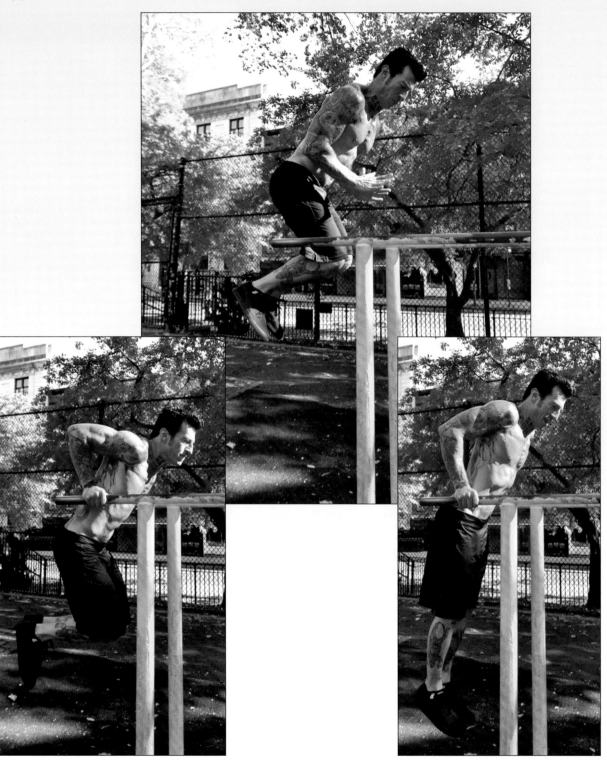

180 POWER DIPS

If clap dips get easy, rest assured that you have one helluva powerful upper-body. But—as ever, with calisthenics—you can always make things harder. The *180 power dip* adds extra explosiveness and agility into the dip. Can you push up explosively enough to spin in mid-air and catch the bar again? I don't know if a *360 power dip* is possible, but I've never seen one.

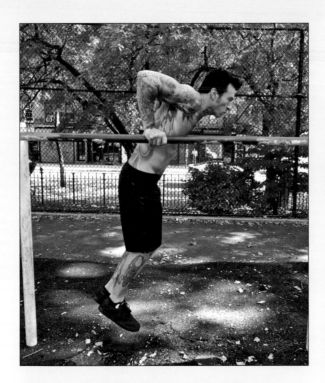
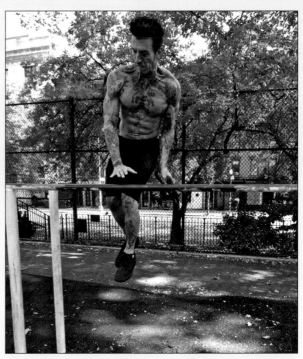

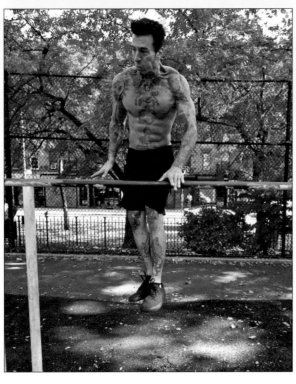
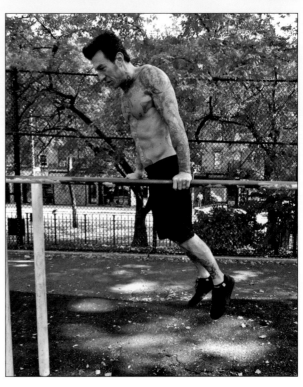

SWING DIPS

Swing dips take things even further, and build total-body power and coordination. Swing your legs forward at the bottom of the dip, and as you straighten your arms, swing your legs and entire body back. By the time your arms are locked out, your trunk and legs should be virtually horizontal. This position only lasts a split-second before the swing back down.

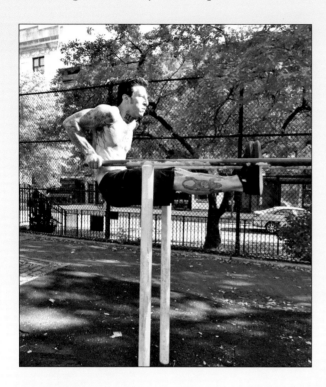
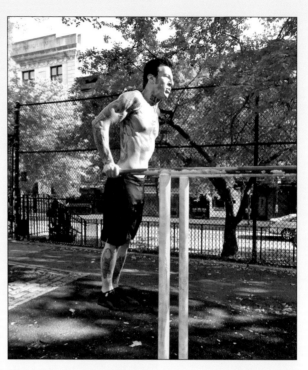

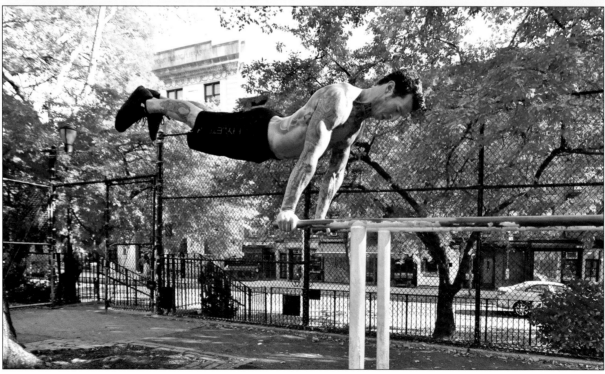

GOING BEYOND

When an athlete aces the muscle-up *perfectly*, their first instinct is to try and do it slower. A perfectly slow, momentum-free muscle-up really is a sight to behold—but if it's power you're after, *slow* is the opposite of what you want. (That's not to say you can't work on this version as part of your *strength* goals, right?)

UNDERHAND MUSCLE-UPS

There are other variations of the muscle-up which make more sense to me when training for power. One of these is the *underhand muscle-up*. A normal muscle-up uses an overhand (palms away from you) grip, but the underhand version throws new power demands on the body, particularly the grip and biceps. The unusual position also makes the press at the top a lot tougher.

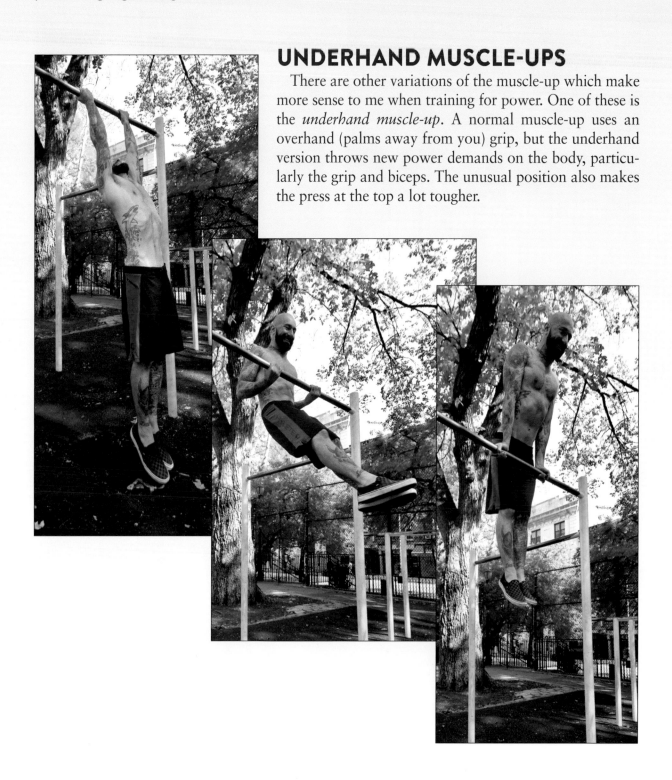

ARCHER MUSCLE-UP

Once you've perfected the underhand version, a great way to make the muscle-up more demanding is to perform it *asymmetrically*—with one arm out a little so it can't assist with the pull/push as much. This is the *archer muscle-up*.

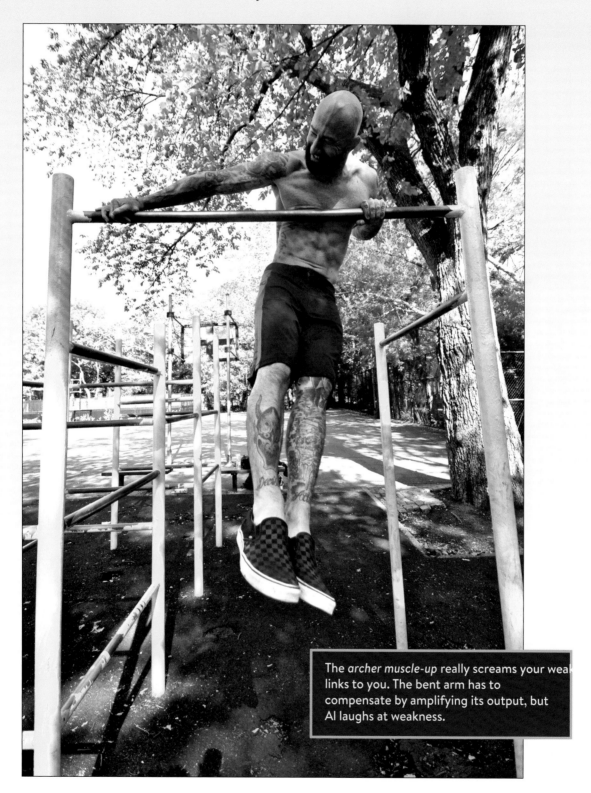

The *archer muscle-up* really screams your weak links to you. The bent arm has to compensate by amplifying its output, but Al laughs at weakness.

FULL KIPS

Another alternative in power building is to work on the *full kip*. You have already worked on *swing kips* as a key part of the muscle-up chain (and every exercise in it) to gain some momentum to help you pull up. But—if you harness enough body-power—*you can perform an extreme kip straight up and over the bar*. It might look a little like a muscle-up—you begin hanging and end up over the bar—but your arms remain fairly straight throughout. Your body movement powers you up!

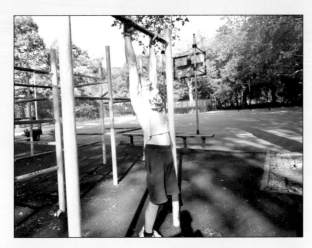 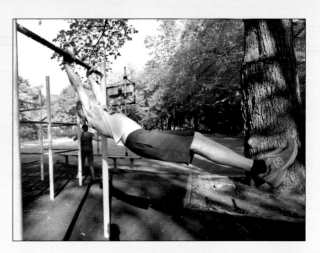

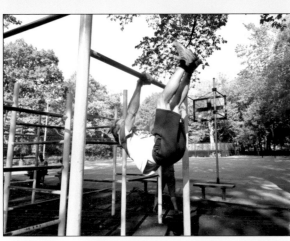 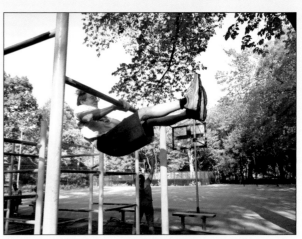

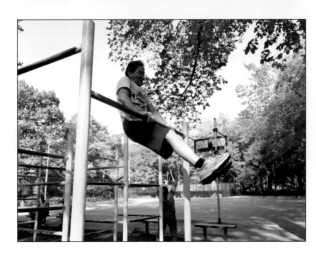 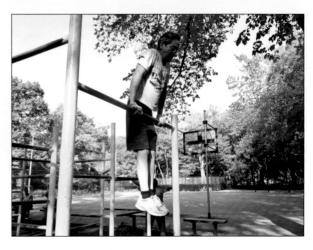

SMALL SPACE DRILLS

Following are three useful speed and power techniques you can utilize in your routine for variety, as ancillary work or to train your muscles from different angles. They are all solo drills, and they require zero equipment. Unlike the progressive exercises in the chains, most of the following drills can be performed rhythmically for higher reps, and can work well when used with any of the chains in this book. In this sense, they can also work as warm-ups or finishing exercises in an explosives session.

SIDEWAYS POP-UPS

Get into a pushup position. Bend the arms, and pop-up your entire body, landing around six inches to the side of where you started. This simple drill is a great example of how different power pushups can be combined in a single set: you can go left, right, left, back, and forwards using this technique. You can also throw in other stuff like *clap pushups*.

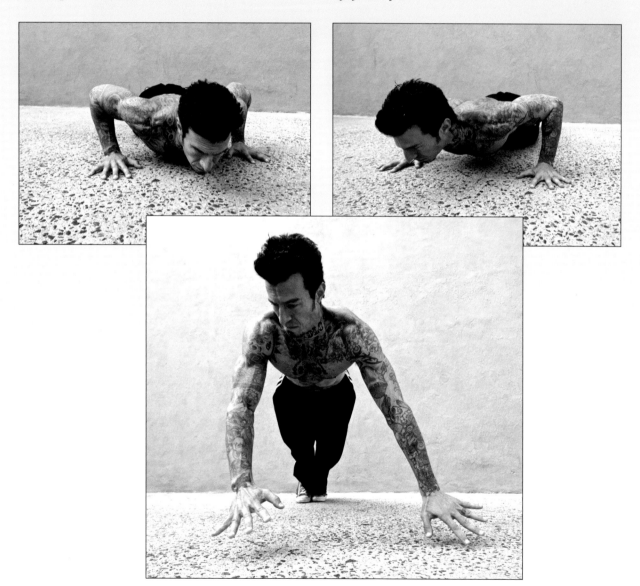

PIKE SLAPS

Lay down, and balance on your butt. Explosively raise your torso and legs, slapping your insteps with your hands at the top of the movement. Bob down and immediately repeat, bouncing back up. All explosive pulling work requires steely abs, and this is a fantastic movement for building super-powerful abdominals—more painful than it looks if you try for high reps. But don't sacrifice speed!

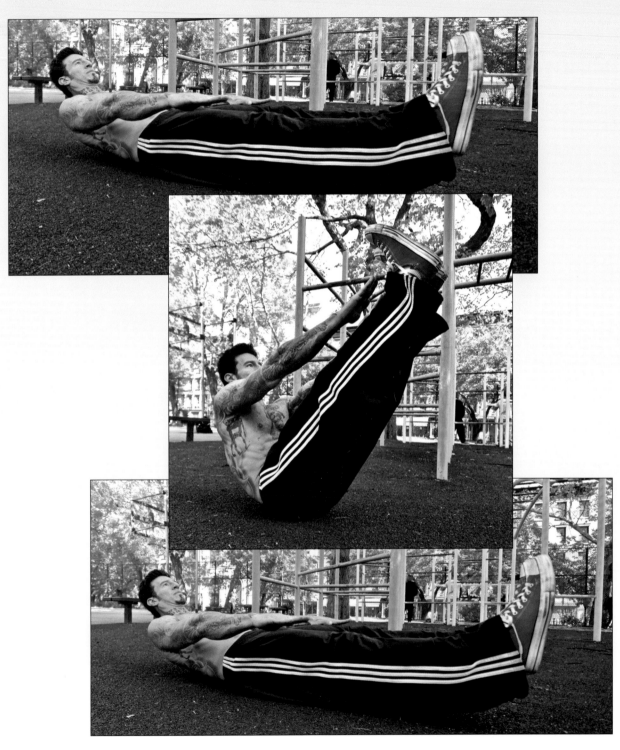

EXPLOSIVE CALISTHENICS

JUMP KICK

Assume a fighting stance, one leg in front of the other. Quickly snap up your back leg in front of you, and utilize that momentum, to whip up your other knee. At the peak of the movement extend the lead knee into a kick. A useful, fairly low-stress exercise for healthy hips, and a good way to raise the legs unilaterally, which is fairly rare in most small space drills.

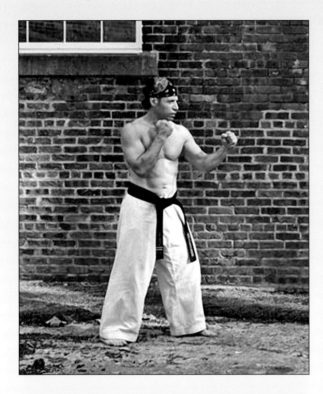 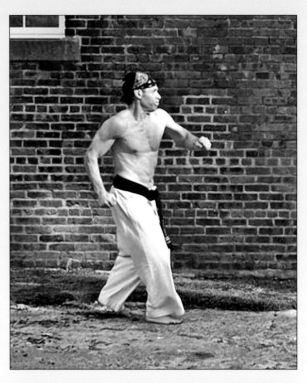

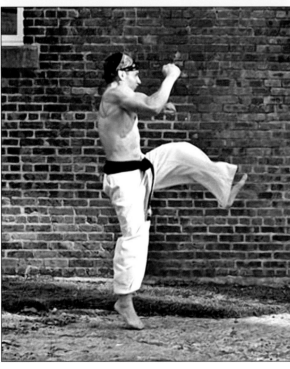 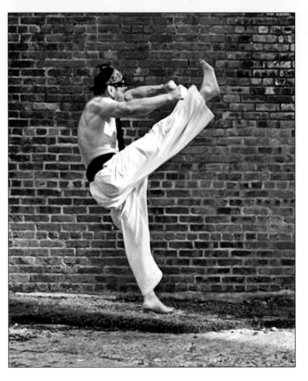

LIGHTS OUT!

Some calisthenics techniques are dependent mostly on *skill*. The *free handstand* is a good example; most athletes can support their bodyweight with their hands—say, against a wall. But very few of these people can hold a free handstand effortlessly; they got the *strength*, but they lack the *skill*. Conversely, some bodyweight exercises are dependent mostly on strength. If you are *strong* enough, a pullup will be easy for ya—even if you have crummy coordination, timing, balance or whatnot.

The bad news is that the muscle-up requires both—strength *and* skill. Unless you have plenty of body-power, *plus* the deadly accurate "groove" of this particular movement, you don't have much hope of getting it done. But the rewards of the muscle-up are incredible. For one, the *pulling* action to get over the bar works as a beautiful balancer to plenty of explosive *pushing*. (You have been doing your *power pushups*, right?) It's also functional, builds total-body explosiveness and acts as a wonderful base exercise for further explosive bar work, if you want to get more gymnastic in your approach.

Is it easy? *No*. Can you learn it if you break it down into enough steps? *Yes*—I promise you. It's like any skill, in that sense. So let's quit wasting time and head for the bar.

PART III

PROGRAMMING: THEORY & TACTICS

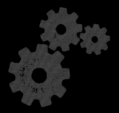

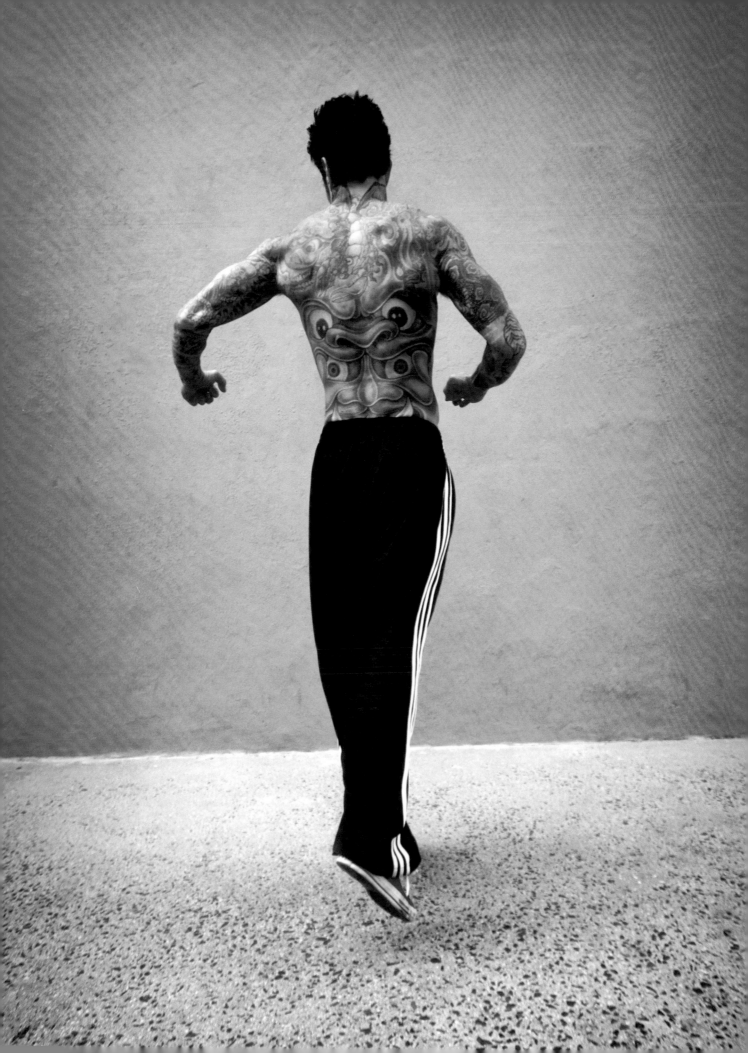

10
MAKING PROGRESS
THE PARC PRINCIPLE

Awesome. You are now proud possessor of six sets of exercise "chains": series of technical progressions which lead you from an easy technique (step 1) all the way to an ice cold, badass Master Step (step 10). If you can work your way up through the steps to the Master Steps, you will become the most explosive, powerful athlete you know. The most explosive, powerful athlete you can probably *imagine*. Trust me—you will meet virtually nobody who can match you if you become master of the Explosive Six!

So the next question is: *how do I move upwards through these chains?* Great question, kid. Have a cigar. Let's talk about it. By the end of this part of the book, you'll be a goddamn Programming Overlord of the Explosive Arts.

PROGRESSION STANDARDS FOR THE EXPLOSIVE SIX?

The first **Convict Conditioning** book was about building muscle and power using bodyweight-only training. In that book, I introduced the concept of *progressions*; the idea that an easy exercise should lead to a harder exercise. How do you know when to move up to the next exercise? Simple—I included a set of *progression standards*. For example, if you are working with *full pushups*, you train hard until you can do two sets of twenty *perfect* reps. When you can do that, you are qualified to move up to the next exercise in the chain—*close pushups*, with the hands touching.

This strategy for slowly building capacity through meeting a series of pre-determined targets works *incredibly* well in strength-building. If you do it right, it's practically foolproof. Of course, I didn't invent this idea. It's a very ancient approach to training, called *double progression*. The "double" refers to the fact that you progress in two ways—first in *reps*, then when you meet your target, in *load* (i.e., harder exercises). This method is very, very ancient. It's definitely in the Bible. Probably.

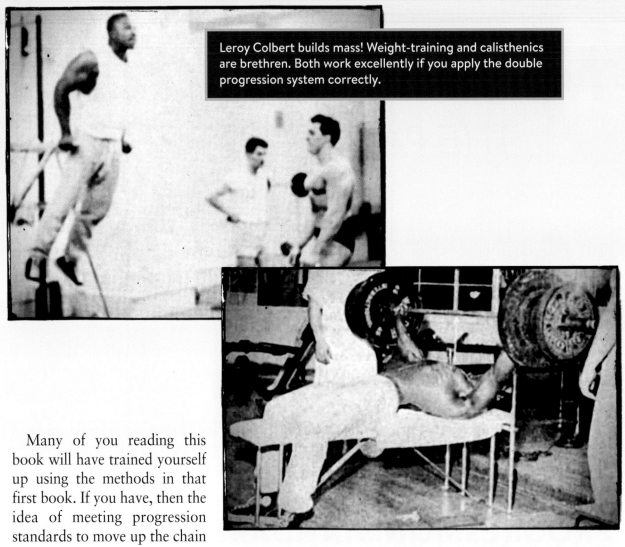

Leroy Colbert builds mass! Weight-training and calisthenics are brethren. Both work excellently if you apply the double progression system correctly.

Many of you reading this book will have trained yourself up using the methods in that first book. If you have, then the idea of meeting progression standards to move up the chain will be like bread-and-butter to you. You will understand it backwards. You will probably also be expecting me to follow the same protocol in this book. You might be expecting me to say something like: *perform two sets of ten in the half kip, before you move up to the kip-up*.

Well, I'm not going to hit you up with that kind of thing. Rep-building works real well for strength and bodybuilding workouts, but when you are rolling with fast, power techniques, it just won't cut it. Why? Three simple reasons:

1. REPS BUILD EXHAUSTION, NOT POWER

When building man-beef, you are looking to *exhaust* the energy in your muscle cells. When you do this, those cells get all nutjob-survivalist, and stock up extra chemicals in case the threat happens again—that's how your muscles pack on mass, over time. Exhausting your muscles is pretty simple—you are constantly looking to add reps in your exercises! More and more. That's just one reason why having rep targets is so damn productive.

But when you are training for power, your goal isn't *exhaustion*—it's super-quick, snappy movements. *Crisp speed* and *exhaustion* are mutually exclusive. So working to build up your reps is a mistake.

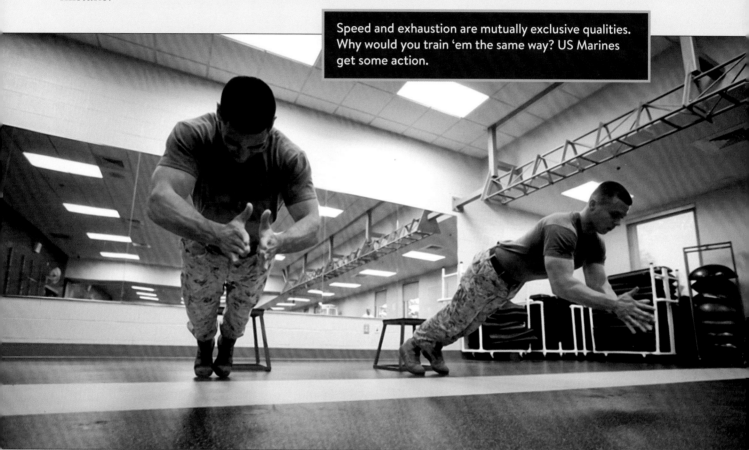

Speed and exhaustion are mutually exclusive qualities. Why would you train 'em the same way? US Marines get some action.

2. ADDING REPS IN EXPLOSIVES CAN INCREASE INJURY RISK

The strength-mass techniques in *Convict Conditioning* are steady, safe movements. Techniques like *pushups* should be performed with a 2-1-2 cadence—i.e., *two* seconds down, a *one* second pause at the bottom, then *two* seconds up. This means that as you do your reps, your muscles fatigue *slowly* and (crucially) *smoothly*, until eventually your form begins to get too uneven, and you stop. Since your muscles are in control of every inch of your movements, there is very little chance of injury when you train this way.

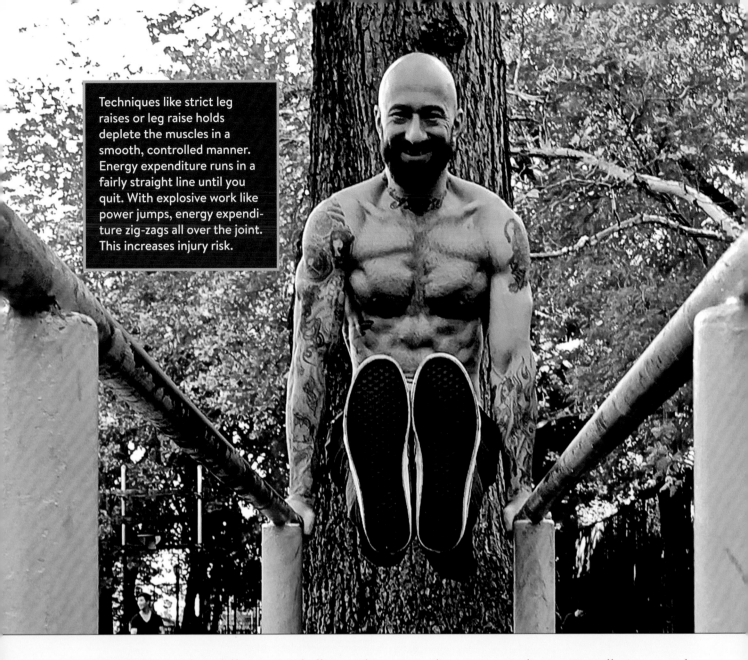

Techniques like strict leg raises or leg raise holds deplete the muscles in a smooth, controlled manner. Energy expenditure runs in a fairly straight line until you quit. With explosive work like power jumps, energy expenditure zig-zags all over the joint. This increases injury risk.

Explosive work is different. It's *ballistic*. This means that your muscles aren't really in control for a large proportion of your movements. Take a back flip as an example—after the first explosive push, momentum and gravity begin to play a huge role. Sure, with effort you can direct yourself to some degree, but the techniques are much faster and more complex than simple strength moves. If something goes wrong, you only have a fraction of a second to readjust. The more reps you perform, the more fatigued you become, and the more your mental concentration is diluted. This makes control of your movements—especially self-correction, if things go wrong—much tougher.

For this reason, you should avoid struggling to build up your reps, to meet rep targets. You should only ever do as many reps as you feel will keep your technique *completely perfect*. Always push for *greater perfection*. Never for *more reps*. That would be counter-productive.

3. ADDING REPS ENCOURAGES THE WRONG KIND OF PSYCHOLOGY

Lastly, the whole idea of *reps* is designed to work with a systematic system where *load increases* need to be mathematically quantified—typically barbell training or calisthenics strength methods. With explosive bodyweight training, we are really not looking to increase the load—we are interested in increasing the efficiency, speed, power and complexity of our movements. We *can* monitor this, but only by gauging the "cleanness" of our movements. Rep targets have jack to do with this; and if you are thinking "reps", you ain't thinking "clean", right? So rid yourself of the old mindset of simply upping reps. It won't work here. We need something new!

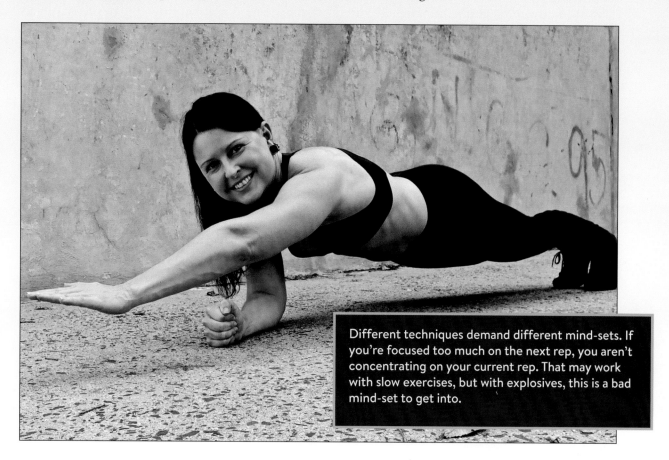

Different techniques demand different mind-sets. If you're focused too much on the next rep, you aren't concentrating on your current rep. That may work with slow exercises, but with explosives, this is a bad mind-set to get into.

Hopefully you hard-asses out there who were born and raised on double progression have maybe read the previous couple pages, and forgiven me for not including rep targets or similar progression standards in this book. But you're pretty smart (that's why you're reading this, dude) so your next question is probably gonna be: *if I'm not trying to hit a certain number of reps, how will I know when to move up from one step to the next in the chain?*

HOW TO KNOW WHEN TO MOVE UP A STEP: A WALK IN THE PARC

If you have been payin' attention to the three reasons to avoid rep goals listed in this chapter, then you probably have a pretty good grasp of what your attitude here should be. You should not be focusing on *how many reps* of an exercise you can pump out—instead, you should be focusing on *how well* you can perform that exercise. Long story short: *when you have mastered basic competence in a technique, you can move up to the next step.* Not before.

Now, I know what you're thinking. Terms like "competence" and "mastered" are pretty subjective terms...they can mean different things to different athletes. You're right. That why I'm going to spell out the four key components of *competence* in explosive training, to zone in more on what I really mean. When I'm explaining these concepts to students, I sometimes use the acronym PARC to help them remember the four concepts. (When *parkour* was invented in France, it was originally spelled "parcours", meaning *course*, or *journey*. Think of the PARC in *parcours*, to help you remember.)

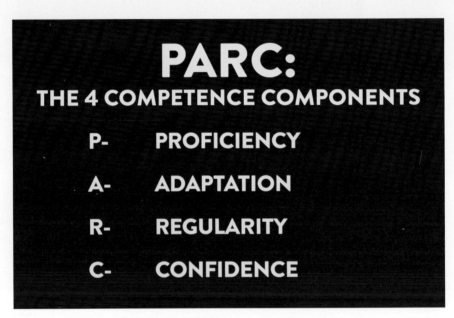

PARC:
THE 4 COMPETENCE COMPONENTS

P- PROFICIENCY

A- ADAPTATION

R- REGULARITY

C- CONFIDENCE

Let's look at these four a bit more in-depth.

PROFICIENCY

Proficiency basically means being able to do something *right*. When you perform the techniques in this book, you perform them as I describe them, or pretty damn close. If you perform a *muscle-up*, you swing and kip, rotate your arms to pull-over, and push yourself up over the bar. You tick all the basic boxes, and you do it cleanly and efficiently. *Proficiency* does not mean *total perfection*. You do not need to be a world-class gymnast as you perform these moves, expecting a perfect "10" score from obsessive, lifelong coaches. Nobody is scoring you, nobody is judging you on some *theoretically* ideal aesthetic form. Your task is to *get the job done*, and build speed and power. If this elbow or that foot is slightly out—nobody cares, so long as you don't hurt yourself. Strive for excellence, but *never* lose your freedom!

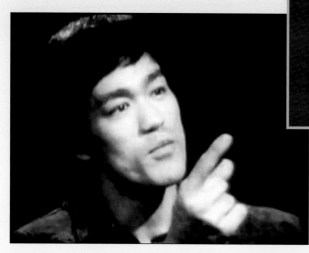

ADAPTATION

This has to do with your *body's* capacity to cope with the skill in question. Many folks can quickly achieve the nervous ability to pick up a particular technique, but their body lags behind. *The spirit is willing—and able—but the flesh is weak.* Sure, a handful of unconditioned trainees will be able to (barely) pull off a *front handspring*, first time of asking. But when they do it, they feel like their shoulders are being yanked out of their sockets; they pull a muscle in their abs; hurt their wrist; and they are in agony the next day. They certainly have done nothing good for their joints, and there's no way they should continue at this kinda pace. If your body really yells at ya or gets dinged up by working with a certain step, then you're *not ready* to move to the next step—even if, technique-wise, you can manage that step. In fact, you're probably best going back a few steps, and working with moves that don't hurt you. And don't skimp on those warm-ups, either (see page 295).

REGULARITY

This is a big one. Managing to pull off a *back-drop flip* (step 8) correctly *one time* does *not* qualify you to zoom forward and attempt *running front flip* (step 9)! This is especially true if you are working with rotating motions, and you are only able to perform the technique correctly once out of every ten attempts! Don't get me wrong; even Olympic gymnasts trip or fumble when performing their movements—sometimes even basic techniques. We all screw up from time-to-time, and this is particularly true with the fast, complex demands of explosive calisthenics. That's just part of being human. But—*as a rule of thumb*—if you can't pull off a technique nine times out of every ten attempts (with a rest in-between), you haven't mastered it enough to be able to move to harder exercises.

CONFIDENCE

This is the mental sense of self-assurance which can only really come from having successfully and safely performed a technique many times. You step up to perform the movement, and you *know* that you can get it—and not just *barely*, but well, and with *room to spare*. If you are anxious before every repetition of a move, you have not achieved competence in that move. You should stay on that step. But hey—that's not a bad thing, necessarily. That means you have more to learn from this exercise. Great! Never forget that moving up a step is *not* what *builds* speed, skill and power—it only *demonstrates* speed, skill and power. It's the careful, consistent effort put into the moves *you can already do* that builds these things.

APPLYING PARC

It will be real helpful for you to absorb the philosophy of PARC early on in your training, so you can coach yourself and gauge how and when to move forward. Watching others train is a great way to do this, but nothing beats simple *self-awareness*. Here are some examples of the application of PARC:

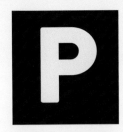

PROFICIENCY

Proficiency is easy to determine—if you understand the movement and are honest with yourself. In a proper *kip-up* (page 126), the athlete should be rock solid at the end of the movement. If you fall over backwards, you are not *Proficient*. Keep training.

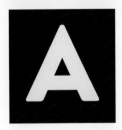

ADAPTATION

If you manage to achieve a *front handspring* (page 156) every few days, but wind up wracked with pain and strained abs each time you try it, then your body has not *adapted* enough. Consider moving back a step or two, or performing supplementary exercises to improve your conditioning.

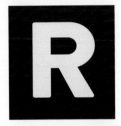

REGULARITY

If you are working on *suicide jumps* (page 62), and—following a warm-up—you can only properly get over the bar every other time you attempt the move, you lack *regularity*. Keep training.

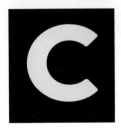

CONFIDENCE

If you psych yourself up for a *back handspring* (page 194) but you're terrified you are going to break your neck, something has gone badly wrong and you lack *confidence*. Never move ahead a step in these circumstances, and consider moving back a step.

Four easy-to-apply concepts. I can't make it any simpler than this, dude. If you follow them, your training will be easier, you will be safer, and you'll progress faster in the long run. Ignore them, and injury and burn-out is on the horizon. I've shown these progressions to many, many guys who have tried to use short-cuts and bypass PARC. The smart ones all come back to it eventually.

Why not be smart from the get-go?

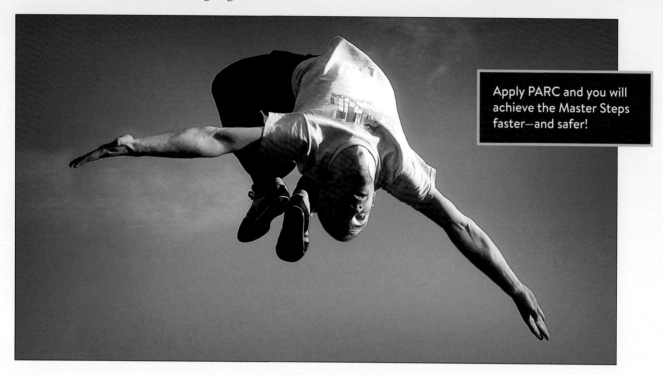

Apply PARC and you will achieve the Master Steps faster—and safer!

LIGHTS OUT!

One of the toughest things about explosive training is that there is no objective, cut-and-dried method for knowing when it's safe and sensible to move up a step. But that's also one of the things that makes it so damn cool. In applying PARC, you are relying on your *discrimination* and *common-sense*—combined with some measure of healthy risk-taking. These qualities are all components of what I've called *body wisdom*—the *sine qua non* of a true calisthenics master.

Read this chapter again, and come to really understand the PARC concepts. Appreciate them so deeply that you could write a page about them without notes, or explain the four ideas fully to a training buddy. Don't just randomly try out the techniques in this book. If you do, you're likely to get injured, and I don't want that. Begin at the beginning, establish a baseline of ability, and find a level of explosive techniques you can safely work with and benefit from over time. Use a systematic program. And as you begin to grow in power and ability, apply the PARC rule to decide whether to move to the next step.

I trust ya. You got this, kid.

11

POWER AND SKILL
TWIN TRAINING METHODOLOGIES

I advise *two* different training approaches for the chains in this book:

- *Power training, and;*
- *Skill training.*

Which one you use depends on which chain you are working on.

WHY TWO DIFFERENT METHODS?

A huge amount of articles and books have been written about different training approaches, so I'll keep this short and sweet. Broadly speaking, there are *two* different types of exercise in this book; exercises that mostly build *basic power* (strength x speed) and exercises which also require sophisticated *movement skills*. (There is overlap, but these broad categories are valid.)

The *vertical leap* is an example of a *basic power move*—it doesn't take a huge amount of *skill* to perform. You just drill it over and over again to build power, strengthen the joints, and generally improve your explosive performance. The *back flip* is an example of a *skill-based movement*. Sure, it still requires a lot of power, but it also requires that your nervous system has actually *learned* the movement. It's not just about "physical" conditioning—there are definitely a lot of athletes who have the physical equipment (power, speed, joint strength) to pull off a back flip, but they can't actually do it—they don't have the *skill*.

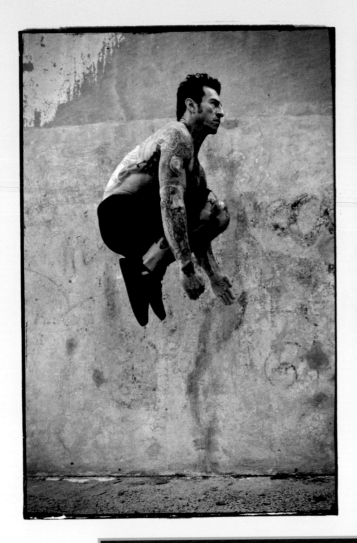
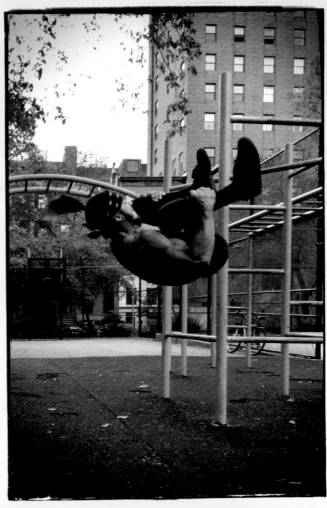

Jumps are fairly simple and can be used to build *power*. More sophisticated techniques like flips also build agility and can be seen as *skill* movements. You should try and train each category differently.

	POWER MOVES	**SKILL MOVES**
MOVEMENT TYPE	• Simple (typically up-and-down)	• Complex (typically involve rotation, partial rotation, or multiple movement angles)
ATHLETIC QUALITIES	• Speed-strength • Linear performance • Joint integrity	• Coordination • Equilibrium • Timing
AREA TRAINED	• Muscles • Muscle-nerve connection • Joints	• Nervous system • Brain • Mind

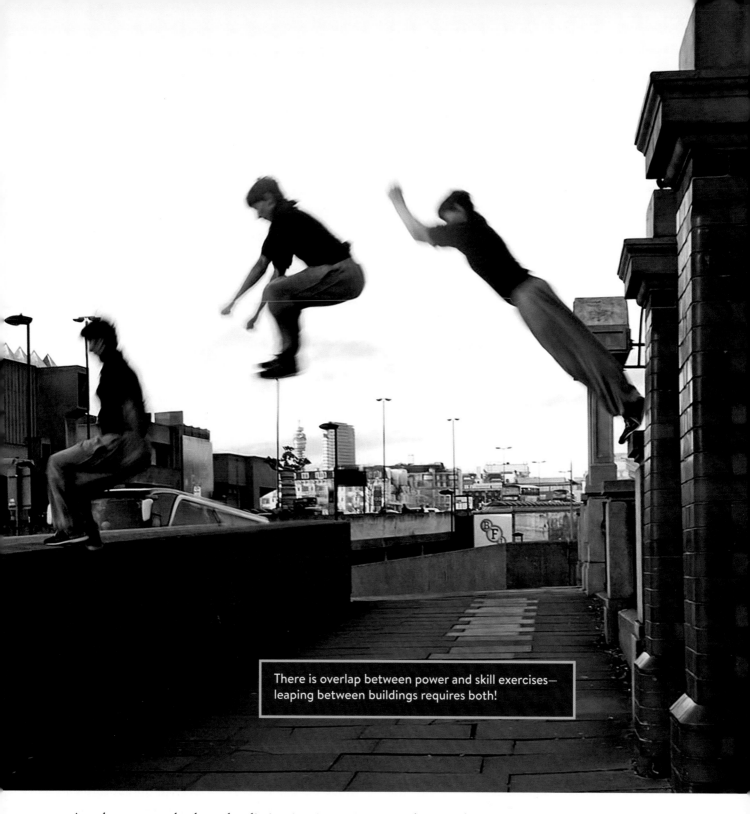

There is overlap between power and skill exercises—leaping between buildings requires both!

Another way to look at the distinction is to use an analogy with *computing*. Basic power drills involve work on the muscles, soft tissues, nerves and even bones. They build better *hardware*. Skill movements are also conditioning the nervous system, brain and mind. They upgrade the *software*. For the best system you can get, you need both, right? You begin by building a great *hardware* unit—adding to it and improving over time—and you can then start uploading superior software.

WHICH IS WHICH?

The six major movement types in this manual are not interchangeable. You should view *jumps* and *power pushups* as your basic power exercises. *Kip-ups*, and *front* and *back flips* should be viewed as skill exercises. *Muscle-ups* are a more balanced blend of skill and power, but I would tend to train them as a skill exercise if you want maximum explosiveness. (The dip progressions included as an ancillary exercise to muscle-ups are neither strictly power nor skill. Train them as you would any regular *strength* movement—low to moderate reps with low sets).

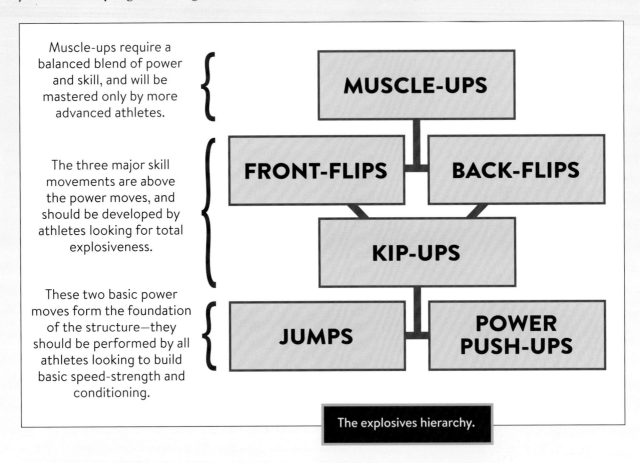

Muscle-ups require a balanced blend of power and skill, and will be mastered only by more advanced athletes.

The three major skill movements are above the power moves, and should be developed by athletes looking for total explosiveness.

These two basic power moves form the foundation of the structure—they should be performed by all athletes looking to build basic speed-strength and conditioning.

MUSCLE-UPS

FRONT-FLIPS   **BACK-FLIPS**

KIP-UPS

JUMPS   **POWER PUSH-UPS**

The explosives hierarchy.

POWER AND SKILL METHODS: A SUMMARY

Over the next couple chapters I'll spell out the practical differences between training for *power*, and *skill work*. For now, I'll just outline the fundamental ideas. The basic principle is that when predominantly training the *muscles* and the *joints* (power training), you are working with aspects of your anatomy which take *time* to adapt to that stimulus—if you train for power, you'll find that after a day or more of rest, you can come back stronger. When you are working for skill—as long as your body is conditioned to it—you are really training the *brain* and *nervous system*. Up to a point, these areas adapt almost instantly.

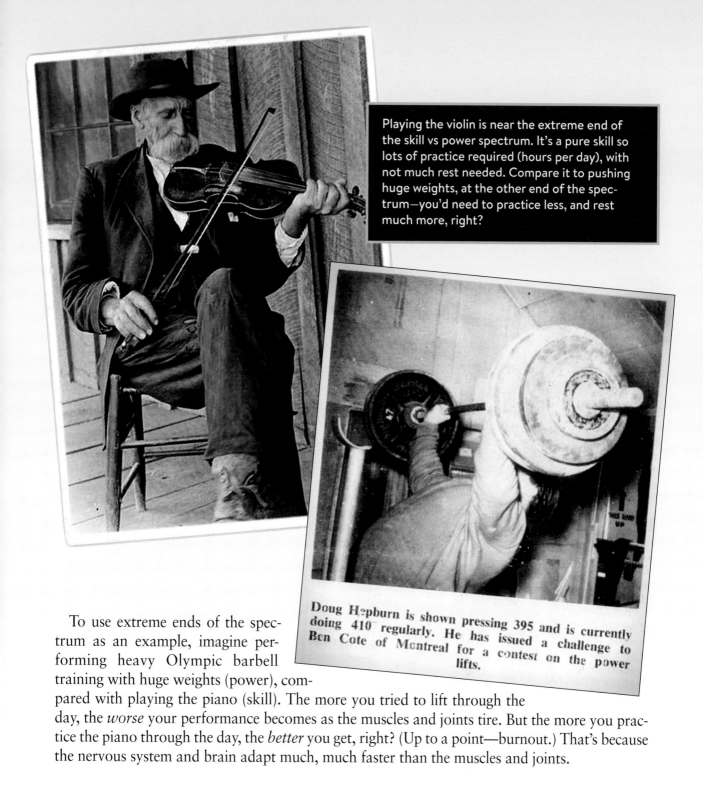

Playing the violin is near the extreme end of the skill vs power spectrum. It's a pure skill so lots of practice required (hours per day), with not much rest needed. Compare it to pushing huge weights, at the other end of the spectrum—you'd need to practice less, and rest much more, right?

Doug Hepburn is shown pressing 395 and is currently doing 410 regularly. He has issued a challenge to Ben Cote of Montreal for a contest on the power lifts.

To use extreme ends of the spectrum as an example, imagine performing heavy Olympic barbell training with huge weights (power), compared with playing the piano (skill). The more you tried to lift through the day, the *worse* your performance becomes as the muscles and joints tire. But the more you practice the piano through the day, the *better* you get, right? (Up to a point—burnout.) That's because the nervous system and brain adapt much, much faster than the muscles and joints.

Ultimately, this means that you should make your power training hard and brief, then rest until your next session, a day or two later. Do what you need to do, then stop. Skill training is different. Do as much as you can! The more you practice your back flip, for example, the better it gets. So get in as many reps as possible. Train it as often as you can—and provided you don't push your muscles and joints too hard during your training, you can actually perform skill work more often than you might think.

By now you will have firmly grasped the fact that, despite some overlap, *power*-based exercises and *skill*-based techniques are essentially different animals. They also need to be approached in diverse ways. I've done my best to summarize the two methods in the table below:

	POWER MOVES: PROGRAMMING	SKILL MOVES: PROGRAMMING
TRAINING PSYCHOLOGY:	Try to get more powerful with every repetition.	Try to make each rep more technically perfect.
REPS PER SET:	For maximum power, use 1-3 reps per set.	For maximum skill, only one rep per set.
SETS PER SESSION:	Varies, but under 20 sets is probably a good upper limit.	Perform as many sets as possible without "burnout".
FREQUENCY:	Perform a session of power moves once every few days.	You can perform a session of skill moves every day, or even several times per day.

LIGHTS OUT!

Understanding the ins-and-outs of different training methodologies can be complex—but the take-home message of this chapter is real simple. The backbone of your power training should be *jumps* and *power-based pushups*. They are simple to perform, condition the body, and build oodles of strength-speed in the upper-and-lower body. On top of these basics, you need to add skill-based movements, which allow you to express your power in a more sophisticated (typically more *agile*) manner. You need to train both categories (power *and* skill) of technique differently.

How do you do this? The next chapter will teach you my method for building *power*. The chapter after that, chapter thirteen, will teach you the best way to train to develop the *skill* movements.

12

POWER BUILDING
THE RULE OF THREE AND THE RULE OF SIX

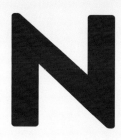ot all of the Explosive Six were created equal. The skill-agility techniques—e.g., *kip-ups* and *flips*—may look incredibly sexy, but they can only be approached by an athlete who has the raw *power* to attempt them. What do I mean by raw power? Well:

- the leg spring to launch the body high enough;
- the midsection snap to tuck the legs up; and
- the shoulder and arm power to increase momentum (and forcefully push the body off the floor in some major steps).

You don't build this kind of power by playing around with exotic flips and kips. You build it *before* you attempt the skill-agility work, by hard, consistent training on *jumps* and *power pushups*.

LINEAR IMPROVEMENT, NOT RACING THOUGH STEPS!

Even after reading these words, too many athletes will approach the jump/power pushup chains in the wrong way. What do I mean by this? Take jumps as an example. I mean they'll try the easy jumps, then try the harder ones, all the way up to the Master Step, then figure that they've "beaten" the chain.

This is not how it works.

If you want to be an explosive athlete, you need to be working with the jump chain (or similar techniques) for your entire career. Do you imagine you have "beaten" the *vertical leap* (step 3) just because you can *perform* it? No way! Keep getting *higher*! Basketball superstars work with these exercises day-in, day-out with for *years*, trying get higher and higher, knowing they will continually build more power as they do so. The same goes for the power pushups. *Linear improvement* on these basics is the name of the game. Sure, move up through the steps, but don't just blindly try and race to the Master Steps—that's fairly easy. Your goal is to use these exercises as *tools* to continue building power and joint integrity throughout your entire career.

If the skill-agility exercises (the flips and kip-ups especially) are your racing *vehicles*, think of the basic power moves (jumps and power pushups) as your *fuel tank*. The more consistently you train with 'em, the bigger and more turbocharged your vehicle. But no matter how much you try and work on the skill stuff without putting in the groundwork on power moves, your progress will suck. You'll be like a speedster running on empty.

INJURY BULLETPROOFING

Consistent work on the jumps and power pushups won't just increase muscle *power*—it'll also improve the capacity of your muscles, soft tissues and even your bones to *handle* these forces. Athletes who haphazardly throw acrobatics into their training continually suffer twisted knees, bad hips, sprained ankles and foot pain. You can avoid almost all this if you commit a modest period of time practicing the jump chain, to condition these areas.

Likewise, I've heard of several cases where guys (it's always guys) are playing about with handsprings, who break an arm, typically the *radius* in the forearm. This happens simply because the bones and soft tissues (the *shock absorbers*) just aren't conditioned to high-power movements. The cure is simple: careful, consistent improvement in the power pushup series. I don't want any of you hurting yourselves, okay? Prepare your bodies adequately before throwing yourselves around!

POWER PROGRAMMING BASICS

So enough with the lecturing, already. How should you program the basic power moves? I'll say up front that I'm not a big fan of the complex charts and graphs you find in many plyo manuals. If you want to peruse those and apply them to the techniques in this book, go ahead. For me, I'm a much bigger fan of *simple engineering*—and I always teach my students *two* basic rules when it comes to programming power basics. Use these two elementary rules in your training, and I promise you your power will take off like a goddamn ramjet. These two rules are called the *rule of three*, and the *rule of six*.

THE "RULE OF THREE"

When it comes to rep-ranges, my advice regarding the power exercises in this book couldn't be simpler. I call it "the rule of three".

THE RULE OF THREE
If you are working for speed-power, never go over 3 reps per exercise.

There you are. It's that simple. If you wish to progress through the Explosive Six power chains, when training on the various steps, you can use 1-rep sets. You can use 2-rep sets. You can use 3-rep sets. Never use more reps than that.

Why such low reps for speed? Remember that your body becomes better only by doing what you tell it to do. Try this thought-experiment: if you warm up well and perform ten non-stop *squat jumps*, is your body fastest on the first jump, or the last jump? Well, if you did your warm-up right, it's fastest on the *first* or *second* jump. By the tenth rep, fatigue toxins have built up in your muscles, energy has been depleted, and that jump is the *slowest* jump. The same is true for all explosive power movements. *Don't waste your time teaching your body how to do slower movements.* Quit after the first few reps, and you will teach your body to move with pure power!

Safety is another consideration. When you are exploring high-velocity moves—like jumps and backflips—your goal should be to perform them with *proficiency* (the P of PARC—page 264). Your goal should *not* be high reps. Using high reps on explosive exercises like these increases the likelihood of screwing up and making a mistake—which could lead to injury. You are more likely to make an error on rep 10—when you are getting tired and losing focus—than on reps 1-3.

So stick to reps 1-3!

ATHLETE QUESTION #1:
Are 3 measly reps enough to force my body to adapt?

Yes. Think of it this way—some of the elite powerlifters and weightlifters become the strongest human beings on the planet on a diet of very low-rep sets. If they can use low reps to make their physiological systems change to build that level of strength, why shouldn't it work for speed-strength? For sure, if you want to build muscle or endurance, you need more reps to force your body to adapt in the way you want. But for speed and power, three is enough.

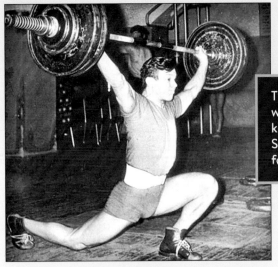

The speed-strength used by Olympic weightlifters is not a million miles away from the kind of speed-strength needed in the Explosive Six. Olympic weightlifters often use low-rep sets for maximum power, just as you should.

ATHLETE QUESTION #2:
But what if I want to build endurance? What if I want to look cool, busting out a dozen clap pushups?

And the answer to that is; *well, if that's what you want, you're not working for speed-power, are you?* You're working for *endurance*, in which case, of course you should jack up your reps. But if you want speed, explosiveness, and quickness, stick to low reps—3 or less. If you want to move up the progressions as quickly as possible this requires building speed-strength, so stick with the rule of three.

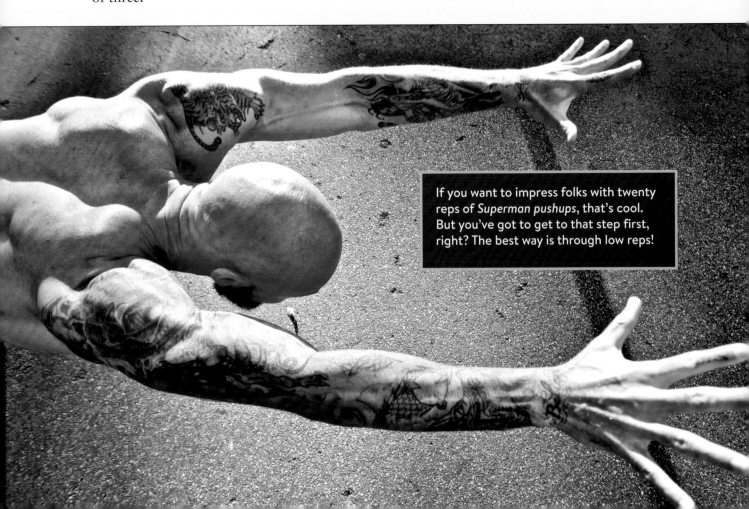

If you want to impress folks with twenty reps of *Superman pushups*, that's cool. But you've got to get to that step first, right? The best way is through low reps!

THE "RULE OF SIX"

While the *Rule of Three* determines your *rep* range for your sets; the *Rule of Six* determines the *total number* of reps you perform for each exercise. To apply it, you just remember to use a total rep number which is a *multiple of six*.

This is a great way to approach your total number of reps per movement:

THE RULE OF SIX

- Beginners should be looking at 6 working reps per exercise

- Intermediates should be looking at 12 working reps per exercise

- Advanced athletes should aim at 18 working reps per exercise

So how does this work? Simple. Let's say you are working with *squat jumps*. If you are a beginner, you'll be looking at doing six working reps of jumps in your workout. (A *working rep* means any reps you do seriously, *after* your warm up. For a warm-up protocol, check out page 295.)

Now, the Rule of Three told you that you should use 1-rep, 2-rep, or 3-rep sets. So some simple math tells us that we have at least 3 basic options for our training session. You could go:

6x1

Six sets of one rep would give you your six-rep total. This approach—performing "singles" as it is often known—is a great way to train explosives. It allows you to put maximum effort and concentration into each repetition. On the down side, you don't get to exploit that rebound effect (see: *Myotatic Rebound*, page 41) which is so effective on some exercises. Also, a session of singles obviously takes longer than doing multiple-rep sets.

Here's another option:

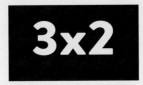

Three sets of two reps. Makes six again, right? (I think.) A classic session of "doubles" which will exploit some rebound, while allowing you plenty of focus and discipline. Tasty way to go.

Then there's:

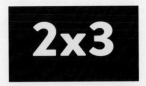

Two sets of three. Three rep sets ("triples") are the bread-and-butter of many explosives athletes and coaches. Triples allow you to really get into a set, without losing focus too much. If you are doing lots of reps or multiple exercises, you always finish and get to the bar quicker, which is always a plus, right?

Then again, there are other ways you could go to get those six reps:

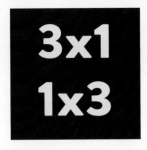

Three sets of singles, followed by a triple. Or:

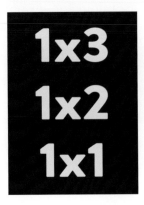

A triple, followed by a double, followed by a single. This is one of many potential "hybrid" options.

So you can see from these examples, that there are plenty of roads to Mecca, my friend. There are lots of different options you can explore to meet your rep goals, as long as you follow the *Rule of Three* (for the reps in a set) and the *Rule of Six* (for total reps of an exercise).

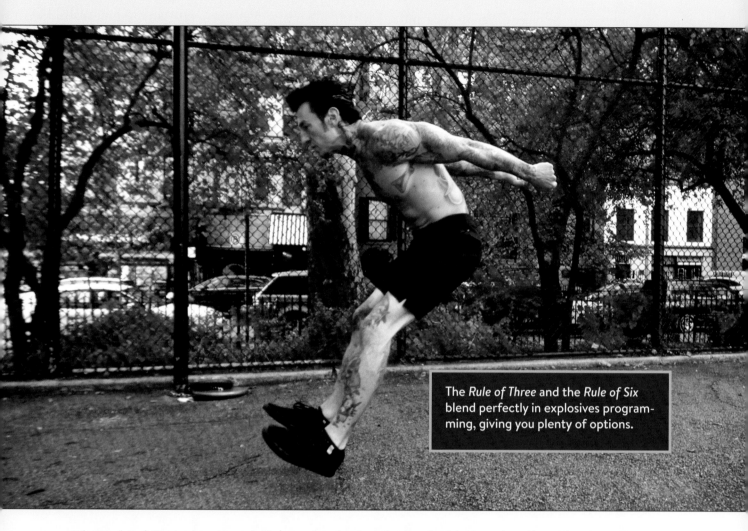

The *Rule of Three* and the *Rule of Six* blend perfectly in explosives programming, giving you plenty of options.

The Rule of Six is time-tested. I've used it for hundreds of athletes, who all got faster and more explosive than they could have believed in their wildest dreams. Why does it work? Partly because it mathematically meshes so easily with the Rule of Three. Partly because it forces athletes to organize their explosives sessions *systematically,* where otherwise there might be chaos. It really does work—use it and you'll see, stud.

ATHLETE QUESTION #1:
Which of these rep-schemes is best?

They are all just as good! As long as you are using the Rule of Three and the Rule of Six, you are doing it right!

ATHLETE QUESTION #2:
Which approach should I be using? Singles, doubles, or triples?

It's up to you. Explore different reps and see which you prefer. They generally all work as well, but for psychological reasons, some athletes prefer singles, some doubles or triples. Have fun with it, and don't forget—you don't need to use the same rep-ranges your whole life. Hell, you can mix them up from session-to-session. Play with triples, singles, hybrids. Mix 'em up! As long as you follow the Rule of Three and the Rule of Six, it doesn't matter, kid. You're winning!

ATHLETE QUESTION #3:
Is 6 reps per exercise enough for beginners?

If there's a question I hear all the time, it's this—is it *enough*? Determined athletes always have this drive to do more, more, more! I admire that—hell, I've been there and done it myself. What you need to remember with explosive training in particular is that *more is not necessarily better*. Explosives are not meant to be cardio or muscle-building—they're designed to stimulate the nervous system, not exhaust you. A *certain amount* of plyometric training will increase your strength, ramp up your speed, and reduce your likelihood for injury. But explosives take their toll on the joints, soft tissues and even the bones—and an excessive amount of it will actually increase your likelihood for injury. Don't forget that most of you will be performing muscular or strength training *as well as this stuff*. Stick to *low-to-moderate* amounts of work *performed well*. You will find that you make progress. Just don't overthink, and talk yourself into failing before you start.

ATHLETE QUESTION #4:
How do I know if I'm a Beginner, Intermediate, or Advanced?

As a rule of thumb:

You are a *beginner* if:
* You are new to explosive training;
* You are experienced, but coming back from a layoff or injury;
* You find the exercise you are working on extremely difficult to perform, even once (sometimes athletes who are tackling very difficult steps should consider themselves beginners)

You are *advanced* if:
* You can easily handle at least step 7 of the chain you are working on:

You are *intermediate* if:
* You do not fit the categories of *beginner* or *advanced*.

As with all generalizations, there will be exceptions to this. It doesn't render the basic ideas invalid, though. Sometimes we have to think "fuzzy".

ATHLETE QUESTION #5:
How long should I rest between sets?

Rest as long as it takes you to get your breath back and get set up for the next set. This typically takes 10-30 seconds. (Thirty seconds, while waiting for the next set, is actually a lot longer than it seems when you just read it!) It should not take more than a minute—remember, you are not fatiguing yourself during your explosives work (the way you would during a muscle-building set). If you need more than a minute to really get mentally prepared, that is acceptable—as long as you don't go over about three minutes, in which case you'll begin to lose the neurological benefits of your previous set. When prepping for the next set, *don't* just slump down on a chair, and never lie down. These things tell your nervous system to begin to change down through the gears. You don't need to run around between sets, but stay on your goddamn feet, okay?

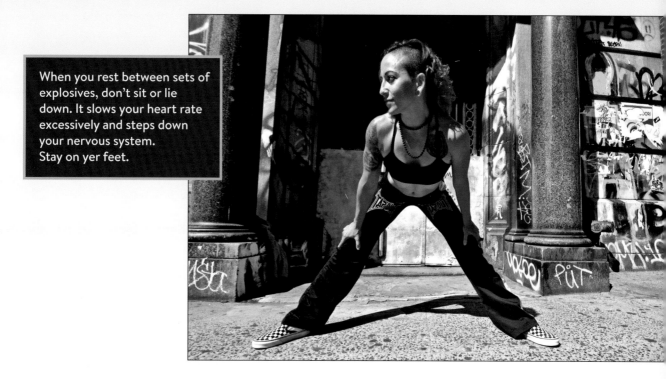

When you rest between sets of explosives, don't sit or lie down. It slows your heart rate excessively and steps down your nervous system. Stay on yer feet.

ATHLETE QUESTION #6:
Which explosive exercises should I perform?

Typically, you should spend most of your power training working with the jumps/power pushups you have reached in the chain. (To find out how to progress properly though the chain, learn the PARC rule in *chapter ten*). That said, *all* of the power movements are of value, and all can be used to generate linear improvement: you can jump higher, clap more times, etc. So you have the choice to use multiple exercises within your set/rep range if you wish.

ATHLETE QUESTION #7:
Are the Rule of Three and the Rule of Six "set in stone", or can I use different protocols?

Yeah, sure you can use other stuff! If any trainer or "guru" tells you that you can only follow his (or her) protocol, run to the hills. If you want to be really elite at bodyweight training—or any training—the truth is you will have to learn to *train yourself*. Unless you are a pro athlete, nobody is gonna be there, babying you from workout-to-workout. You're going to have to master the art of *self-coaching*. Part of this is working faithfully with the protocols of others—to see if and how they work—but also eventually tinkering with those fixed protocols, exploring, experimenting, and coming up with your own stuff.

I advise my students to apply the Laws of Three and Six because they are simple, foolproof, and proven to give phenomenal results. They are the very best I have to give to you. It wouldn't feel right if I gave you anything less. Does that mean that nothing else works, you can't add reps, or that you shouldn't experiment? *Nah!*

LIGHTS OUT!

I've done my best to keep Part III of this book—the "how to" stuff—real simple. (Like me!) But we're a lot of pages in so far, and if you haven't picked up all the finer details yet—*don't panic*. This stuff isn't going anywhere. (Unless you picked this up on the bus while the guy next to you is asleep, in which case, read quicker.)

The most important concepts to take home so far are:

- The Explosive Six chains are not all equal: some are for building basic *power* (the *jumps* and *power pushups*), some are better classed as *skill* movements (the *kip-ups, flips,* and to a lesser degree, the *muscle-ups*)

- The basic power movements and the skill movements should be approached differently, using different programming tactics

- Power movements are essential and should form the backbone of your training—they make the skill movements possible

- Program power movements using the *Rule of Three* and the *Rule of Six*

If you're paying attention—and I know you are—then your next question will be: *how do I program/train for the <u>skill</u> movements*?

That's up next, beautiful.

13

SKILL DEVELOPMENT

TIME SURFING AND CONSOLIDATION TRAINING

The concept of *skill* training introduced in chapter 11—work on complex movements which require a lot of coordination and dexterity, like flips and kip-ups—can be summed up in four points:

CHOOSE THE RIGHT EXERCISE

Skill training works best for exercises where the athlete has the *power level* to perform the movement, but has yet to master the correct *coordination*. When performing an exercise ask yourself: *can I perform this exercise easily and with perfect form*? If the answer is *yes*, you don't need to apply skill training. You can use conventional set x rep schemes, or move up a step to a more challenging exercise.

AIM FOR PERFECTION

The goal of every single rep of skill training is to perform the technique more *perfectly*. The athlete must not be interested in *subjective* goals, like training "hard" or pushing themselves. Nor should they be wrapped up in *objective* goals like going higher or faster: leave that for the power work. Obviously—since form tends to degrade as the athlete tires—this means that for skill work, reps must be low, or single reps. As soon as you get too tired to really perform a skill drill to the best of your ability—when your form begins to collapse—it's time to call it a day. Don't think of skill training as "working out", but "practice". Get Zen.

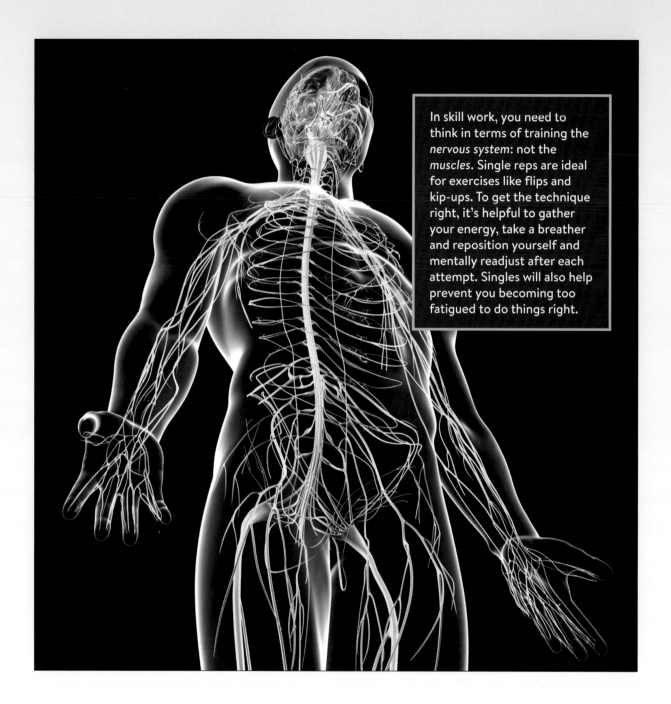

In skill work, you need to think in terms of training the *nervous system*: not the *muscles*. Single reps are ideal for exercises like flips and kip-ups. To get the technique right, it's helpful to gather your energy, take a breather and reposition yourself and mentally readjust after each attempt. Singles will also help prevent you becoming too fatigued to do things right.

AIM FOR HIGH VOLUME

Skill training will increase *power*, but it primarily improves neural *coordination*. The nervous system learns all skills (including acrobatic skills) by *repetition*. This is sometimes known as *Hebb's Law*: in short, the more often you repeat something, the quicker you'll learn it (see also page 314). It follows that (if we are using singles or low reps), to get high volume we need to use a lot of sets). The upshot of this—practice as *often* as you can.

TRAIN "FRESH"

This is related to the previous two concepts. If you want your reps to be as *perfect* as possible, and if you wish to work with a technique *frequently*—often several times a day—you can't exhaust yourself during skill training. This means that you should rest in between repetitions to the degree that your fatigue doesn't build up and tire you to the point where you become stale or your muscles/joints get sore. How long do you wait between reps? Until you feel rested. This can be as little as ten seconds for easier work, or a minute or more for trickier stuff. Of course, you can rest even longer—hours, if you want (provided you don't get warmed-down during the work—see page 295). To really stay fresh, it's also a good idea to have a day or two off from skill work every so often, to let the body recover from any residual fatigue.

There, in a nutshell, you have the core of skill training:

- Always shoot for **perfect** reps
- Only use singles or **very low reps**
- Use a **high amount of sets**
- **Train fresh**—take enough/lots of rest between those sets.

That's the Cliff's Notes on the theory. But how do you apply these four concepts to day-to-day training? Basically there are two methods: *time surfing* and *consolidation training*.

TIME SURFING

In chapter 11, I (hopefully) emphasized to ya that basing training around reps and sets is not as useful for skill work as it is for, say, power work or bodybuilding. This is because *how many reps you can do* is not as important as *getting better at doing those reps*.

So—if you're not scheduling 3 x 10 reps for an exercise, how do you plan your training?

The most basic, efficient way is *time surfing*. This just involves setting by a period of time in your workout—say, five minutes—to practice a technique. Instead of counting sets and reps, you just look at a clock (or set your watch, phone, or whatever), practice, and stop five minutes later. Understand—you do not perform *continuous reps* for five minutes. That would comprise one huge, five minute set! Instead, you perform a rep, take a breather until you feel ready to go again, and perform another rep, and so on.

As an example, let's suppose an athlete is starting to work with the front *flip chain*. After a good warm up (page 296), they start at the beginning, with step 1, *shoulder rolls* (page 146). They take a note of the time, and perform their first repetition. They shake loose, and think about how it felt. After the dizziness goes away, they try for another rep. Not sure they got it right, they try again. Breathing is getting faster now—they take a few deep breaths until they are back to normal. Then they do another rep. This goes on until five minutes is up. That's all time surfing is.

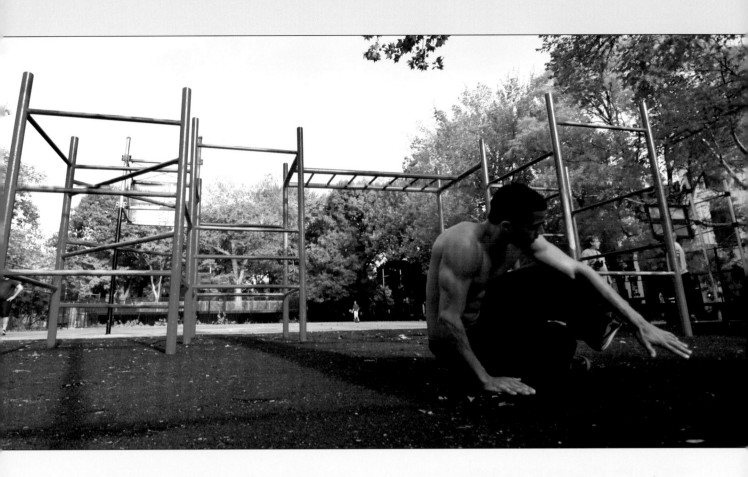

Although it *can* be used with power work, time surfing is a better way to train for a skill. It permits you to be thoughtful, subjective, and explore what you're doing, without recording numbers or worrying about beating your last performance. It allows an athlete to get lots of reps in, avoids fatigue, and dumps the need to do any counting. Like I say, *five minutes* is good for a beginner, but you can stretch the amount of time if you like. Don't get in the habit of watching the clock and trying to squeeze more reps in, though. If you want more reps, add a minute, or however long you want. Just remember that a minute—during training—may actually *feel* a lot longer than it sounds while reading this book. Let's say an athlete is well conditioned, and performs his or her reps with ten second breaks in-between. If you kept up your pace, that's about five reps per minute—fifty reps in a ten minute period. Not bad.

Time surfing works well when:

- You could perform several reps of an exercise, if you wanted
- You are progressing quickly
- You are performing multiple exercises and need to fit them into your program

If you "milk" your training—by not rushing ahead too quickly, and continuing to benefit from exercises you can control *fairly* well—time surfing can give great results, and for long periods of time. But there are negatives to this kind of training (aren't there always?) For one, this method places limits on your practice time: it means you are only allowing yourself a small window of time during your day for practice; with 24 hours in each day, using up just 5-10 minutes might be seen as a bit of a waste by some. Secondly, time surfing only really shines if you can already perform the movements you are working with, fairly consistently. If you are exploring very difficult techniques which you cannot quite "get"—but are on the verge of achieving—then *consolidation training* will probably work better for you.

CONSOLIDATION TRAINING

I described the nature of CT in *Convict Conditioning*:

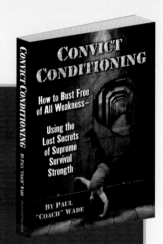

> *If you are really having a problem getting just a handful of reps on a particular exercise, try consolidation training...When you have been working a movement series for a prolonged period, sometimes it can be tough to move from one step to the next...this is not uncommon as you become increasingly advanced. Consolidation training is an excellent way of coping with this situation. Instead of working the new exercise once or twice a week and struggling to improve your reps every time, try working the new exercise every day...Use good form, but don't strain. The name of the game is to spread your effort by performing lots of reps over a period of several days, not to push your muscles hard in any single attempt. If you get excessively sore, back off for a couple of days. Follow this unique protocol for a week or two. As the days pass, the once nearly-impossible technique will gradually seem easier. When you go back to your regular training, you will find that multiple reps are much, much more attainable.*
>
> — **Convict Conditioning**, Chapter 11

Use CT when:

- You are moving up to a particular step/technique you are struggling with
- You can barely even perform a technique once
- Progression is more difficult

Consolidation work is in fact the natural way to train. A lot of people—conditioned by years of weight-training into thinking that workouts *must* consist of discrete sessions of *reps x sets*—think this approach is weird and esoteric. But there's nothing revolutionary or radical about consolidation training. It is, in fact, the most natural way for humans to train. It is the default, intuitive method—but only if we haven't been brainwashed by years of sets and reps. If you look at a kid

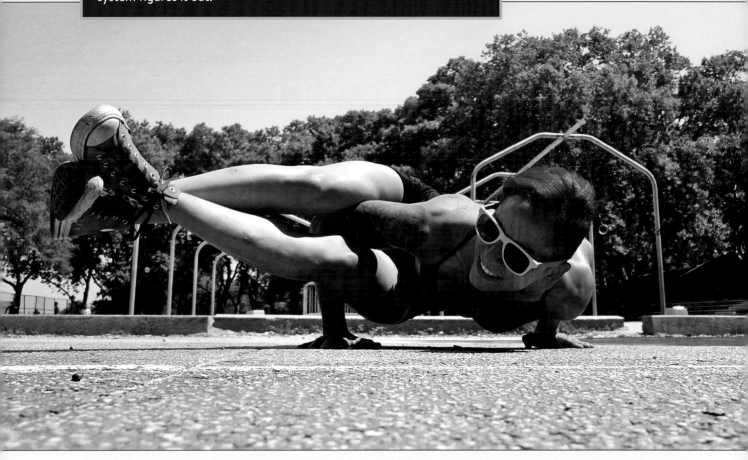

trying to master something difficult—maybe a breakdancing trick, a cheerleading stunt or a parkour technique—they won't do it a bunch of times in a row, then come back a few days later. They will go into the yard, try it a few times before school, and fail. Then they'll maybe try it a few times during recess. Then they'll give it a shot a few times in their room at night. Eventually—if they keep this up, maybe taking the odd day off to let their mind and body rest up—they'll get the hang of that move. This all builds up to lots of reps, and, ultimately, that's the only way us humans learn anything. It's also similar to the way young animals learn during "play".

There are drawbacks to CT, however. Since it's unstructured, it requires good instincts (*body wisdom*) to pull off, without under- or over-doing it. Choosing to train several times a day, while not really time-consuming, can be a pain in the ass if you have a busy daily schedule (like work, school, domestic stuff, and so on). Lastly, CT works best when you are focusing on one, maybe two movements. The more you add in, the more any adaptation gets diluted, and the more likely your nervous system is to suffer from mental logjam. So using it exclusively for all chains of the Explosive Six would either be very difficult or totally counterproductive.

LIGHTS OUT!

As I pointed out in chapter 11, most of the chains in this book (namely the kip-ups, flips and muscle-up chains) don't really suit the typical in-gym sets x reps approach. Instead, the two methods put forward in this chapter—*time surfing* and *consolidation training*—work better.

Both time surfing and CT have their benefits, but they also have negatives: time surfing limits your practice time, and CT doesn't fit well into a fixed program. For this reason, most athletes will wish to *blend* both approaches together in their daily training. I'd advise most athletes to use the time-surfing method to neatly fit the bulk of their practice into a clean program, and then augment that schedule with some multiple daily CT sessions when they come up against a tough movement, or when they want to progress a bit quicker.

For those hungry hombres out there who want even more, I'll outline some black-and-white programming approaches in the next chapter.

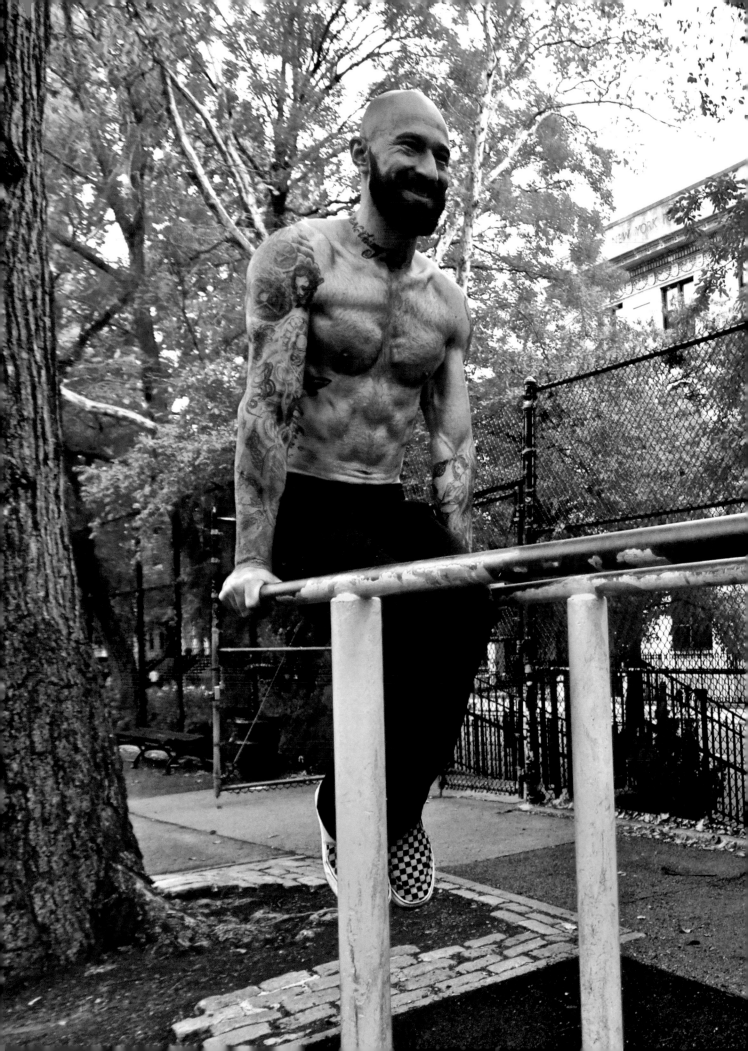

14

SAMPLE PROGRAMS
SESSION TEMPLATES

In *Convict Conditioning*, I kept program templates to a minimum. It seems that these days, program templates are all folks want to talk about. Back in my time, all we thought about was *training!* We were adding reps, improving our techniques, breaking records and learning new skills. We barely noticed that we even had a "program"!

I think handing folks a bunch of programs is a bad idea in the long run; as I explained in the first book, the most important thing an athlete can learn is the art of *self-coaching*. That begins (and pretty much ends) with your own sweat. You work out, and learn as you go. That attitude might make me sound like some kinda old school troglodyte, but so be it.

FOCUS ON *PROGRESSIONS*, NOT TEMPLATES

The coaches, experts and athletes who really "got" *Convict Conditioning* were the folks who understood that the progressions were the key to the whole thing—not the workouts. As long as you grasp the principles of productive training, you can use the progressions in a gazillion different types of programs: for mass, wiry strength, joint functioning, etc. There is nothing magical about a workout template, no matter what goddamn genius invented it. Only the athlete can make the magic, with their concentration, effort, consistency and body wisdom. Focus on getting better, and the program will happen by itself.

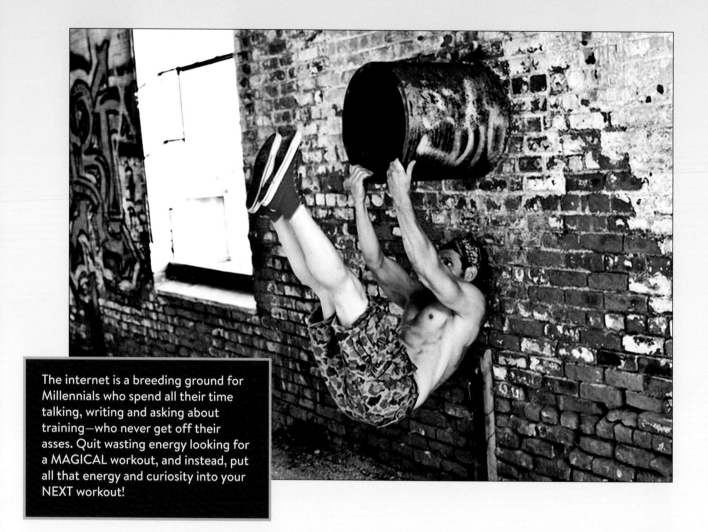

The internet is a breeding ground for Millennials who spend all their time talking, writing and asking about training—who never get off their asses. Quit wasting energy looking for a MAGICAL workout, and instead, put all that energy and curiosity into your NEXT workout!

If it's true that workout templates were not so crucial in *Convict Conditioning*, then that holds much, much truer for the contents of *this* book. The majority of the exercises in this book are *skill-based* progressions—this means that the typical workout-template method of performing a few sets of multiple reps every few days is not going to cut it. *Consolidation training*—where you work these movements on a more ad hoc, frequent basis—is more efficient. Consolidation training just *can't* be shoe-horned into your average fixed workout template—it requires flexibility, intuition, discretion. If you've been reading the last few chapters (you did, right?) you'll understand that what I'm saying is true.

Nevertheless, I can do my best to give you a few pointers. In this chapter I'm going to present some fundamental—and hopefully applicable—approaches to training plans that will fit different goals and objectives.

WARM-UP PROTOCOL!

Be aware: The following program templates only describe "work sets": the sets you do as the main part of your workout, *after* warming up.

Warming up is essential before *any* hard training, but it is *even more* important when you are performing high-velocity movements. You need to ensure that your muscles are warm and pliable, your joints freshened up, and your reflexes tuned in.

Warming up also gradually lowers *neurological inhibition*: shifting up through your "power" gears will makes you stronger. That's why warm-up attempts are so crucial in sports like powerlifting or Olympic weight-lifting—it makes the athletes stronger.

How much you warm up depends on various factors: your condition, your age, the temperature, and so on. A good warm-up protocol might include:

- Joint rolling exercises

- A few minutes of higher-rep exercises to heat the entire body: many of the *small space drills* in the various chapters would work well for this, as would some animal-type movements (see *Bonus Section 2*)

- Stretching out any tight areas with tension-flexibility exercises

- A few easy sets of the type of movement you are going to perform for your work sets. This might involve 2-3 sets of steps from lower down the chain you are working on. You still can keep your reps low here, provided you did some higher-rep "heating" work earlier.

CONSOLIDATION TRAINING

You should always perform some kind of warm-up before explosive work—this is even true is you are performing consolidation training throughout the day. Sure, you shouldn't do prolonged warm-ups, as the multiplied volume through the day might exhaust you: but you can explore joint loosening exercises, plus a few "easy" reps prior to the drill you want to work on.

PURE POWER

DAY 1:	Jump work	3 sets of 2
	Power pushups	3 sets of 2
DAY 2:	Off	
	Repeat	

All sets given are work sets. Prior to this, the athlete should warm up thoroughly.

For athletes who are new to explosive work, it doesn't get simpler than this. Combine the two basic power moves in a single, low volume session. It can even be completed (after a warm up—see previous page) prior to a strength workout, cardio workout, or sports training. As you make progress, begin to up your volume (see page 279).

VARIATIONS:

• The sets and reps given above are just a suggestion. Tinker with your sets and reps according to the *Rule of Three* and the *Rule of Six*.

• This is an ultra-low volume program for total beginners. As you gain conditioning, build up your sets and reps. Bear in mind, however—always—that explosive training is NOT an endurance sport. Keep your reps crisp, fresh, and turned up to maximum power. When you start to tire, you're done.

• If this makes you too sore—explosives can be tough—throw in another day of rest.

• A slightly different variation would be to alternate exercises; on Day One, do jumps, Day Two, power pushups with either rest on Day Three, or skip a fixed rest day and instead take a day off whenever you feel a bit stale.

SACRED TRINITY

DAY 1:	Jump work	6 sets of 2
	Kip-up work	5-10 mins
DAY 2:	Power pushups	6 sets of 2
	Kip-up work	5-10 mins
DAY 3:	Off	
	Repeat	

I advise athletes to gain a good level of proficiency with *jumps* and *power pushups*—say, reaching step 6 of both chains—before interspersing skill work from the other chains. When you do begin employing skill work, I suggest that *kip-ups* are the first chain you explore. Why? Three reasons: first, kip-ups teach great basic agility skills; they involve partial *rotation* of the body, *hip flexing* (pulling the knees towards the head) and *waist snap*. Second, this chain is fairly easy on the body, compared to the others. Thirdly, it's the *easiest* of the skill chains—if you can't do a kip-up, you don't stand a hope in hell of performing a *flip*, or even a good *muscle-up*. This program allows you to continue your power training, while getting lots of kipping practice—six sessions of kipping over eight days. That should help you progress nice and fast. (Note that I don't give a repetition range for skill work—just a suggested *time surfing* period. See page 287).

VARIATIONS:

- *Less work:* for those who need it, an extra rest day can be inserted between each session.

- *More work:* for workhorses who desire more frequency, skip the rest day and work four days in a row before taking a day off. This may be too much, however.

4-LEAF CLOVER

DAY 1:	Jump work	6 sets of 2
	Kip-up work	5-10 mins
DAY 2:	Power pushups	6 sets of 2
	Front flip work	5-10 mins
DAY 3:	Off	
	Repeat	

Once athletes have gotten to grips with power work, and are getting the hang of the *kip-up*—perhaps step 6 or 7—if they wish to begin mastering more of the Explosive Six, then they can start adding new drills into their routines. It's a good rule of thumb to begin making progress with the *front flip* chain before the *back flip* chain, because even though (in my opinion) a well-executed front flip is harder than a good back flip, the earlier stages of the front flip are a bit easier because of the fear factor: many beginners are more intimidated by going head over heels *backwards*. The above approach has the athlete swap one session of kip-ups—you should be experiencing diminishing returns by now, anyway—and add in some early front flip training.

VARIATIONS:

- There's always room for flexibility in any good program. If you love the kip-up and want to perform it more often, you can always perform a few single repetitions—say five—of your current kip-up step, prior to the front flip work.

- Those of you who want more practice could take the above suggestion further and perform a 5 minute kip-up session, followed by a 5-10 minute front flip session on both Day One and Day Two. But beware of biting off more than you can chew—overload causes burnout real fast.

"25s"

DAY 1:	**Any chain**	**5 sets of 1 rep** **Every 2 hours** **(10 hours max)**

Repeat, taking days off as necessary.

All sets given are work sets. Prior to this,
the athlete should warm up thoroughly

Who says you need to work on *all* of the Explosive Six? What if you only want to learn *one* of the skills? (There are reasons you might want to do this—say you are a wrestler and want to master the *back handspring* as an explosive compliment to your bridging workouts. Or maybe only one chain lights your fire? Whatever.) A good method of doing this is to apply *consolidation training* in a very specific way—you begin at the beginning of the chain, and start with step 1. You warm up a little and perform five single reps of step 1—five times per day, spread apart by at least two hours. This is 25 reps per day. When you can hit all 25 reps in acceptable form, you move to the next step. Take a day off as and when you need one.

VARIATIONS:

- Why not mix and match? This method would also work if you were trying to improve quickly in *two* chains—you could just alternate chains each hour. (More than two chains might be too much.)

- This approach is just regimented *consolidation training*, so there are obviously plenty of ways to tinker with the math, depending on the difficulty of the step you're working on, your conditioning level, and your available time. Some options are:

  — 3 reps every hour (over a 5 hour period)   = 15 reps
  — 5 reps every hour (over a 5 hour period)   = 25 reps
  — 3 reps every hour (over a 10 hour period)   = 30 reps
  — 5 reps every hour (over a 10 hour period)   = 50 reps

2-DAY SPLIT

DAY 1:	Jump work	6 sets of 3
	Power pushups	6 sets of 3
	Kip-up work	5 minutes
	Back flip work	10 minutes
DAY 2:	Off	
DAY 3:	Jump work	6 sets of 3
	Power pushups	6 sets of 3
	Front flip work	10 minutes
	Muscle-up work	10 minutes
DAY 4:	Off	
	Repeat	

All sets given are work sets. Prior to this, the athlete should warm up thoroughly.

Eventually athletes dedicated to building maximum explosive power, speed and agility will want to work with all six explosive chains in this book. While it's not impossible to work with all six chains in a single session—Olympic gymnasts may work on a *dozen* movements each session—I think for most athletes this would be overkill, causing physical burnout and mental logjam. In most cases you're better off splitting the six chains over two sessions and really focusing on three exercises per time.

VARIATIONS:

- This approach is still compatible with *consolidation training*. You can apply this program while still inserting mini-sessions of a particular chain throughout the day (see "25s", previous page). That variation works very well if you are "stuck" on a particular step, which requires extra practice.

THE MUSCLEMAN

Jump work	(5-10 mins) before legs/squat
Power pushup	(5-10 mins) before chest low-speed pushups
Kip-up work	(5-10 mins) before midsection/ leg raises
Front flip work	(5-10 mins) before shoulders/ handstand PUs
Back flip work	(5-10 mins) before back/low back/bridging
Muscle-up work	(5-10 mins) before lats/upper-back/pullups

All sets given are work sets. Prior to this, the athlete should warm up thoroughly.

I suspect that most readers of this book will not *only* be interested with developing explosive power—most will already be training in strength or bodybuilding. A great way to integrate explosives into a pre-existing routine is to *begin your body-part training with some explosives work, and then follow with your regular strength/bodybuilding exercises.* Beginning with moderate-volume explosives—far from exhausting you before your strength/bodybuilding sets—will actually *increase* your strength during your regular workouts, due to "charging" your nervous system (*neural innervation*). Many old-time strongmen did jumps before heavy squats, for just this reason. Adding explosives into an already vigorous training schedule can be pretty demanding, so make sure you ease into it—a new chain here, an extra set there. Most strength athletes/bodybuilders use "split routines" designed to target limited body areas each session, to increase recovery: lobbing in explosives, which typically work the entire body, can throw a wrench into that careful planning. The only solution is to go carefully, and if your progress is slowing up, or if you are feeling fatigued/aches and pains, slow up. Remember, you can always insert extra rest days or just skip some explosives mini-sessions now and again.

JOHNNY KUNG FU

DAY 1:	Jump work	6 sets of 3
	Kip-up work	5 minutes
	Back flip work	10 minutes
	Front flip work	10 minutes
DAY 2:	Power pushups	6 sets of 3
	Muscle-up work	10 minutes
DAY 3:	Off	
	Repeat	

All sets given are work sets. Prior to this, the athlete should warm up thoroughly.

This is a more advanced approach for an experienced explosives athlete working with all six chains of the Explosive Six. There's higher frequency here, as well as a little more specialization to allow for that frequency—Day One contains jumping skills (*jumps, kip-ups, flips*) Day Two is more upper-body power (*power pushups, muscle-ups*).

VARIATIONS:

- This would work great for an athlete who has already reached the Master Steps—specialist work (from the *Going Beyond* section of each chapter) could be incorporated after the Training listed above. (It would also work as is, as a maintenance program for a guy or gal who has reached all the Master Steps and is focusing on other qualities).

- As ever, if you start getting stale in your movements, add a random rest day. Despite the specialization, there's always plenty of overlap when working with explosives. Some athletes might do better with a day off after each session, if adding impromptu off days isn't enough.

LIGHTS OUT!

I can understand why an intelligent person would want to use an intelligent training program. I get it. But please don't waste any time (like so many seem to) looking for a *perfect* or *magical* training program. The magic comes from the athlete; it's their effort, their instincts, their consistency and dedication. The *program* is secondary, always. As Bruce Lee said, training is not really an objective pursuit: it's *subjective*. Its main motor is the human mind, the spirit. These are delicate, mercurial things, which need to be accommodated. If you want longevity in this game, you need to remember this; be creative, and kind to yourself. Be free, be flexible. Every 6-8 weeks, change something in your program. Keep it fun, interesting. The great Bill Pearl always used to say that there was no one workout that would look after an athlete their whole lives: the man was right.

All great programs are not really "routines" but *approaches*; you can mix the variables—sets, reps, exercise order, frequency—to suit your life, your instincts or needs. Maybe you work out in a commercial gym, or you need (or wish) to follow a conventional 7-day plan. Great—just add to or cut a day from the programs in this book. Folks often talk to me about the programs in my previous books like they were *Holy Scripture*. Boy—do they give me too much credit! And worse, they don't give enough to *themselves*. Take charge. Trust yourself. Give yourself permission to just train to the beat of your own drum. You'll do fine, kid.

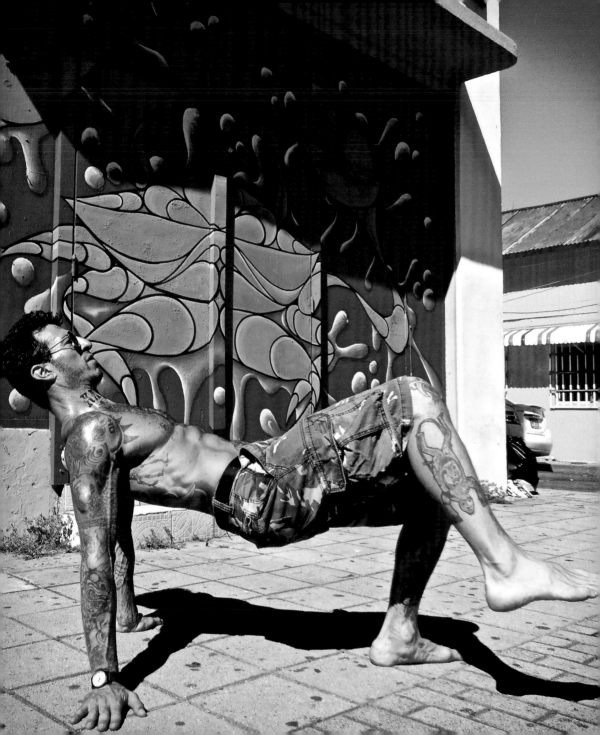

BONUS MATERIAL

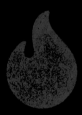

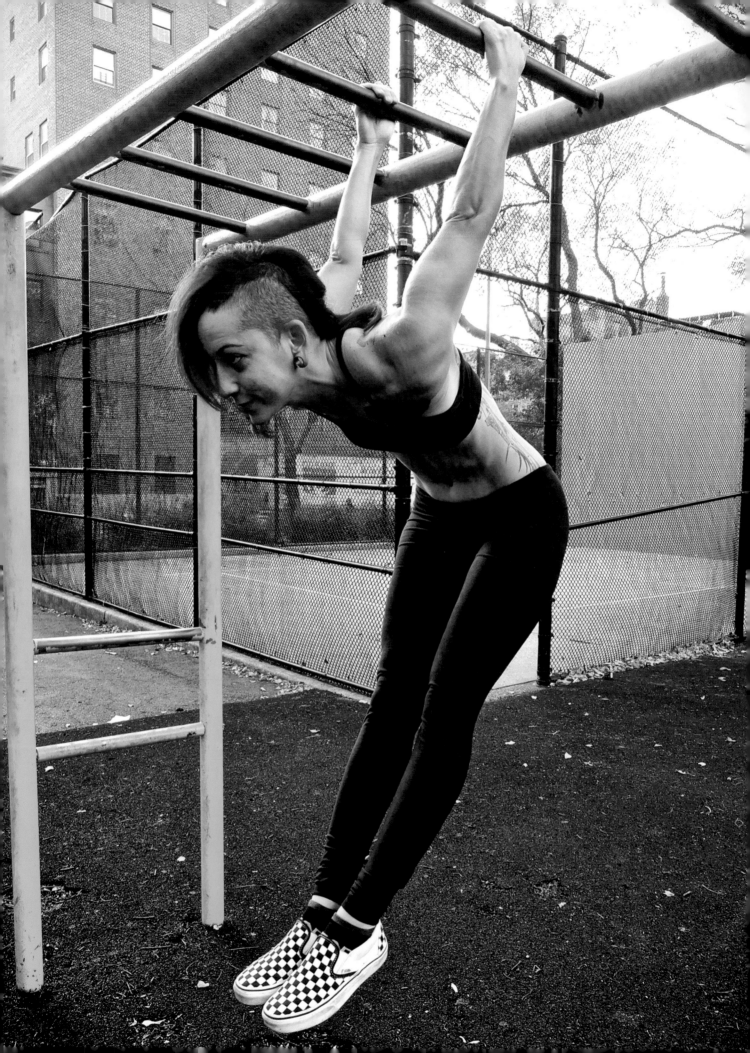

BONUS SECTION 1

ADVANCED SPEED TRAINING: "COACH" WADE'S TOP TEN TRICKS AND HACKS

I f you've read through this manual, you'll now know the best way possible to become a more explosive athlete—by becoming elite-level at a handful of classic bodyweight movements which require huge power, awesome speed, and epic agility and reflexes. You'll know the finest progressions to use while training in these exercises, and you'll also have some programming approaches under your belt.

Most authors would stop there—quit while they're ahead. Not me. I'm too dumb. Plus, I like writing for you guys too much. That's why I had to slip in just one more chapter before bedtime; and in this chapter I'm going to be giving you my top ten tips and tactics for becoming faster than a speeding bullet!

Some of these ten ideas are pretty fundamental and anyone with any common sense will understand that they must be adopted by any athlete who wants to really amp up their quickness. Others are a little more abstruse...some are downright wacky. You choose. If just *one* of these here ideas helps you in your training, or evolves the way you mentally approach your training, then it was worth writing it.

Let's go:

SUPER-SPEED TACTIC #1: HACK THE SPEED CYCLE!

Nope, the *speed cycle* isn't something you head for in the gym so you can chit-chat to that hot fox wearing lycra on the bike next to you. The speed cycle is a theoretical process by which we do super-fast stuff—like dodging a punch, jumping to catch a Frisbee, or even leaping over a moving vehicle. You need to understand this process first and foremost if you want to maximize your speed training. Why? Because it contains components most athletes automatically bypass.

Let's look at the stages of the speed cycle:

STAGE I	Pre-Perception Awareness	
STAGE II	Perception Speed	
STAGE III	Recognition Speed	
STAGE IV	Decision Speed	
STAGE V	Movement Speed	

I. PRE-PERCEPTION AWARENESS

This is the first stage of fast movement, where you become aware of the *possibility* that you may have to move fast. Let's say, you are in a dive bar in Detroit wearing a *Red Wings Suck!* T-shirt, when some big toothless hockey fan squares up to you. If you have any brains at all, you'll begin to realize the *possibility* that you may be assaulted, even though it *hasn't actually happened yet.* This is *pre-perception awareness.* This stage involves *sensory awareness* of your environment, but also a trained or intuitive *mental processing* of what you are experiencing. This stage may not exist at all in some circumstances, where you have to react to something you couldn't predict—say you were walking along and out of nowhere a brick flies at your face. But those circumstances are fairly rare.

II. PERCEPTION SPEED

This is where you first become cognizant of the event that requires you to move fast—the punch flies towards your face, for example. This occurs through the senses, primarily the visual, although depending on the circumstances your other senses can be a big help too.

III. RECOGNITION SPEED

After your eyes lock onto the fist moving towards them, it takes a tiny fraction of a second for the brain to actually realize what *exactly* is happening. Believe it or not, we can easily interpret a fast-moving hand in several different ways: *is this huge man falling over? Is this guy going to pat me on the shoulder, or give me a high-five?* Etc.

IV. DECISION SPEED

Okay, now you recognize that you're being attacked. You need to *decide* the best thing to do about it. All of this happens very, very fast of course; forget what you saw in the *Sherlock Holmes* movie where Robert Downey Jr. perfectly plots out every stage of his bare-knuckle fight. No prolonged upper-cortex mental decisions are made. It's a nearly-immediate brainstem thing. *Do you dodge? Do you block? Do you try and hit the other guy first?*

V. MOVEMENT SPEED

Great—your brain decided that blocking the punch by *raising your arm and leaning back* was the right course of action. All that remains is for your body to actually *do that*. Movement speed is about how quick the nervous system/muscles can actually move and do what they're told to.

* * * * * * * * *

There are various different formats of this progress, and some use different terms for the stages, or more complex stages. If you prefer you own interpretation, that's cool.

What's most interesting about this paradigm for me, is that fact that most athletes who want to be fast spend up to 100% of their training time exclusively on stage V: building greater *movement speed*. That's awesome, but it's also pretty misguided—athletes who do this are missing out on the other four stages. Damn, that's 80% of what makes you truly fast!

The solution? Find ways of training the other four stages, and build them into your workouts. The next few speed tactics will focus on this concept, and give you some prime ideas on how to do just that.

SUPER-SPEED TACTIC #2: EXPLOIT GRETZKY'S LAW!

Wayne Gretzky was one of the all-time greatest hockey players ever to set foot on the ice—maybe *the* greatest. He had a bunch of incredible qualities, but possibly most impressive was his lightning speed: and remember, hockey is as fast as hell to begin with.

Whenever he was pressed on what made him so damn good, Gretzky had a stock reply:

> *A good hockey player plays where the puck is.*
>
> *A great hockey player plays where the puck is going to be.*
>
> — Wayne Gretzky

Think about how this relates to the speed cycle: it has nothing to do with reaction time or movement speed. It's about *anticipating* what's going to happen next, *before* it happens—this relates to stage I: *Pre-Perception Awareness*.

Anyone can apply this to any sport, or any situation where they need to be fast. Instead of just passively waiting to "react" to something, you try to actively *predict* that event ahead of time—even just a split-second ahead of time—so your reaction time will be that much quicker, making you faster than the next guy. This is true of combat, emergency situations, but also all sports: tennis, basketball, wrestling, you name it.

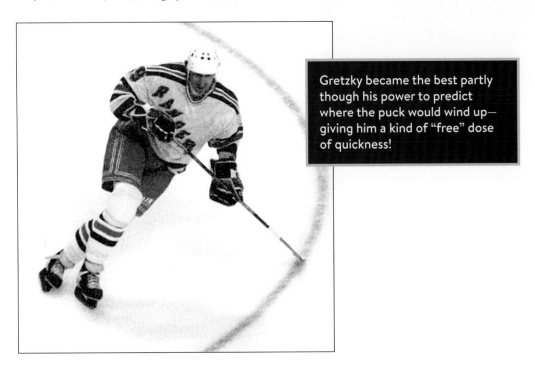

Gretzky became the best partly though his power to predict where the puck would wind up—giving him a kind of "free" dose of quickness!

How do you get better at this? Three points: *sensory openness*, *mental focus*, and an *understanding* of the situation in front of you. The first two you can pick up more or less immediately if you try; the third is about *study*. Study your game, the environment you're in. Study your opponent. If you can put some energy into these things, you are much more likely to pick up tiny cues and clues as to what's going to happen next. In sparring: *is your opponent shifting his weight onto his back leg, ready for a front kick?* In tennis: *is your competitor looking to your left, to place a shot there?* Etc. There are too many variables to spell out here, but depending on your sport or situation you should be able to work them out yourself.

This is the most logical and primary way of getting faster: but very few athletes ever seem to work on this aspect. Most people are too used to instinctively 6 than 6 making rapid predictions. Like animals, we just instinctively respond when the adrenaline kicks in; we rarely step up to that human potential of ours and unlock the power of our brains.

...If it was so key to Wayne Gretzky's speed, it's worth thinking about, right?

SUPER-SPEED TACTIC #3:
TRAIN THE SENSES!

If the last tactic relates to the first stage of the speed cycle, this one relates to the second stage: *Perception Speed*.

The overall health and efficiency of our senses play a crucial role in our total speed: if we *see* an "event" slower, we react slower. A large component of total speed is *reaction time*: and if you are reacting, you are reacting to some external event, be it a punch, a kick, a missile, an upcoming obstacle, whatever. The vast majority of these "events" are *visual* in nature; we see them, and our vision tells us to judge when and how to react. We are often so wrapped up in the idea that speed is all about a fast *muscular system*, that we rarely train the *perceptual system*: the five senses.

Martial artists—particularly aficionados of the traditional, classical systems—may be an exception. The older arts contain various methods for training the different senses, and all athletes can learn a lot from them. All you need to train your senses is your imagination, but here are a few ideas to get you started:

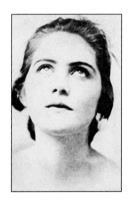 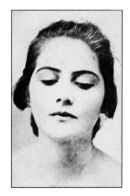 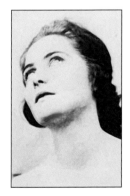 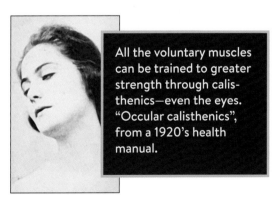

All the voluntary muscles can be trained to greater strength through calisthenics—even the eyes. "Occular calisthenics", from a 1920's health manual.

VISUAL

There are numerous exercises designed to increase eye health—the old yoga technique where you stare at a candle to nullify the blinking instinct is just one. Another is to follow a "circuit" of a figure-8 with your eyeballs; do it ten times, then rest and repeat. Over time, the muscles of your eyes will get faster, improving your perception speed. You can train your peripheral vision by something as simple as watching TV sitting side-on; look straight ahead, and see what you can pick up. As the nerves in the sides of your eyes strengthen, you can alter your angle even further.

AURAL

Everything is so goddamn *loud* these days—TVs, radios, and the cinema actually rattles your fillings. The French philosopher Rousseau predicted that as

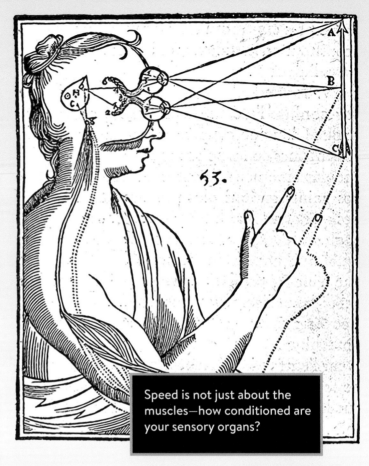

Speed is not just about the muscles—how conditioned are your sensory organs?

our technology makes things easier for us, our natural senses would decay accordingly. It's true—most of us keep our vision fixed for hours at a time, to a TV, laptop, whatever. Weak hearing is epidemic these days. Our ancestors were hunter-gatherers who had to attune to the slightest rustle of a leaf, or even bending of grass, to locate predators or quarry. You can train your hearing back to the Paleolithic default setting with specific techniques. Build the muscles and tissues of the eye by looking around when you walk—focus on different objects at different distances to keep the lenses pliable and fresh. Turn your TV down until you can barely hear it. When it becomes audible, repeat the process. *Sensory mediation* is a more advanced method; sit in silence for a while. Soon you'll discover that the world around you isn't "silent" at all: you'll hear creaking walls, water moving in the pipes, birds outside, people in the distance. Over time you can refine your hearing to ridiculous levels with this technique. *Sonic location* is another good skill to drill: place something quiet—say, a laptop with a whirring cooling fan—some distance from you. Then spin around until you lose your bearings. Pause and listen until you can work out exactly where the device is, relative to you. Knowing where slight sounds emanate from—especially if they are out of your line of sight—is also useful in combat, for obvious reasons.

KINESTHETIC

We don't often think of movement or *touch* as a speed-sense, but we can potentially react much faster to *touch* than we do to *sight*. Many security personnel and bodyguards use a contact technique Geoff Thompson calls "the fence", where they gently put their hand out in front of their chest; the second an aggressor touches their fingertips—and therefore comes within attacking range—they strike. Ancient *wing chun* masters took tactile reflex training to the level of a science, with a practice called *chi sau*. Was it a coincidence that Bruce Lee—considered one of the fastest men of this, or any other era—learned wing chun as a kid? I don't think so.

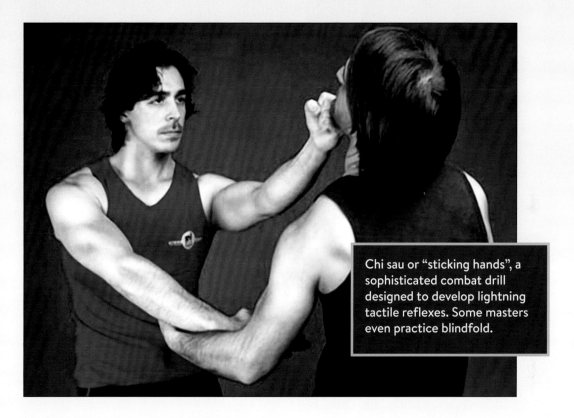

Chi sau or "sticking hands", a sophisticated combat drill designed to develop lightning tactile reflexes. Some masters even practice blindfold.

OLFACTORY/GUSTATORY

Can your senses of *smell* or *taste* help you get faster? Just maybe. Mammals all sniff the air to get a sense of their surroundings; reptiles like snakes stick out their tongues to (literally) get a taste of the action. Many species can pick up pheromones or hormones from other creatures which send specific messages of attraction, fear or even potential violence. Sure, perhaps human beings can't consciously pick out those variables in our environments any more, but trust me—those senses didn't go anywhere. They just manifest as "gut feelings" about people or situations. Most civilized folks struggle to ignore their instinctive reactions to people and things. *Don't.* Learn to listen to your instincts and trust them, wherever you are. Even today, it could mean the difference between life and death.

SUPER-SPEED TACTIC #4: EXPLOIT REFLEX CHANNELING!

Go to an FBI training school and you'll see that the bulk of the crisis training there is about drilling the same techniques—based on time-worn tactics—again and again. They do this for two reasons. The first is based on a scientific principle called the *Yerkes-Dodson Law*. This law states that, at a higher level, *there is an inverse relationship between arousal and performance*. In other words, when you are extremely emotionally excited—which is what a crisis or a critically important event does to you—your performance (including your *speed*) goes down the toilet. When this happens, you can't *think* your way out of things. You need to have already programmed your behaviors into your reflexes to get the job done without "you" being present.

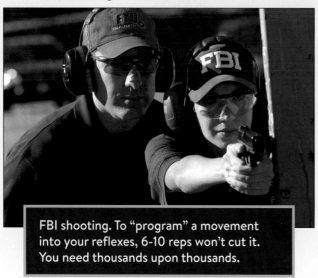

FBI shooting. To "program" a movement into your reflexes, 6-10 reps won't cut it. You need thousands upon thousands.

How do you "program" your reflexes? This has to do with another bit of science called *Hebb's Rule*. This is sometimes known as the *law of repetition*, and—to paraphrase—it states that *neurons that fire together, wire together*. In other words, if you want to program your nervous system with certain automatic behaviors—whether it's blocking a punch, serving well at tennis, or shooting a bad guy—the best way to make it sink into your nervous system is to drill it. What do I mean by "drill"? There is an old story in kung fu, of a student who wanted to master a certain kick for combat. He asked his *sifu* how to achieve this, and the master told him to perform the kick in mid-air *a thousand times* to be able to do it correctly just *once*. Then, when he could kick correctly, he would have to practice the same kick against a solid target a thousand times. Then he would practice the kick against a solid-but-moving target a thousand times. Then he would have to perform the kick a thousand times perfectly in sparring—only then would he be ready to perform the kick *once* in a real fight! That's what I mean by *drilling*. The move becomes part of you.

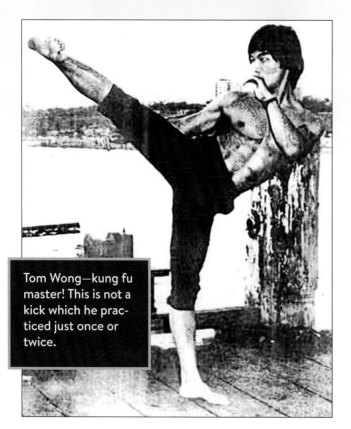

Tom Wong—kung fu master! This is not a kick which he practiced just once or twice.

What does all this have to do with speed? It has to do with the third and fourth stages of the speed cycle: *recognition speed* and *decision speed*. Maximum speed at these stages cannot come from the mind or thoughts—it has to come from the brainstem and nervous system: the automatic reflexes. The only way to have the best reflexes in there is to program them in: by drilling. Build that speed-software into your nervous system by thousands and thousands of reps in training, and you'll be unbeatable!

SUPER-SPEED TACTIC #5: UTILIZE THE PLYOMETRIC EDGE!

Too many athletes (and even coaches) confuse *plyometrics* and *explosiveness training*. Many athletes working with jumps or power pushups assume they are doing "plyo"—they ain't. The two are not the same.

Plyometrics is a neologism drawn from the Greek words *plio* meaning "more" and *metric* meaning "measurement". Plyometrics as a training method was a special "secret" Soviet technique created by Yuri Verkhoshansky in the late sixties. Used properly, plyometrics refers to any exercise which causes the muscles to stretch under force a fraction of a second before contracting again; and this was originally done by rapidly "loading" the muscles with stretch-energy via gravity. The typical example was the *depth jump*, where the athlete jumps down off an object—which would rapidly force the muscles to stretch, when the athlete hits the ground—then *immediately* jumps back up.

Verkhoshansky developed this method to help track athletes. He believed that the sudden fall would "shock" the muscles and nervous system, causing them to respond defensively by firing back with extra power. (Verkhoshansky didn't coin the term *plyometrics*; that was made-up by an American athlete, Fred Wilt, witnessing the Soviets train. The method was originally called "shock training".) The method works, at least partly, by activating the *myotatic* (stretch) *reflex*. Modern exercise ideologists have expanded on this, by throwing in theories like "the stretch shortening cycle" and concepts like "muscle spindles" and "golgi tendon organs".

So—how can you apply the idea of plyometrics to the exercises in this book? The key is to begin each rep with a *fall*; you then immediately explode back up, after a small dip (which is the bending of the joints). You can apply this concept best to the power stuff, the jumps and explosive pushups. There are two ways to apply it. In the first (and flashiest) method, you jump down off a box, and jump back up (maybe even onto another box, or in mid-air).

You can apply the same idea to pushups; begin in the pushup position with your hands on two boxes either side of you, then drop off the boxes and explode back up off your hands onto them. Some athletes can get an unreal height doing this.

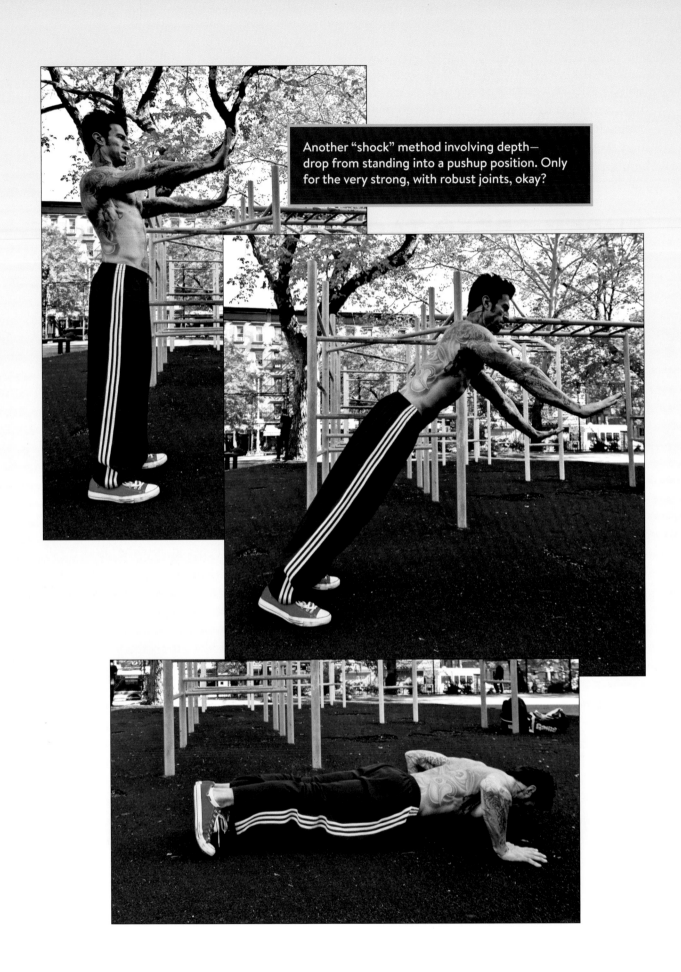

Another "shock" method involving depth—drop from standing into a pushup position. Only for the very strong, with robust joints, okay?

EXPLOSIVE CALISTHENICS

The second (and simpler) method is to perform multiple reps, with no rest in-between those reps. Think about it—if you jump up from the ground, that first jump is not truly plyometric, because it's not preceded by a "shocking" drop. However, if you land from that first jump, and *immediately* perform a second jump, you can access the drop/shock forces of the landing from the first jump: therefore the second rep (and every one following) can be *plyometric*, provided you don't pause during the set. You can do the same for pushups—use the fall from the first rep to immediately "charge" your second rep.

It's a good idea to take a short breather to mentally focus and readjust between reps on exercises like flips and kip-ups. But you should *not* apply the rebound principle for your multiple reps on jumps and pushups if you can. Knock them out machine gun-style. Hit your first rep hard as possible, then the second you land, use the rebound and elastic forces in your muscles to immediately bounce back up. Verkhoshansky nailed it: shock training *does* work, and it *will* increase your explosive speed.

SUPER-SPEED TACTIC #6: LOSE WEIGHT!

This one's a no-brainer—but surprisingly few students of calisthenics take it seriously. I'm not saying that a calisthenics master needs ripped abs—that depends on the last few percent of body fat being stripped away, and an athlete can easily be at their best when they are not emaciated that way. That said, carrying twenty, thirty, forty, or even more than fifty pounds of excess blubber (like most Americans are today) is a big no-no.

Movements like *back flips*, *kip-ups* and *muscle-ups* are damned hard even for light athletes. Carrying a bunch of extra weight will make them virtually impossible. Sure, I know: there are some tubby athletes who can perform these moves—if you haven't seen it happen, you can if you look hard enough. But just think how *incredible* these guys could be if they jettisoned all that extra weight! Wow. Plus, imagine how much unnecessary extra force it transfers to the joints during explosive movements. A *lot*.

Calisthenics—even explosive work—is really just *movement*. Nobody (provided they can move) should be restricted from taking part. Even if you are very obese, you can begin some kind of calisthenics training. (With your doc's permission of course. How sad is it that I have to say that to avoid getting my ass sued, huh?) Just begin with the earliest steps you can perform without hurting your body; anything is better than nothing. Progressive calisthenics is the perfect discipline to go alongside weight loss, because it doesn't prioritize excessive calories/protein intake (like bodybuilding or weight-training) and it doesn't exhaust you so much that you become ravenous and undo all your hard work (think cardio/endurance sports). I have always argued, too, that calisthenics has a "subconscious effect"—when you force your body to move its own weight, your brain realizes that fact and adjusts your metabolism and appetite accordingly. Dieting sure is easier with a side of calisthenics, in my opinion, and in the opinion of many others.

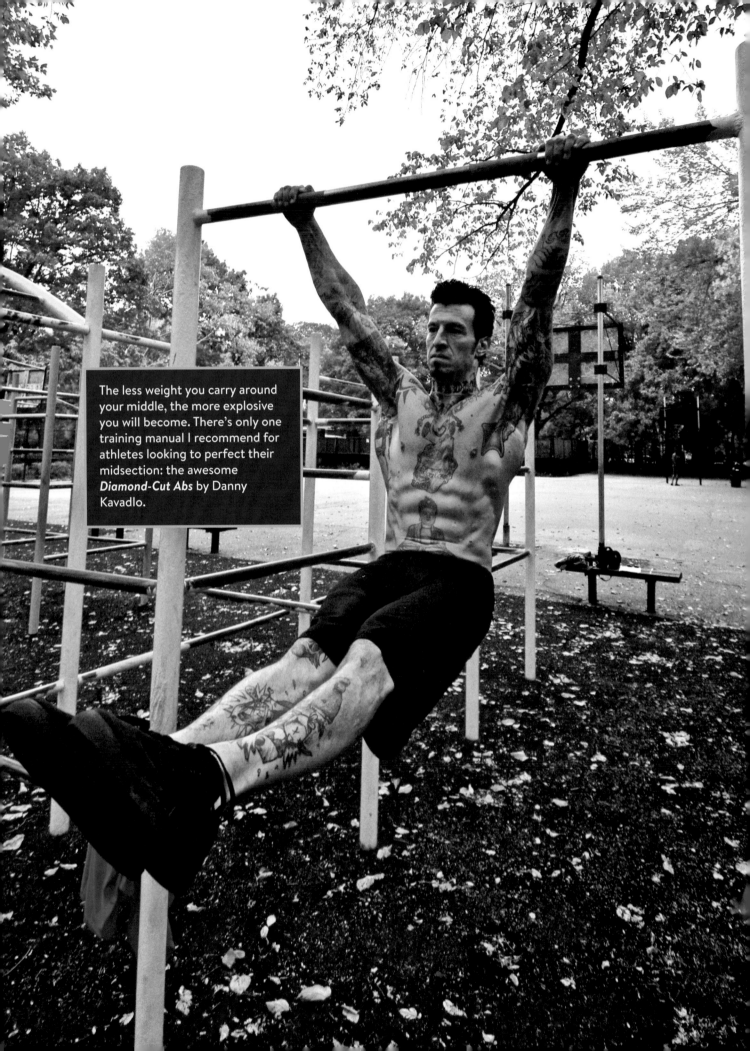

The less weight you carry around your middle, the more explosive you will become. There's only one training manual I recommend for athletes looking to perfect their midsection: the awesome *Diamond-Cut Abs* by Danny Kavadlo.

And how should you diet? Damn, diet books are always the biggest sellers in any bookstore, so you probably don't need me chirping in. I gave my full outlook in *Convict Conditioning 2*, but the principles are nothing special:

- Don't be obsessive—ever. Be flexible with food choices
- Eat a balanced diet (some carbs and some protein at each meal, and a blend of meat, dairy, vegetables, fruit and cereal)
- Reduce basic portion sizes to lose bodyweight
- Eat 3 x per day (possibly with a snack or two)
- Don't eat several hours before bed, and try and go to sleep on an empty stomach

This advice is nothing mind-blowing or esoteric, but it's pretty much the opposite of the usual fitness junk advice, which says:

- Be as strictly disciplined as possible—*junk food will kill ya!*
- Focus primarily on large amounts of protein, plus supplements
- Count calories/grams of macronutrients
- Eat 6-8 times a day
- Never go without food for more than a couple of hours, or your muscles will drop off and you'll become fatter!

If you want to follow the usual "health and fitness" advice, go for it. But be warned that it has only made our nation heavier and poorer, while making the supplement companies that much better off.

SUPER-SPEED TACTIC #7: OPTIMIZE JOINT HEALTH!

One reason older folks move slower is that they condition themselves to it—literally, they *program* themselves to move slow by moving slow all the time. They could potentially move much faster, but their bodies are limited by the software they're running. The reason so many older people program themselves to move slowly like this is that they have painful joints. If you really want to be fast—young or old—you must, must take care of your joints. Some general thoughts on this:

NO PONDEROUS WEIGHTS

Yeah, I know squatting four-figures is all the rage in some gyms, but you *will* pay for it later. My opinion—bodyweight-only is the best method for joint health and longevity. Nature's way wins, hands down!

CULTIVATE SUPPLE STRENGTH

I discussed this elsewhere—I also call it *tension-flexibility*. Use calisthenics methods to stretch and bend your joints under the body's own power and load. This strengthens the joints, draws blood to the soft tissues, healing them, and retains an ideal range-of-motion. There's a reason NFL guys go to *yoga* for rehab.

PROGRESS SLOWLY

One reason the old-timers used to build strength *slowly* was that they believed the muscles grow and develop quicker than the joints (the tendons, soft-tissues, cartilage, etc). I totally agree with this. Work in new exercises slowly, and progress at a sensible speed. Once your joints "catch up" to your muscles, you'll be surprisingly bulletproof.

TRAIN YOUR WEAK POINTS

Joint injuries constantly cause further injuries because athletes inevitably over-protect injured areas, causing further strength asymmetry. A chain always snaps at its *weakest* link—never its *strongest* link. So remove your weak links!

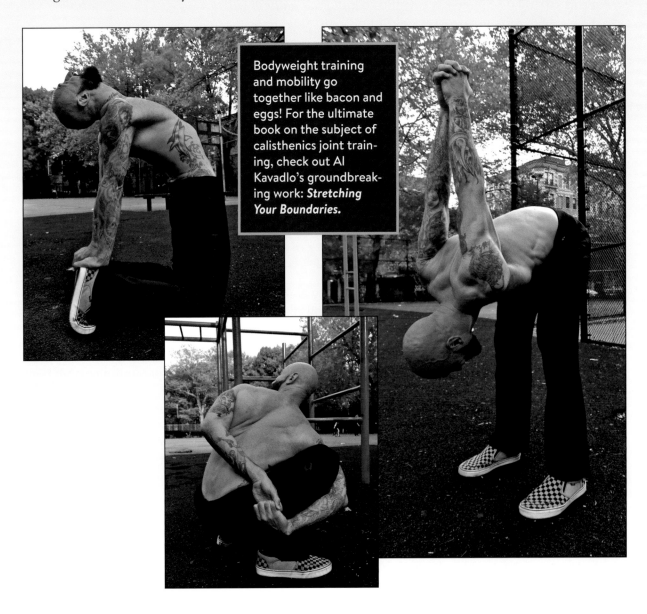

Bodyweight training and mobility go together like bacon and eggs! For the ultimate book on the subject of calisthenics joint training, check out Al Kavadlo's groundbreaking work: *Stretching Your Boundaries.*

SUPER-SPEED TACTIC #8: EXPLORE B-BALL DRILLS!

This is another training methodology drawn from prison experience. I've known a number of cell athletes who, to hone their reactions and movement speed, work solo with a basketball. It might sound nuts, but it makes a lot of sense. If you're spending a lot of time in a cell, your reflexes rust up like you wouldn't believe. You probably don't get any team sports, and you get no time to play on the Xbox. So how do you hone your reactions? Time tested b-ball drills.

The kind of drills you perform are limited only by your imagination. I could fill another book with 'em. You can catch, twist, drop, duck, jump, bend, bounce, and on and on. Here are a few basic drills to give you some flavor.

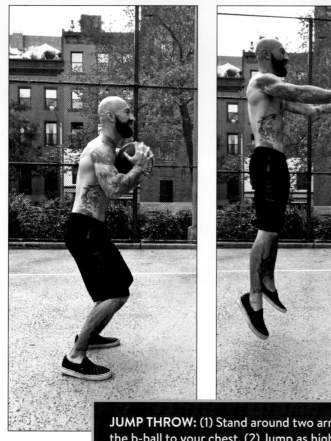
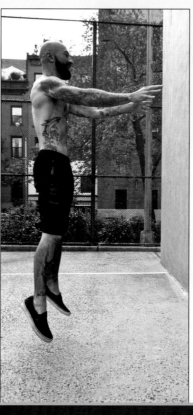
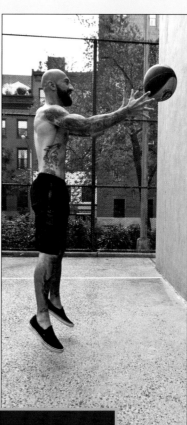

JUMP THROW: (1) Stand around two arm's lengths from the wall, holding the b-ball to your chest. (2) Jump as high as you can: the second your feet leave the ground, throw the ball at the wall. (3) You need to catch the basketball on the rebound *before* your feet hit the ground again.

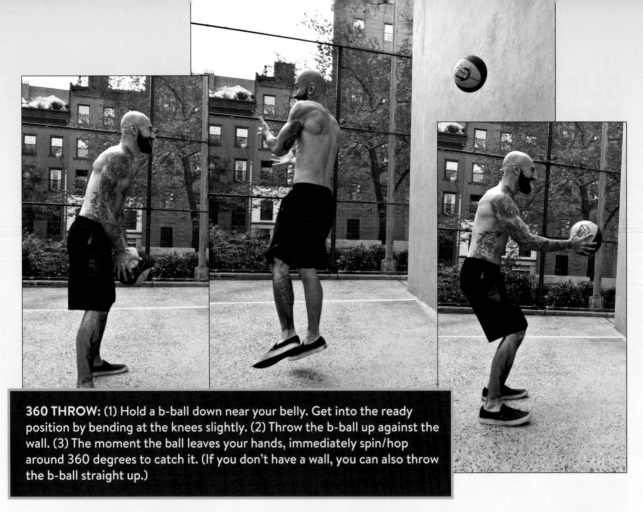

360 THROW: (1) Hold a b-ball down near your belly. Get into the ready position by bending at the knees slightly. (2) Throw the b-ball up against the wall. (3) The moment the ball leaves your hands, immediately spin/hop around 360 degrees to catch it. (If you don't have a wall, you can also throw the b-ball straight up.)

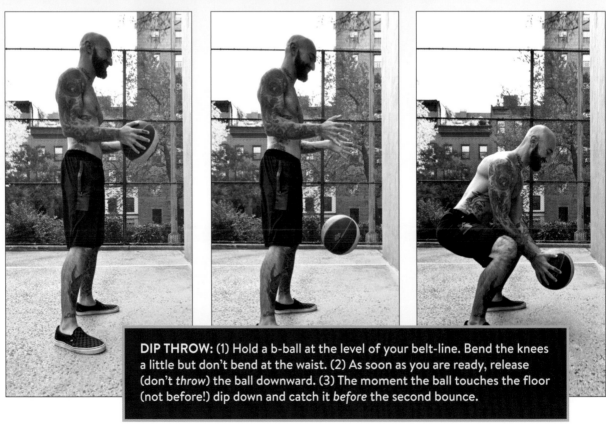

DIP THROW: (1) Hold a b-ball at the level of your belt-line. Bend the knees a little but don't bend at the waist. (2) As soon as you are ready, release (don't *throw*) the ball downward. (3) The moment the ball touches the floor (not before!) dip down and catch it *before* the second bounce.

SUPER-SPEED TACTIC #9: MASTER THE SPEED ILLUSION!

There's a famous maxim by the great master of strategy, Sun Tzu:

> *When we are near, we must make the enemy believe we are far away;*
>
> *when far away, we must make him believe we are near.*
>
> — Sun Tzu, *The Art of War*

I used to have a buddy who was a huge Kempo nut, who always used to tell me that—even in his late fifties—he could kick the ass of much, much younger guys in sparring, because he was *smarter* than them. This thought stuck with me for years. What did he mean by *smarter*? He was talking about using his body positioning *to make his opponents think he was further away than he really was*—then BANG! When he lashed out with a strike, it seemed like it was faster than lightning. In fact, the strike was probably slower than the punches and kicks coming from the guys he was fighting, but it *seemed* faster because it had less distance to travel due to his sneaky posture.

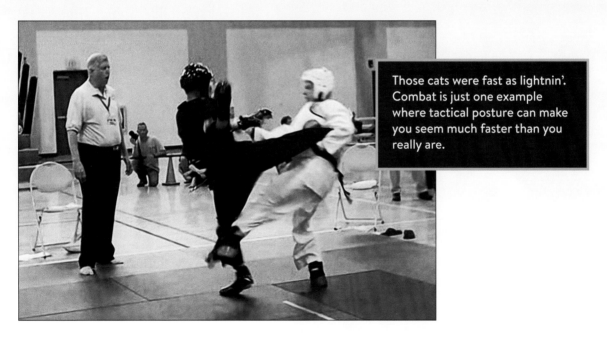

Those cats were fast as lightnin'. Combat is just one example where tactical posture can make you seem much faster than you really are.

Of course, this is not really about *being* faster than the next guy—only *seeming* that much faster than you really are, which amounts to the same thing. The iconic martial arts writer Loren Christensen calls this tactic the "illusion of speed", and he explains the art and science of this approach beautifully in his legendary book *Speed Training* (1996). I'd advise all fighters interested in the details of this strategy to get their hands on the book—the moment it came out it became the classic of the genre, and it hasn't been toppled since, in my opinion.

As ever, I'm using the example of speed in *combat*, but this basic strategy—Sun Tzu's strategy—is applicable to any other areas where you use speed against an opponent: football, basketball, hockey, etc. If you can use various cues to fool your opponent as to your direction/positioning, you can come out of nowhere to dazzle them with your *apparent* speed.

However brutal or physical your discipline, the *smart* approach works better than you might imagine.

SUPER-SPEED TACTIC #10: THINK FAST, KIMOSABE!

Think fast? Is that joke?

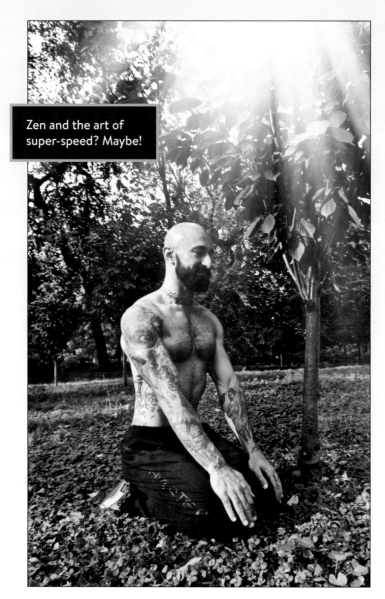

Zen and the art of super-speed? Maybe!

Nope—I'm deadly serious. By thinking you are fast—and thinking about speed generally—you will *literally* become faster.

I've already mentioned Christensen's martial arts bible *Speed Training* in this chapter. In closing the manual, Christensen notes how radically his own movement speed had increased as a result of all his research during the writing process. Much of this, he states, was due to the fact that he was putting his money where his mouth was, and experimenting hard with speed techniques in the dojo. So far, so reasonable, right? But then—out of the blue—Christensen hits you with something that sounds so bizarre, it almost seems as if the author himself has trouble accepting it:

In my book *C-MASS*, I described the phenomena of *neurological inhibition*. This is the idea that the human body is physically capable of much higher levels of performance that we can usually consciously access. So why can't we access it? Because the nervous system deliberately puts "blocks" on your abilities, in order to prevent your body from damaging itselves or burning out. But, via the mind, the brain can manipulate those subconscious blocks. Just by *watching* super-fast movements, or even *thinking* about moving very quickly, we convince the nervous system that moving real fast is actually something we can do safely. As a result, the blocks get lifted.

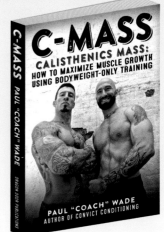

Lift those mental blocks! Watch the fastest humans in the world do their thing. Speed them up, digitally—your subconscious won't know the difference! Imagine yourself moving with lightning speed, again and again. Picture yourself as dynamite—think of the words *fast* and *loose*. Banish words like *slow* or *rusty* from your mental vocab. Cultivate a positive, speed-based *mindset*. If your performance needs improving, never say to yourself: *I'm too slow!* Say: *I can go faster!*

...And you know what, kid? You will.

LIGHTS OUT!

If there's a take-home message on really maximizing your speed, it's this: *keep training faster*. We can talk about scientific laws and biological ideas and whatnot, but it's really not weird or esoteric. You need to move efficiently and perform lots and lots of reps, all the while *thinking* you are fast, and trying to move as fast as you can. Accept no limits.

Let's finish with a quote from one of the truly great speedsters—the legendary Bruce Lee. At a martial arts seminar, the movie star was harassed by an eager fan who was desperate to improve his punching speed. He kept on asking whether Bruce could help him—if he could share any "secret" tips or advice.

With the whimsical-but-wise deadpan expression he was famous for, the master replied simply: *Sure. Punch faster.*

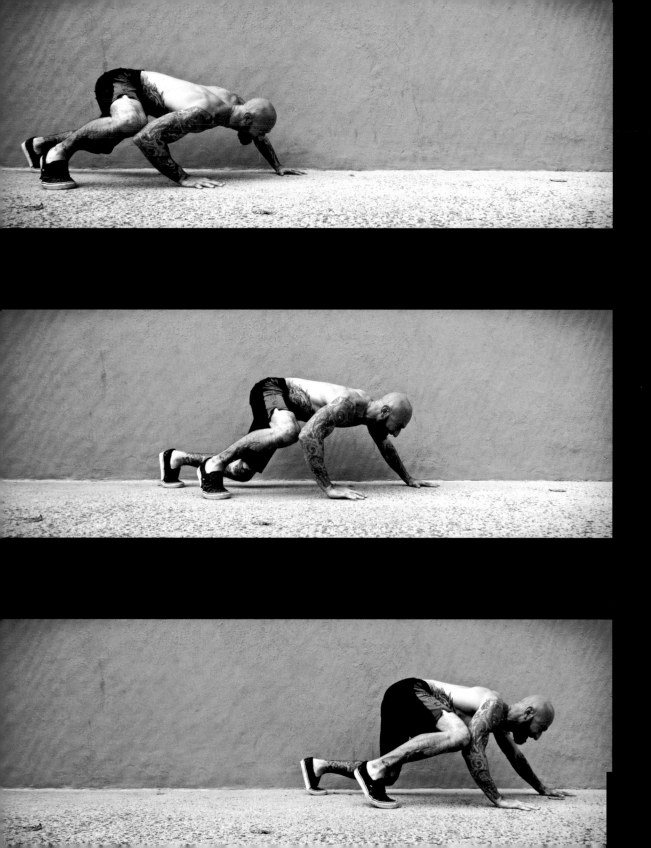

Bonus Section 2
ANIMAL AGILITY DRILLS

Wait! We're still not done yet, kid. I'm convinced that any bodyweight book on speed, power and agility would be incomplete without including some of the most interesting and unusual movements found in calisthenics: *animal drills*.

I've included the major ten animal-type movements in this final bonus section. The majority of them are quadrilateral crawling movements, but some are bipedal or performed hanging. There are scores of animal movements, but the bulk of them are just variations of these basics that have been tinkered with (feel free to mix and match to make your own creations). Bear in mind also that each of these techniques can be performed going *forwards*, *backwards* or *sideways* to work the muscles in totally different ways; so you actually have at least 30 different movements here.

Mimicking animal movements to promote strength and fitness is nothing new. The practice can be traced back to ancient kung fu forms—conceivably even further (Paleolithic cave paintings exist showing men adopting animal postures). Animal drills are a true "wild card", an *x-factor* to add to your power and strength training. Conventional exercises—like jumps, pushups, pullups—tend to be *linear*. The body goes up and down. In animal drills, the body tends to move in an *asymmetrical* manner—one leg/arm before the other. This exposes the body to *lateral* and *torque* forces which develop the small muscles that criss-cross the trunk and hip/shoulder girdles, increasing strength and efficiency and going a long way to reducing risk of injury. This type of movement also promotes total-body coordination and dexterity.

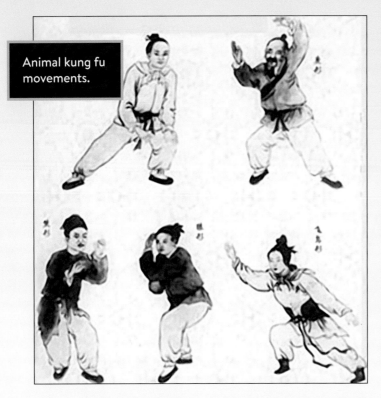

Animal kung fu movements.

For these reasons, you may want to experiment with the following drills in your workouts. They work well as warm-ups or finishing movements, or you can sling one (or two, or three) of these in the middle of your workout to break things up and add variety.

It's difficult to count reps on these techniques, so just focus on the movements, stretching and tensing the muscles. Go until you are good and warm, and not much further. A good rule of thumb is: *keep springy*. These are not good endurance exercises: don't keep going on and on, until you are exhausted and crying, longing for death. It's not a Jerry Lewis Telethon.

BEAR WALKS

This is a great "crawl" or all-fours walk for beginners and experts alike. You can bend your legs, but keep your arms straight and try to keep your butt high in the air without rounding your spine too much. Walk on, young master—it's a great, simple workout for the arms, abs, and chest. The bent-over position also trains the hamstrings, glutes and spine.

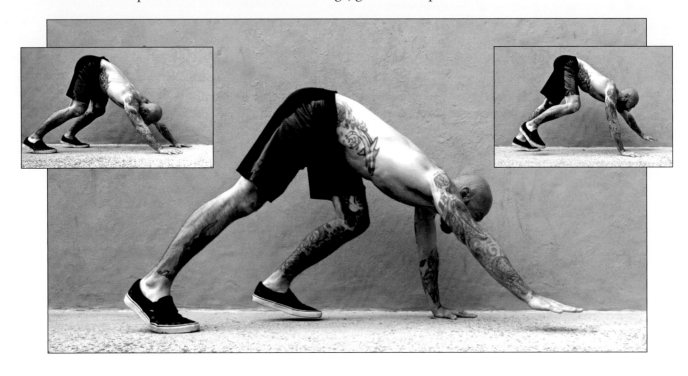

PANTHER STALK

I've heard some folks call this wriggly beaut *Spider-man crawls*. Get down low on all-fours, and "stalk" forwards, touching the knee to the elbow on the same side—that's the key to really activating the "lateral chain" on this exercise. Try to keep your butt down if you can. You can also perform this exercise with your entire body as close to the ground as possible, without touching (except for the palms and toes). This variation is sometimes called the *crocodile* (*below*).

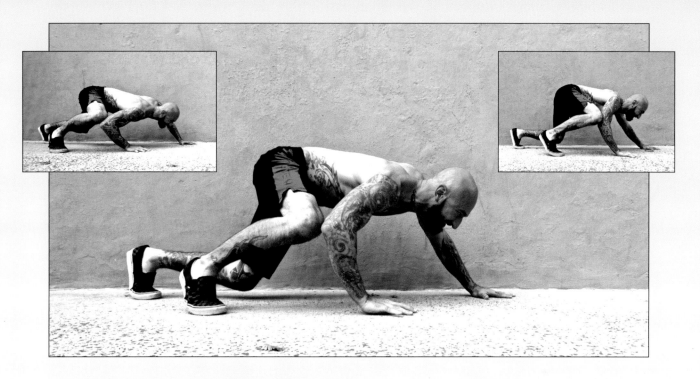

VARIANT: CROCODILE WALK

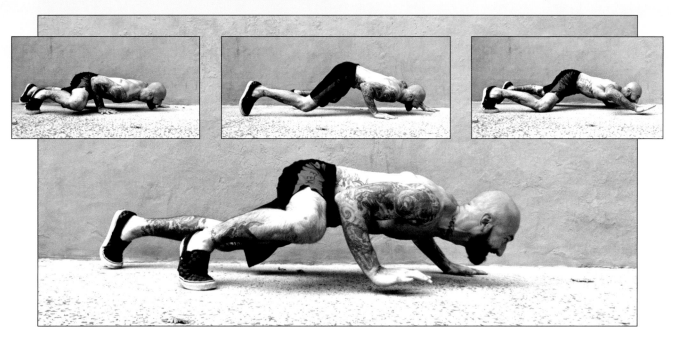

DOG SPRINT

We don't need to shoe-horn any artificial sense of technique in here—let nature take the lead. Did you ever try to run on all fours as a kid? You were getting a killer workout, and you never realized. Do it now! You'll notice that if you really try to run fast, your hands will take point, followed by the legs; you extend your body, pushing through the legs, and repeat. You will probably "lead" with one side—that's cool. This is very similar to the way a dog runs full tilt. Despite our years as bipeds, humans can actually get pretty fast at this: the world record for 100 meters is 16.87 seconds by Kenichi Ito. Some folks can't run that fast on two damn legs.

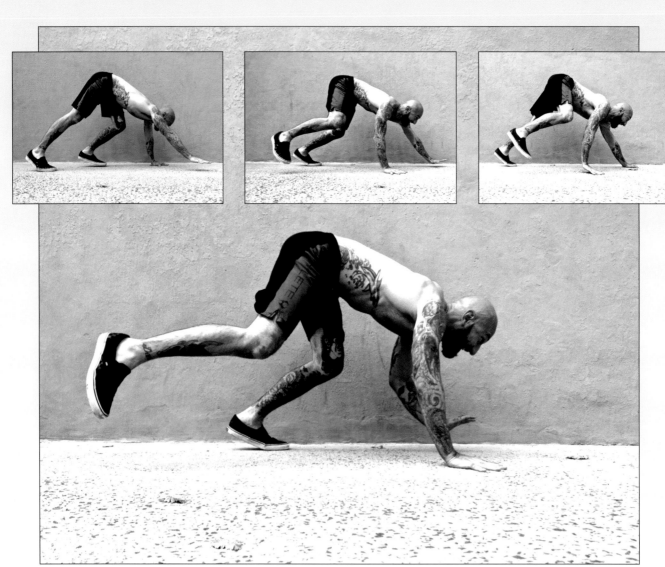

LOCUST JUMPS

This one is a wonderful total-body warmer. Get into a pushup position with the legs close together. Bend the arms until your chest is a few inches from the ground, and just hop forward in short little jumps. Try to cross the room this way if you can, with only the palms and toes making contact with the ground. Don't panic if that sounds confusing: this sucker's probably tougher to describe than it is to do. This exercise—like so many great calisthenics techniques—has always been a favorite in India, but it became more popular in the West in the sixties after the late, great B.K.S. Iyengar described it in his epic manual *Light on Yoga*.

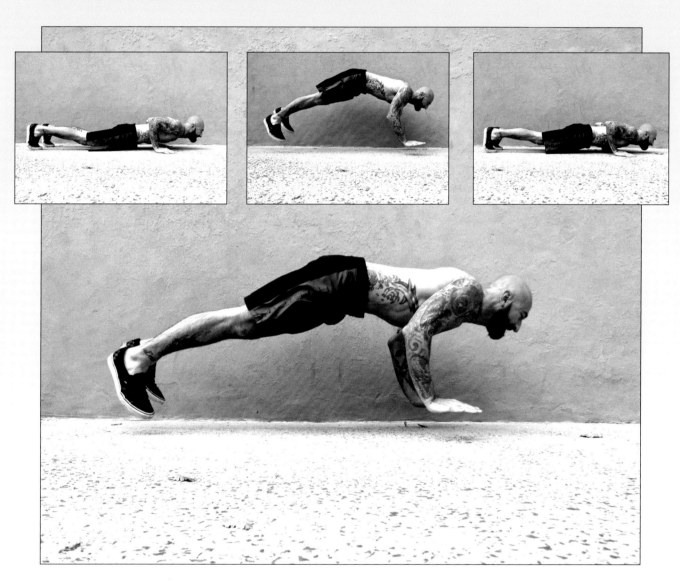

CRAB WALK

The *crab walk* is an important animal drill, because it is performed *prone*—ass down. Walking like this is a fantastic workout for the back muscles, particularly the muscles around the shoulder-blades: the triceps also get a blast. Keeping the body upright is a challenge for the trunk muscles. The crab walk is a great reminder that these drills can be performed forwards, backwards or side-ways—diagonally is fun, too. Each direction feels totally different. A more advanced variation can be performed by walking in a *bridge hold* (*opposite*).

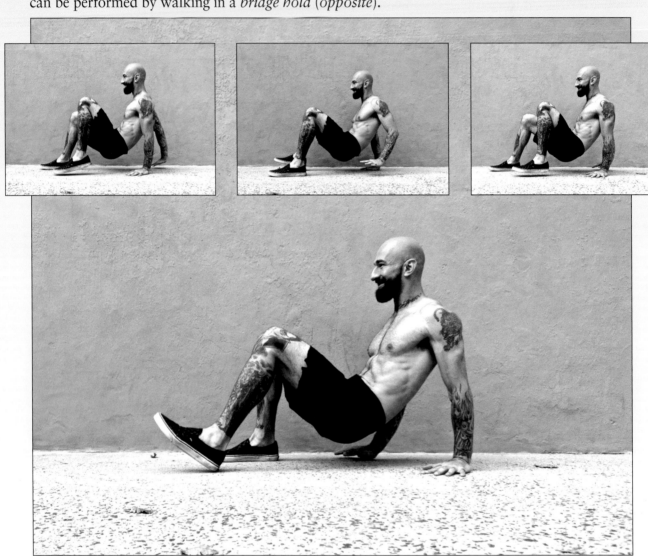

VARIANT: ADVANCED CRAB WALK

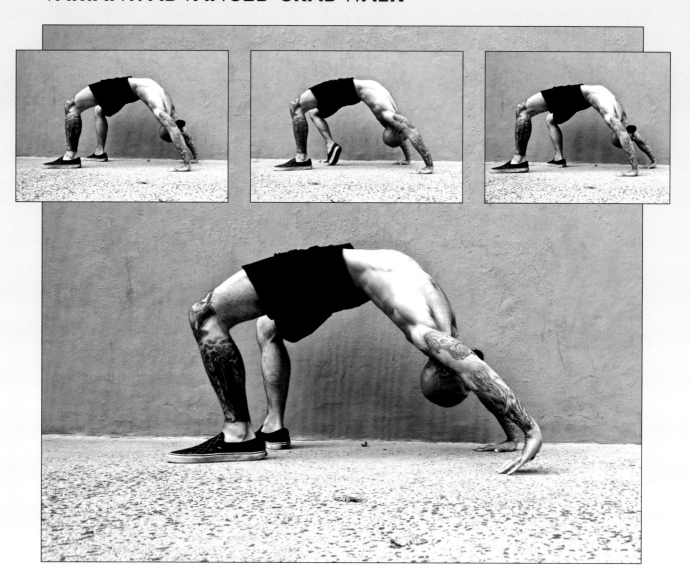

DUCK WALK

This animal drill is a *bipedal* technique: it's performed on two limbs, unlike crawling work. Squat down as deep as you can, and walk around, keeping as low as possible. This builds tension-flexibility in the hips, thighs, knees and ankles. A very, very valuable movement drill, and a great example of how calisthenics basics (the *deep squat*) can be toyed with in ways that radically improve mobility and joint health. Experts can even get pretty fast in this movement.

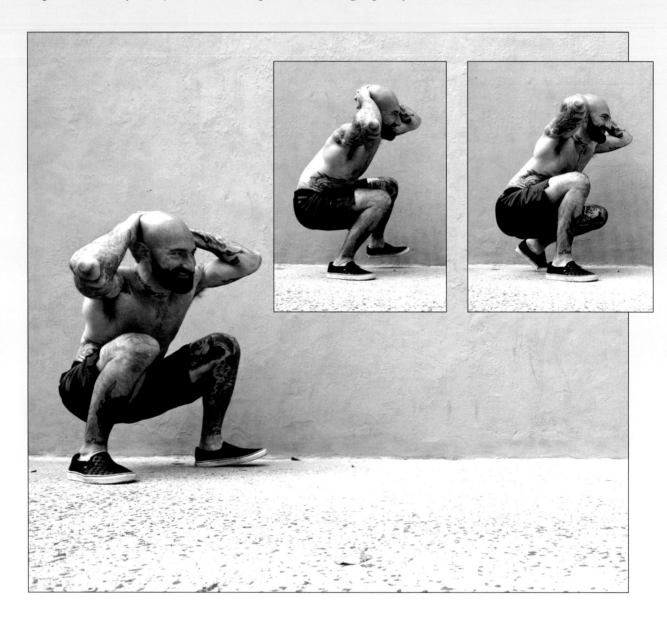

KANGAROO HOP

    This little jump is a companion movement to the *duck walk*. Instead of walking in a deep stance, you jump from spot-to-spot. Remain springy during this one by keeping on the balls of your feet. For a harder stretch, drop onto your heels (*below*). Keeping your arms behind your head is an advanced variation which will really build good balance, too. If that position is too tough, you can place your hands on the floor to steady yourself in-between jumps.

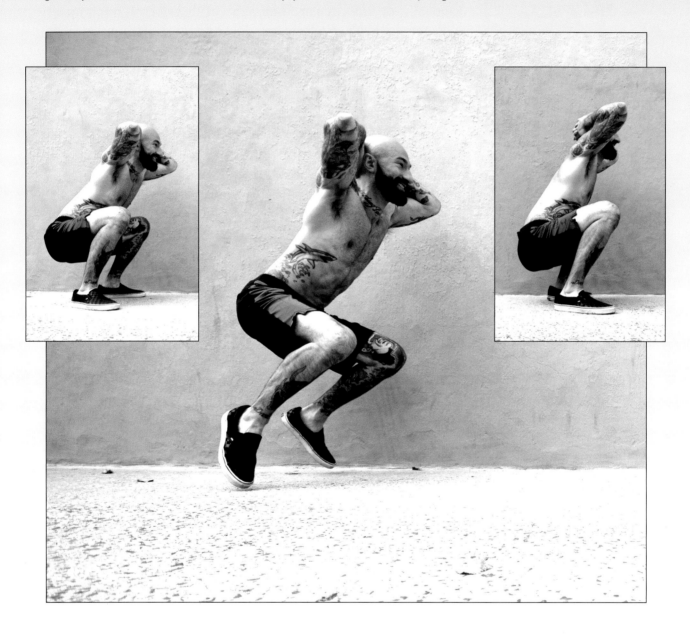

CHIMP SWING

Who said animal drills have to take place on the *ground*? Plenty of animals move around in trees (*arboreal locomotion*, kiddo). Let's get in on the fun—and the benefits. A basic, easy start is to just hang down from a horizontal bar and *swing*. You can swing backwards or forward, or from side-to-side (*shown*). You can also try swinging diagonally, or in a circular fashion. See if that doesn't reach upper-body muscles in places where you didn't know you had places.

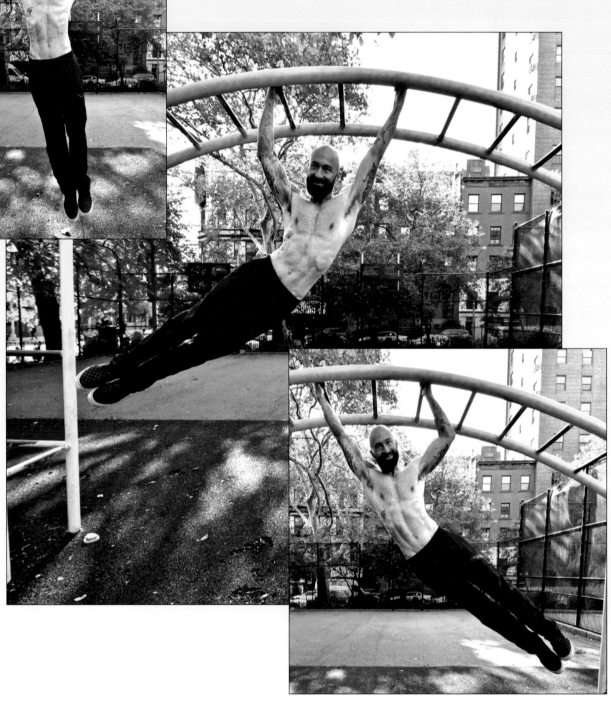

BAT-FLIPS

Ever seen a bat hanging from a tree by its feet? Well, you aren't dangling upside-down for this one, but the idea's there, right? Hang from a bar, and bring the knees up for a little momentum; quickly use that momentum to flip your hands over. Then reverse it. Wonderful explosive grip work, working the forearms, elbows, shoulders and even the abs. (For more variations, check out the grip training chapter in *Convict Conditioning 2*.)

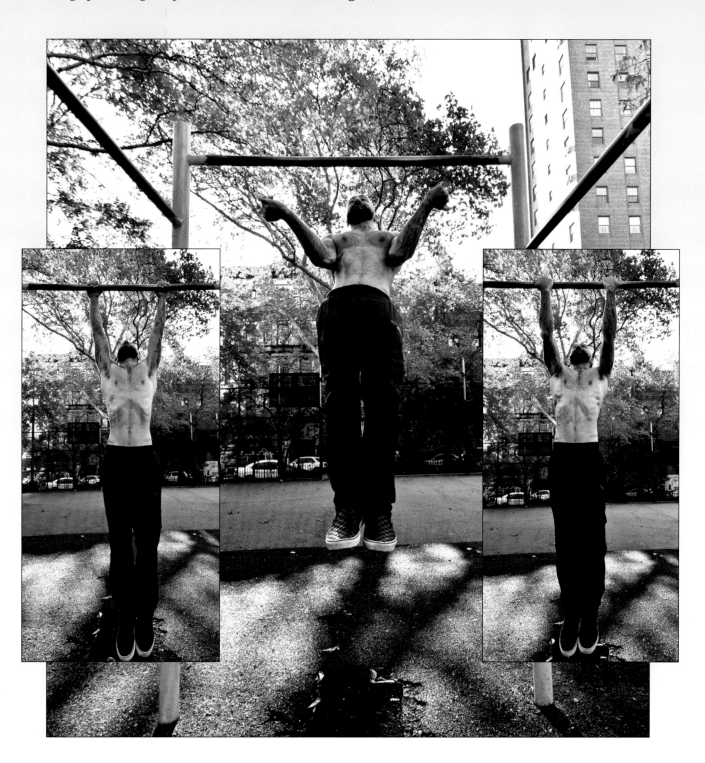

MONKEY TURNS

Here's a more complex hanging exercise; it requires extra strength, especially in the grip and small muscles, since for some of the drill you are hanging one-handed. With an overhand grip, reverse the grip on one hand (making it underhand). Let go with the overhand grip, turning to face behind you as you grip again with an underhand grip: repeat in reverse. This version is designed for a straight horizontal bar, but if you have access to a big jungle gym or monkey bars, then you can freestyle on those (*as seen on opposite page*).

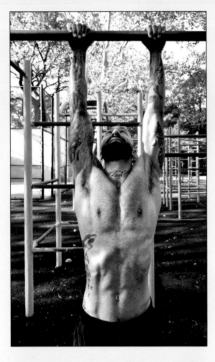
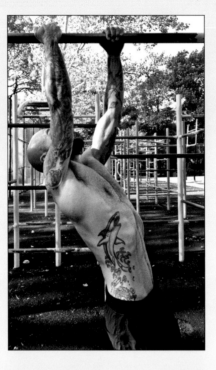
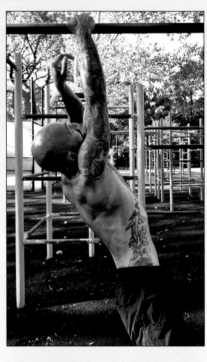
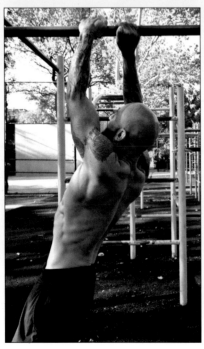
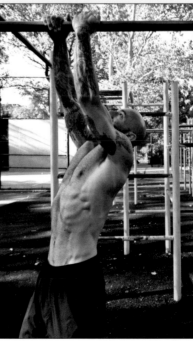
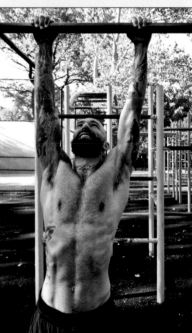

EXPLOSIVE CALISTHENICS

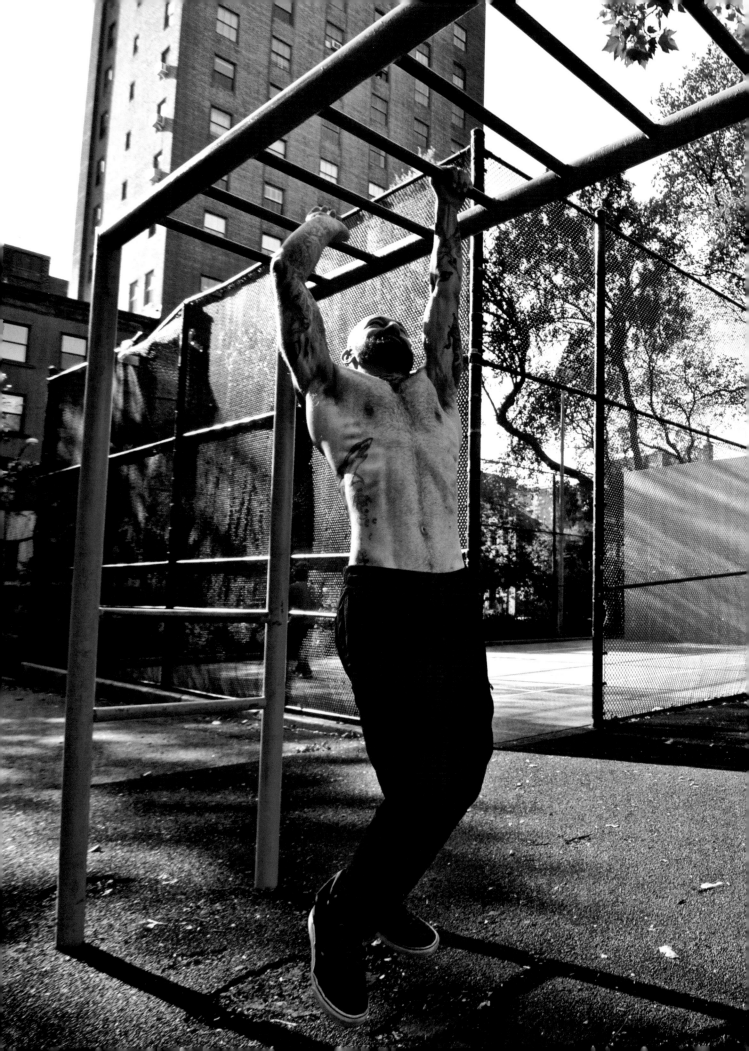

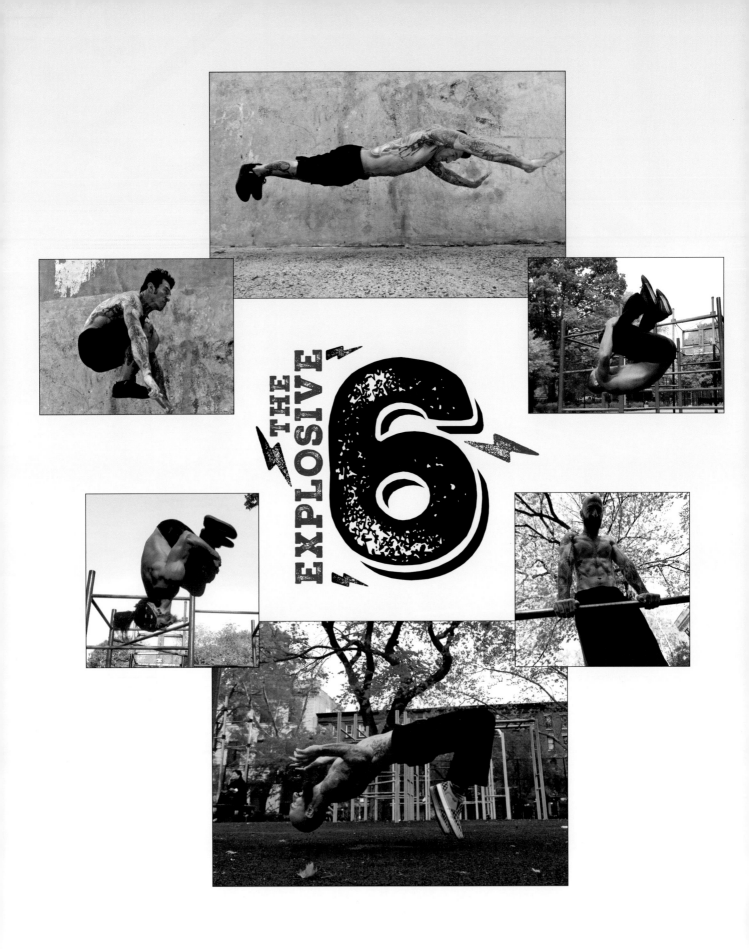

THE EXPLOSIVE 6

EXPLOSIVE CALISTHENICS

THE EXPLOSIVE 6

COMPLETE PROGRESSION CHARTS

1 2 3 4 5 6 7 8 9 M

POWER JUMP CHAIN

STEP 1	STRAIGHT HOP	**STEP 6**	SLAP TUCK JUMP
STEP 2	SQUAT JUMP	**STEP 7**	TUCK JUMP
STEP 3	VERTICAL LEAP	**STEP 8**	CATCH TUCK JUMP
STEP 4	BLOCK JUMP	**STEP 9**	THREAD JUMP
STEP 5	BUTT-KICK JUMP	**MASTER STEP**	SUICIDE JUMP

POWER PUSHUP CHAIN

STEP 1	INCLINE POP-UP	**STEP 6**	HIP-STRIKE PUSHUP
STEP 2	KNEELING PUSH-OFF	**STEP 7**	CONVICT PUSHUP
STEP 3	POP-UP	**STEP 8**	HALF-SUPER
STEP 4	CLAP PUSHUP	**STEP 9**	FULL BODY POP-UP
STEP 5	CHEST-STRIKE PUSHUP	**MASTER STEP**	THE SUPERMAN

KIP-UP CHAIN

STEP 1 ROLLING SIT-UP	**STEP 6** HALF KIP
STEP 2 ROLLING SQUAT	**STEP 7** KIP-UP
STEP 3 SHOULDER POP	**STEP 8** STRAIGHT LEG KIP-UP
STEP 4 BRIDGE KIP	**STEP 9** WUSHU KIP-UP
STEP 5 BUTT KIP	**MASTER STEP** NO-HANDS KIP-UP

FRONT FLIP CHAIN

STEP 1 SHOULDER ROLL	**STEP 6** FRONT HANDSPRING
STEP 2 PRESS ROLL	**STEP 7** FLYSPRING
STEP 3 JUMP ROLL	**STEP 8** BACK-DROP FLIP
STEP 4 HANDSTAND ROLL	**STEP 9** RUNNING FRONT FLIP
STEP 5 BACK-DROP HANDSPRING	**MASTER STEP** FRONT FLIP

BACK FLIP CHAIN

STEP **1**	REAR SHOULDER ROLL	STEP **6**	MONKEY FLIP
STEP **2**	REAR PRESS ROLL	STEP **7**	BACK HANDSPRING
STEP **3**	BRIDGE KICK-OVER	STEP **8**	1 ARM BACK HANDSPRING
STEP **4**	SIDE MACACO	STEP **9**	4 POINT BACK FLIP
STEP **5**	BACK MACACO	MASTER STEP	BACK FLIP

MUSCLE-UP CHAIN

STEP **1**	SWING KIP	STEP **6**	CHEST PULLUP
STEP **2**	JUMPING PULLUP	STEP **7**	HIP PULLUP
STEP **3**	KIPPING PULLUP	STEP **8**	JUMPING PULLOVER
STEP **4**	PULLUP HOP	STEP **9**	BAR PULLOVER
STEP **5**	CLAP PULLUP	MASTER STEP	MUSCLE-UP

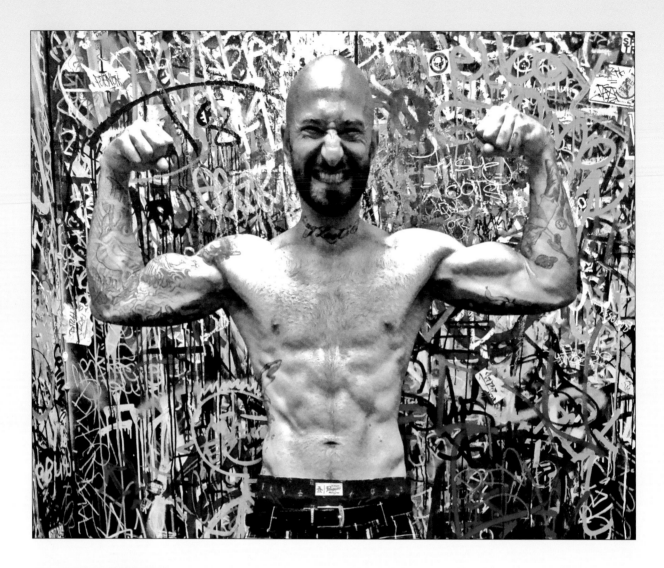

AL KAVADLO

Al Kavadlo is probably the planet's most recognizable bodyweight athlete. For my money, he is the world's greatest calisthenics coach, too. He is the Lead Instructor of Dragon Door's internationally-acclaimed *Progressive Calisthenics Certification* (PCC). Al is also the best-selling author of the training manuals **Raising the Bar**, **Pushing the Limits**, **Stretching your Boundaries** and the now-classic **We're Working Out!** Al can be found at *www.AlKavadlo.com*.

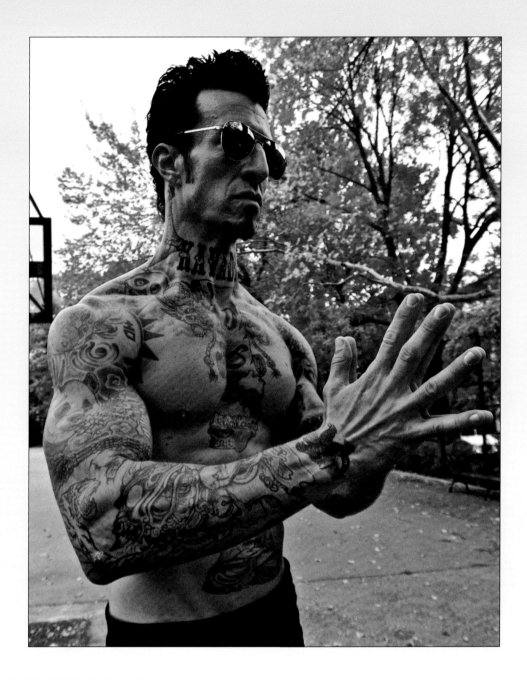

DANNY KAVADLO

Danny Kavadlo is one of the world's most established and respected personal trainers. He is currently the only athlete to achieve the Master Instructor rank with Dragon Door's *Progressive Calisthenics Certification* (PCC). Danny is also the author of the critically-acclaimed books: *Everybody Needs Training* and *Diamond-Cut Abs*. Danny's unique motivational style has earned him a huge number of fans, and that number is growing by the day. The man's website is *www.DannyTheTrainer.com*.

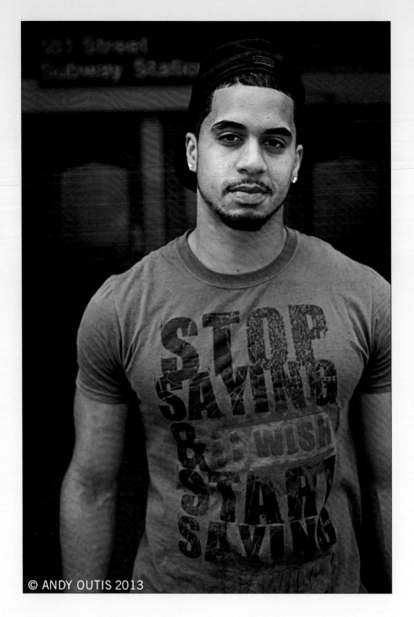
© ANDY OUTIS 2013

JOSE "VERTICAL" JIMENEZ

Vertical has been training parkour for over nine years now and through parkour he was introduced to *Barstarzz* or *Street Workout*. A huge fan of calisthenics, Vertical started training with the Barstarzz in 2009 and in the same year he became an official member. Being a practitioner of parkour, Vertical was able to become a stuntman for movies, films, commercials, shows, and many other gigs. "I am extremely grateful for the path that I have chosen for my life. I am currently still training and getting stronger, faster, better every day."

Barstarzz.com

https://www.youtube.com/user/Verticalmotionpk

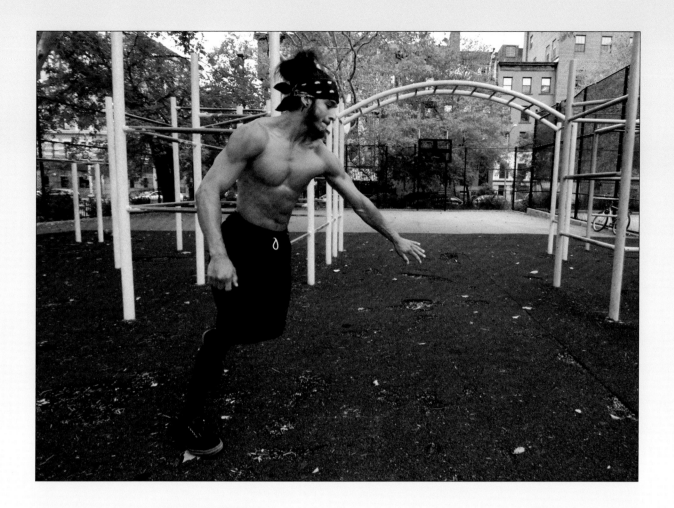

LUCIANO ACUNA JR.

"I was always a monkey playing in the parks and jungle gyms, jumping and flipping off of anything and everything." With his friends, Luciano used to perform mini "shows" at the park from the ages of 11-14. From a young age, he played all kinds of sports. One of his greatest achievements was choosing to be a senior "walk-on" wrestler. Subsequently, he had a 16-0 record in the year of 2007 with his Grand Street Wolves Wrestling team; this was the epic year they became the Undefeated City Champions. After graduating, Luciano continued his acrobatic training where he discovered a movement called parkour/freerunning. This is also how he came across extreme calisthenics and street workouts. After falling in love with these disciplines/movements, it opened up an opportunity to start a career, and Luciano used these mixed talents to do modeling and filming gigs. While having side gigs, he was part of the *New York Knicks Acroback Tumblers* at Madison Square Garden. From there he got into the stunt world, which has thus led to his current careers as professional stuntman, actor, model, acrobat, and American Ninja Warrior competitor. Luciano plans on spreading wellness and athletic education by reopening the new *BKLYN BEAST* facility before 2016. The facility will have all kinds of instructional classes and open sessions for all ages, all in a safe environment to train and evolve from human beings to human BEASTS.

www.bklynbeast.com • *instagram.com/luckyluciano112*

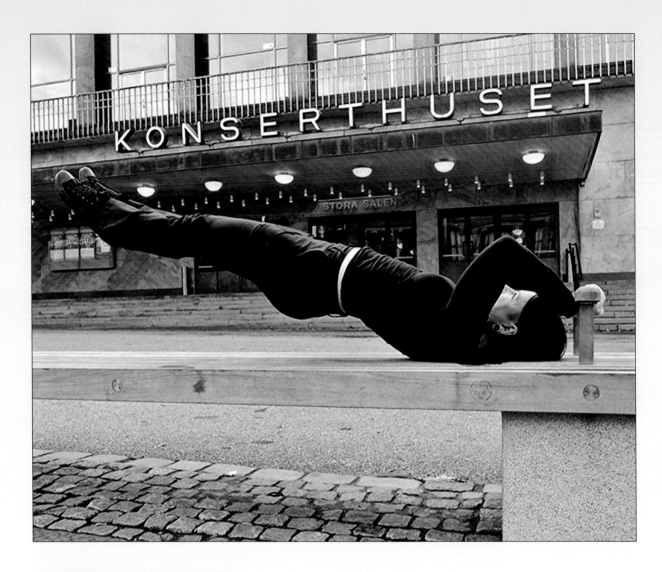

ADRIENNE HARVEY

Adrienne Harvey (Senior PCC) also deserves a heads-up here, as an invaluable figure in Dragon Door's *Progressive Calisthenics Certification*. Very few athletes really *get* progressive bodyweight training the way Adrienne does. Adrienne is also a highly sought-out personal trainer and popular figure in the fitness world. She is an RKC Level 2 certified kettlebell instructor, CK-FMS, and maintains the website *www.GiryaGirl.com*.

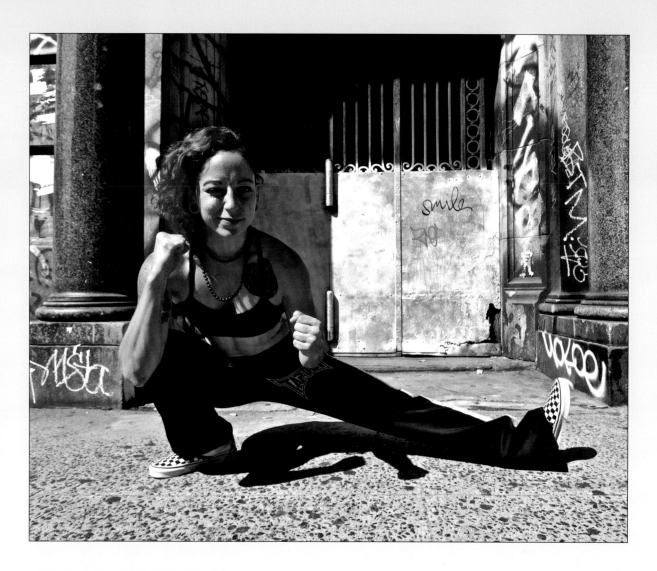

GRACE MENENDEZ

The totally badass Grace Menendez PCC was kind enough to donate some shots to the project. Grace is a Cuban Yoga teacher, personal trainer and is currently the reigning Calisthenics Queen of NYC! Connect with her at: *www.DieselGrace.com*.

PHOTO CREDITS

Director of Photography: Al Kavadlo

Original photos by: Al Kavadlo, Danny Kavadlo, Grace Menendez, Adrienne Harvey, Michael Polito and George Pruitt.

For the truly excellent image on page 304, I'm hella grateful for the kick-ass photographic skills of Danny's beautiful wife, Jennifer. Jen, you always deliver the best shot in the book. Thank you!

Al's buddy, the *amazing* Bob Rothchild was kind enough to bust out the wonderful full kip you see on page 252. Sir, you're a goddamn inspiration. Thanks!

The uber-cool Michael Polito also acted as a model—many thanks my friend. Michael is a legit black belt, so was the perfect choice to demo the jump kick!

The wonderful twisting flip image in chapter 7 was kindly provided by the awesome graphic designer Ray Dak Lam. The athlete was Jacob Jung. Thank you, Ray! Check out the man's fantastic portfolio at *www.behance.net/raydak*.

The parkour railing jump image in chapter 3 is attributable to Marco Gomes, and has been cropped.

The parkour jump image in chapter 4 is attributable to THOR (Parkour Foundation Winter) and has been cropped.

The parkour flip image in chapter 7 is attributable to "Rich Tea" and has been cropped.

The back flip image in chapter 10 is attributable to Andree Magill and has been cropped.

The parkour leap image in chapter 11 is attributable to Tony Hisgett and has been cropped.

The Wayne Gretzky image in Bonus Section 1 is attributable to Rick Dikeman and has been cropped.

The wing chun image in Bonus Section 1 is attributable to Ebmastr and has been cropped.

The Tom Wong image in Bonus Section 1 is attributable to Tom Wong and has been cropped.

The sparring image in Bonus Section 1 is attributable to Whorah and has been cropped and recolored.

All other images in this book have been either deemed to be in the public domain or utilized in the spirit of Fair Use.

ACKNOWLEDGEMENTS

In the dedication I called John Du Cane the *world's greatest innovator in fitness*. I wasn't just blowing smoke when I said that. The top three hottest trends in modern fitness are probably intermittent fasting, bodyweight strength, and kettlebell training. John brought intermittent fasting to the world's attention when he published Ori Hofmekler's groundbreaking **Warrior Diet**; he made kettlebells famous by teaming up with Pavel Tsatsouline and manufacturing the monsters; and goddamn if he isn't also the brains behind the cutting-edge bodyweight strength revolution, founding the international *Progressive Calisthenics Certification* (PCC) project. God bless you my friend, for everything you have given to me, my family, and the world.

It's bull to tell you that Al and Danny Kavadlo were just *models* for this book. In reality, this work was a *collaboration* between myself and them. They took photos, provided encouragement, and improved *everything* I sent them. As ever, Al—despite being decades younger than me—offered me invaluable instruction, advice and guidance on multiple key aspects of this book: he was even involved in the design stage. Very few readers of this manual will understand what these men give to bodyweight—for free—on a daily basis. Their massive success renews my faith in the fitness world. A student of mine once jokingly referred to me as "another Kavadlo brother", and he had no idea how much that meant to me. Thanks, my brothers.

Derek Brigham: you are undoubtedly the greatest graphic designer on the scene today. Given the hundreds of images, notes and errors you patiently waded through—and turned into gold—you are probably a candidate for sainthood, also. God bless ya, Big D. Check the genius at: *www.DBrigham.com*.

My profound thanks goes out to all the CC fans who asked for this book—if it hadn't been for you folks, I *promise* you this book would not have seen the light of day. Thank you for believing in me: this one is for all of you.

And finally, to Joe Hartigen: thank you for everything you taught me. I apologize for not doing justice to your wisdom.

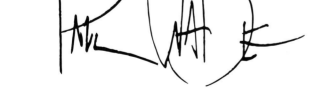

Get Harder, Stronger, More Powerful and Ripped to Shreds—with PCC, the World's Premier Bodyweight Exercise Training Program

Based on the teachings of Convict Conditioning founder, PAUL WADE… led by AL and DANNY KAVADLO

PCC
PROGRESSIVE CALISTHENICS CERTIFICATION

The Progressive Calisthenics Certification Workshop (PCC)

Dragon Door's Progressive Calisthenics Certification (PCC) provides you the world's most comprehensive training in the core principles and fundamentals of bodyweight exercise for strength and conditioning.

Master the cutting-edge bodyweight exercise progressions developed by *Convict Conditioning* founder **Paul Wade**—and earn the right to teach this acclaimed system to athletes, martial artists, trainers, coaches and all men and women dedicated to the cultivation of supreme strength and rugged toughness.

Discover how to generate tigrish power, enhance your co-ordination and balance, protect your joints, transform your physique, build steel-like tendon integrity and blowtorch fat from your body.

» **Boost your value as a coach or personal trainer.** Not only are the movements extraordinarily cool—and adjustable to any skill level—they are also amongst the most effective, functional techniques on earth.

» **The PCC represents the ultimate bodyweight cert, and whatever your field or specialization**—from strength training to rehab, bodybuilding to team sports—you will come away from this three-day cert with vast resources of training knowledge unavailable anywhere else.

CONVICT CONDITIONING

How to Bust Free of All Weakness—Using the Lost Secrets of Supreme Survival Strength

BY PAUL "COACH" WADE

Find a PCC Workshop in your area:
www.dragondoor.com/workshops/pccworkshop/

24 HOURS A DAY ORDER NOW 1-800-899-5111
Visit: www.dragondoor.com

The Best Training Resolution You Can Make: Log Yourself—All Year Long!

The Fastest Way to Make Physical Progress a Guarantee— Besides Dedicated, Skillful Practice—Is to Keep a Training Log

We've all heard the phrase 'the spirit is willing but the flesh is weak'. And never was this more true than in the quest for strength!

So, what are the two golden keys, or secrets to bending the flesh to the spirit's desire?

The first secret is the system—and the system is dedicated, organized application over time. And in the hard world of strength that means keeping track of your goals and measuring your progress. When it comes to serious training, you keep a log or you fail. The sins of sloppiness, haphazardness, laziness and disorganization lay waste to our dreams of physical achievement—and sabotage the best intentions to beat our flesh into righteous steel. We invite you to exorcize the demons of weakness from your flesh—with a "religious" dedication to tracking and measuring—*Convict Conditioning* style.

The second secret for strength success is inspiration. In this stunning companion to his best-selling bodyweight exercise masterpieces, Convict Conditioning author Paul Wade, goes far, far beyond the traditional log book—by delivering a bucket-load of inspiring stories and jewel-like training tips to push you forward in your quest for ever-greater strength.

This book is the first-ever training log designed specifically for bodyweight athletes. Other logs are structured to contain sections where you detail the amount of weight you used, the type of equipment or machine you worked out on, even what your heart-rate was and what vitamins you took today. You won't find any of this distracting information in this log. It's a log for pure, unadulterated, hardcore bodyweight training. We provide the inspiration and the structure— you provide the perspiration and bloody-mindedness to seize the plan and make it happen.

There is a window of opportunity awaiting you. The strength gains that have continued to elude you can finally be yours. That window of opportunity lies within these pages and within your heart. Bring it!

By far the best log book we have seen, frankly, is **Paul Wade's *Convict Conditioning Ultimate Bodyweight Training Log***. But don't think that you have to use it just for your bodyweight work. It'll serve just as well to document your progress with kettlebells, martial arts or any other practice.

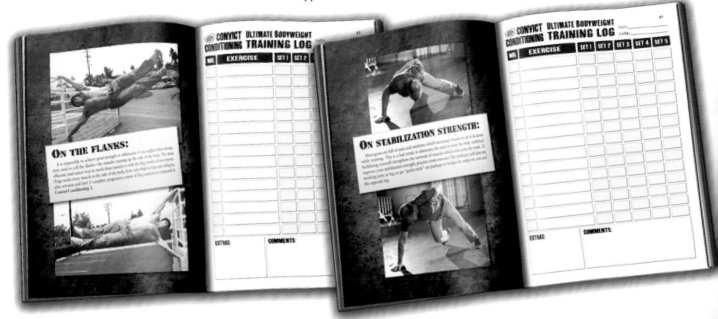

Reader Praise for *Convict Conditioning Ultimate Bodyweight Training Log*

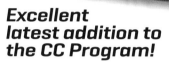

Above and Beyond!

"Not JUST a log book. TONS of great and actually useful info. I really like to over complicate programming and data entries at times. And honestly, All one has to do is fill in the blanks... Well that and DO THE WORK. Great product."
—Noel Price, Chicagoland, IL

A unique training log

"This log book is one of a kind in the world. It is the only published body weight exclusive training log I have personally seen. It is well structured and provides everything for a log book in a primarily body weight oriented routine. The book is best integrated with the other books in the convict conditioning series however has enough information to act as a stand alone unit. It is a must have for anyone who is a fan of the convict conditioning series or is entering into calisthenics." — Carter D., Cambridge, Canada

Excellent Companion to Convict Conditioning 1 & 2

"This is an amazing book! If you are a fan of Convict Conditioning (1 & 2) you need to get this training log. If you are preparing for the Progressive Calisthenics Certification then it's a must-have!!! The spiral bound format is a huge improvement over the regular binding and it makes it that much more functional for use in the gym. Great design, amazing pictures and additional content! Once again - Great job Dragon Door!"
—Michael Krivka, RKC Team Leader, Gaithersburg, MD

Excellent latest addition to the CC Program!

"A terrific book to keep you on track and beyond. Thank you again for this incredible series!"
—Joshua Hatcher, Holyoke, MA

Calling this a Log Book is Selling it Short

"I thought, what is the big deal about a logbook! Seriously mistaken. It is a work of art and with tips on each page that would be a great book all by itself. Get it. It goes way beyond a log book...the logging part of this book is just a bonus. You must have this!"—Jon Engum, Brainerd, MN

The Ultimate Bodyweight Conditioning

"I have started to incorporate bodyweight training into my strength building when I am not going to the gym. At the age of 68, after 30 years in the gym the 'Convict Conditioning Log' is going to be a welcome new training challenge."
—William Hayden, Winter Park, FL

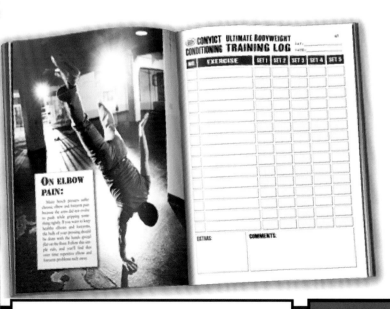

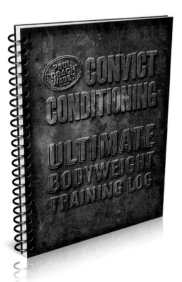

Convict Conditioning Ultimate Bodyweight Training Log

By Paul "Coach" Wade
#B67 $29.95
eBook $19.95
Paperback (spiral bound) 6 x 9
290 pages 175 photos

Beginner   Mid-Level   Advanced

How Do YOU Stack Up Against These 6 Signs of a TRUE Physical Specimen?

According to Paul Wade's *Convict Conditioning* you earn the right to call yourself a 'true physical specimen' if you can perform the following:

1. AT LEAST one set of 5 one-arm pushups each side—with the ELITE goal of 100 sets each side

2. AT LEAST one set of 5 one-leg squats each side—with the ELITE goal of 2 sets of 50 each side

3. AT LEAST a single one-arm pullup each side—with the ELITE goal of 2 sets of 6 each side

4. AT LEAST one set of 5 hanging straight leg raises—with the ELITE goal of 2 sets of 30

5. AT LEAST one stand-to-stand bridge—with the ELITE goal of 2 sets of 30

6. AT LEAST a single one-arm handstand pushup on each side— with the ELITE goal of 1 set of 5

Well, how DO you stack up?

Chances are that whatever athletic level you have achieved, there are some serious gaps in your OVERALL strength program. Gaps that stop you short of being able to claim status as a truly accomplished strength athlete.

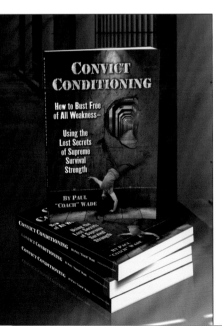

The good news is that—in *Convict Conditioning*—Paul Wade has laid out a brilliant 6-set system of 10 progressions which allows you to master these elite levels.

And you could be starting at almost any age and in almost in any condition...

Paul Wade has given you the keys—ALL the keys you'll ever need— that will open door, after door, after door for you in your quest for supreme physical excellence. Yes, it will be the hardest work you'll ever have to do. And yes, 97% of those who pick up *Convict Conditioning*, frankly, won't have the guts and the fortitude to make it. But if you make it even half-way through **Paul's Progressions**, you'll be stronger than almost anyone you encounter. Ever.

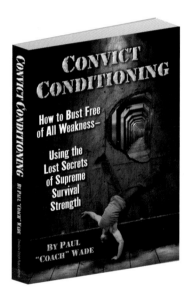

1 Beginner 2 Mid-Level 3 Advanced

Convict Conditioning

How to Bust Free of All Weakness—Using the Lost Secrets of Supreme Survival Strength

By Paul "Coach" Wade
#B41 $39.95
eBook $19.95

Paperback 8.5 x 11 320 pages
191 photos, charts and illustrations

Dragon Door Customer Acclaim for Paul Wade's *Convict Conditioning*

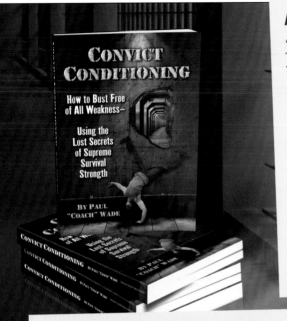

A Strength Training Guide That Will Never Be Duplicated!

"I knew within the first chapter of reading this book that I was in for something special and unique. The last time I felt this same feeling was when reading *Power to the People!* To me this is the Body Weight equivalent to Pavel's masterpiece.

Books like this can never be duplicated. Paul Wade went through a unique set of circumstances of doing time in prison with an 'old time' master of calisthenics. Paul took these lessons from this 70 year old strong man and mastered them over a period of 20 years while 'doing time'. He then taught these methods to countless prisoners and honed his teaching to perfection.

I believe that extreme circumstances like this are what it takes to create a true masterpiece. I know that 'masterpiece' is a strong word, but this is as close as it gets. No other body weight book I have read (and I have a huge fitness library)...comes close to this as far as gaining incredible strength from body weight exercise.

Just like Power to the People, I am sure I will read this over and over again...mastering the principles that Paul Wade took 20 years to master.

Outstanding Book!"—*Rusty Moore - Fitness Black Book - Seattle, WA*

A must for all martial artists

"As a dedicated martial artist for more than seven years, this book is exactly what I've been looking for.

For a while now I have trained with machines at my local gym to improve my muscle strength and power and get to the next level in my training. I always felt that the modern health club, technology based exercise jarred with my martial art though, which only required body movement.

Finally this book has come along. At last I can combine perfect body movement for martial skill with perfect body exercise for ultimate strength.

All fighting arts are based on body movement. This book is a complete textbook on how to max out your musclepower using only body movement, as different from dumbbells, machines or gadgets. For this reason it belongs on the bookshelf of every serious martial artist, male and female, young and old."—*Gino Cartier - Washington DC*

I've packed all of my other training books away!

"I read CC in one go. I couldn't put it down. I have purchased a lot of body-weight training books in the past, and have always been pretty disappointed. They all seem to just have pictures of different exercises, and no plan whatsoever on how to implement them and progress with them. But not with this one. The information in this book is AWESOME! I like to have a clear, logical plan of progression to follow, and that is what this book gives. I have put all of my other training books away. CC is the only system I am going to follow. This is now my favorite training book ever!"—*Lyndan - Australia*

Brutal Elegance.

"I have been training and reading about training since I first joined the US Navy in the 1960s. I thought I'd seen everything the fitness world had to offer. Sometimes twice. But I was wrong. This book is utterly iconoclastic.

The author breaks down all conceivable body weight exercises into six basic movements, each designed to stimulate different vectors of the muscular system. These six are then elegantly and very intelligently broken into ten progressive techniques. You master one technique, and move on to the next.

The simplicity of this method belies a very powerful and complex training paradigm, reduced into an abstraction that obviously took many years of sweat and toil to develop.

Trust me. Nobody else worked this out. This approach is completely unique and fresh.

I have read virtually every calisthenics book printed in America over the last 40 years, and instruction like this can't be found anywhere, in any one of them. *Convict Conditioning* is head and shoulders above them all. In years to come, trainers and coaches will all be talking about 'progressions' and 'progressive calisthenics' and claim they've been doing it all along. But the truth is that Dragon Door bought it to you first. As with kettlebells, they were the trail blazers.

Who should purchase this volume? Everyone who craves fitness and strength should. Even if you don't plan to follow the routines, the book will make you think about your physical prowess, and will give even world class experts food for thought. At the very least if you find yourself on vacation or away on business without your barbells, this book will turn your hotel into a fully equipped gym.

I'd advise any athlete to obtain this work as soon as possible."—*Bill Oliver - Albany, NY, United States*

More Dragon Door Customer Acclaim for *Convict Conditioning*

Fascinating Reading and Real Strength

"Coach Wade's system is a real eye opener if you've been a lifetime iron junkie. Wanna find out how really strong (or weak) you are? Get this book and begin working through the 10 levels of the 6 power exercises. I was pleasantly surprised by my ability on a few of the exercises...but some are downright humbling. If I were on a desert island with only one book on strength and conditioning this would be it. (Could I staple Pavel's "Naked Warrior" to the back and count them as one???!) Thanks Dragon Door for this innovative new author."—*Jon Schultheis, RKC (2005) - Keansburg, NJ*

Single best strength training book ever!

"I just turned 50 this year and I have tried a little bit of everything over the years: martial arts, swimming, soccer, cycling, free weights, weight machines, even yoga and Pilates. I started using *Convict Conditioning* right after it came out. I started from the beginning, like Coach Wade says, doing mostly step one or two for five out of the six exercises. I work out 3 to 5 times a week, usually for 30 to 45 minutes.

Long story short, my weight went up 14 pounds (I was not trying to gain weight) but my body fat percentage dropped two percent. That translates into approximately 19 pounds of lean muscle gained in two months! I've never gotten this kind of results with anything else I've ever done. Now I have pretty much stopped lifting weights for strength training. Instead, I lift once a week as a test to see how much stronger I'm getting without weight training. There are a lot of great strength training books in the world (most of them published by Dragon Door), but if I had to choose just one, this is the single best strength training book ever. BUY THIS BOOK. FOLLOW THE PLAN. GET AS STRONG AS YOU WANT. "—*Wayne - Decatur, GA*

Best bodyweight training book so far!

"I'm a martial artist and I've been training for years with a combination of weights and bodyweight training and had good results from both (but had the usual injuries from weight training). I prefer the bodyweight stuff though as it trains me to use my whole body as a unit, much more than weights do, and I notice the difference on the mat and in the ring. Since reading this book I have given the weights a break and focused purely on the bodyweight exercise progressions as described by 'Coach' Wade and my strength had increased more than ever before. So far I've built up to 12 strict one-leg squats each leg and 5 uneven pull ups each arm.

I've never achieved this kind of strength before - and this stuff builds solid muscle mass as well. It's very intense training. I am so confident in and happy with the results I'm getting that I've decided to train for a fitness/bodybuilding comp just using his techniques, no weights, just to show for real what kind of a physique these exercises can build. In sum, I cannot recommend 'Coach' Wade's book highly enough - it is by far the best of its kind ever!"—*Mark Robinson - Australia, currently living in South Korea*

A lifetime of lifting...and continued learning.

"I have been working out diligently since 1988 and played sports in high school and college before that. My stint in the Army saw me doing calisthenics, running, conditioning courses, forced marches, etc. There are many levels of strength and fitness. I have been as big as 240 in my powerlifting/strongman days and as low as 185-190 while in the Army. I think I have tried everything under the sun: the high intensity of Arthur Jones and Dr. Ken, the Super Slow of El Darden, and the brutality of Dinosaur Training Brooks Kubic made famous.

This is one of the BEST books I've ever read on real strength training which also covers other just as important aspects of health; like staying injury free, feeling healthy and becoming flexible. It's an excellent book. He tells you the why and the how with his progressive plan. This book is a GOLD MINE and worth 100 times what I paid for it!"
—*Horst - Woburn, MA*

This book sets the standard, ladies and gentlemen

"It's difficult to describe just how much this book means to me. I've been training hard since I was in the RAF nearly ten years ago, and to say this book is a breakthrough is an understatement. How often do you really read something so new, so fresh? This book contains a complete new system of calisthenics drawn from American prison training methods. When I say 'system' I mean it. It's complete (rank beginner to expert), it's comprehensive (all the exercises and photos are here), it's graded (progressions from exercise to exercise are smooth and pre-determined) and it's totally original. Whether you love or hate the author, you have to listen to him. And you will learn something. This book just makes SENSE. In twenty years people will still be buying it."—*Andy McMann - Ponty, Wales, GB*

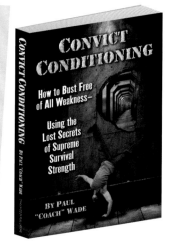

Convict Conditioning
How to Bust Free of All Weakness—Using the Lost Secrets of Supreme Survival Strength
By Paul "Coach" Wade
#B41 $39.95
eBook $19.95
Paperback 8.5 x 11   320 pages
191 photos, charts and illustrations

Beginner   Mid-Level   Advanced

The Experts Give High Praise to
Convict Conditioning 2

"Coach Paul Wade has outdone himself. His first book *Convict Conditioning* is to my mind THE BEST book ever written on bodyweight conditioning. Hands down. Now, with the sequel *Convict Conditioning 2*, Coach Wade takes us even deeper into the subtle nuances of training with the ultimate resistance tool: our bodies.

In plain English, but with an amazing understanding of anatomy, physiology, kinesiology and, go figure, psychology, Coach Wade explains very simply how to work the smaller but just as important areas of the body such as the hands and forearms, neck and calves and obliques in serious functional ways.

His minimalist approach to exercise belies the complexity of his system and the deep insight into exactly how the body works and the best way to get from A to Z in the shortest time possible.

I got the best advice on how to strengthen the hard-to-reach extensors of the hand right away from this exercise Master I have ever seen. It's so simple but so completely functional I can't believe no one else has thought of it yet. Just glad he figured it out for me.

Paul teaches us how to strengthen our bodies with the simplest of movements while at the same time balancing our structures in the same way: simple exercises that work the whole body.

And just as simply as he did with his first book. His novel approach to stretching and mobility training is brilliant and fresh as well as his take on recovery and healing from injury. Sprinkled throughout the entire book are too-many-to-count insights and advice from a man who has come to his knowledge the hard way and knows exactly of what he speaks.

This book is, as was his first, an amazing journey into the history of physical culture disguised as a book on calisthenics. But the thing that Coach Wade does better than any before him is his unbelievable progressions on EVERY EXERCISE and stretch! He breaks things down and tells us EXACTLY how to proceed to get to whatever level of strength and development we want. AND gives us the exact metrics we need to know when to go to the next level.

Adding in completely practical and immediately useful insights into nutrition and the mindset necessary to deal not only with training but with life, makes this book a classic that will stand the test of time.

Bravo Coach Wade, Bravo." —**Mark Reifkind**, Master RKC, author of *Mastering the HardStyle Kettlebell Swing*

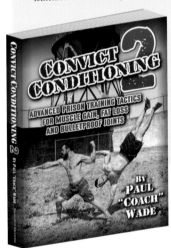

Convict Conditioning 2
Advanced Prison Training Tactics for Muscle Gain, Fat Loss and Bulletproof Joints
By Paul "Coach" Wade
#B59 $39.95
eBook $19.95
Paperback 8.5 x 11 354 pages
261 photos, charts and illustrations

2 Mid-Level

3 Advanced

"The overriding principle of *Convict Conditioning 2* is 'little equipment-big rewards'. For the athlete in the throwing and fighting arts, the section on Lateral Chain Training, Capturing the Flag, is a unique and perhaps singular approach to training the obliques and the whole family of side muscles. This section stood out to me as ground breaking and well worth the time and energy by anyone to review and attempt to complete. Literally, this is a new approach to lateral chain training that is well beyond sidebends and suitcase deadlifts.

The author's review of passive stretching reflects the experience of many of us in the field. But, his solution might be the reason I am going to recommend this work for everyone: The Trifecta. This section covers what the author calls The Functional Triad and gives a series of simple progressions to three holds that promise to oil your joints. It's yoga for the strength athlete and supports the material one would find, for example, in Pavel's *Loaded Stretching*.

I didn't expect to like this book, but I come away from it practically insisting that everyone read it. It is a strongman book mixed with yoga mixed with street smarts. I wanted to hate it, but I love it."
—**Dan John**, author of *Don't Let Go* and co-author of *Easy Strength*

"I've been lifting weights for over 50 years and have trained in the martial arts since 1965. I've read voraciously on both subjects, and written dozens of magazine articles and many books on the subjects. This book and Wade's first, *Convict Conditioning*, are by far the most commonsense, information-packed, and result producing I've read. These books will truly change your life.

Paul Wade is a new and powerful voice in the strength and fitness arena, one that is commonsense, inspiring, and in your face. His approach to maximizing your body's potential is not the same old hackneyed material you find in every book and magazine piece that pictures steroid-bloated models screaming as they curl weights. Wade's stuff has been proven effective by hard men who don't tolerate fluff. It will work for you, too—guaranteed.

As an ex-cop, I've gone mano-y-mano with ex-cons that had clearly trained as Paul Wade suggests in his two *Convict Conditioning* books. While these guys didn't look like steroid-fueled bodybuilders (actually, there were a couple who did), all were incredibly lean, hard and powerful. Wade blows many commonly held beliefs about conditioning, strengthening, and eating out of the water and replaces them with result-producing information that won't cost you a dime." —**Loren W. Christensen**, author of *Fighting the Pain Resistant Attacker*, and many other titles

"*Convict Conditioning* is one of the most influential books I ever got my hands on. *Convict Conditioning 2* took my training and outlook on the power of bodyweight training to the 10th degree—from strengthening the smallest muscles in a maximal manner, all the way to using bodyweight training as a means of healing injuries that pile up from over 22 years of aggressive lifting.

I've used both *Convict Conditioning* and *Convict Conditioning 2* on myself and with my athletes. Without either of these books I can easily say that these boys would not be the BEASTS they are today. Without a doubt *Convict Conditioning 2* will blow you away and inspire and educate you to take bodyweight training to a whole NEW level."
—**Zach Even-Esh**, Underground Strength Coach

Online Praise for *Convict Conditioning 2*

Best Sequel Since The Godfather 2!

"Hands down the best addition to the material on *Convict Conditioning* that could possibly be put out. I already implemented the neck bridges, calf and hand training to my weekly schedule, and as soon as my handstand pushups and leg raises are fully loaded I'll start the flags. Thank you, Coach!"
— Daniel Runkel, Rio de Janeiro, Brazil

The progressions were again sublime

"Never have I heard such in depth and yet easy to understand description of training and physical culture. A perfect complement to the first book although it has its own style keeping the best attributes of style from the first but developing it to something unique. The progressions were again sublime and designed for people at all levels of ability. The two books together can forge what will closely resemble superhuman strength and an incredible physique and yet the steps to get there are so simple and easy to understand."
—Ryan O., Nottingham, United Kingdom

Well worth the wait

"Another very interesting, and as before, opinionated book by Paul Wade. As I work through the CC1 progressions, I find it's paying off at a steady if unspectacular rate, which suits me just fine. No training injuries worth the name, convincing gains in strength. I expect the same with CC2 which rounds off CC1 with just the kind of material I was looking for. Wade and Dragon Door deserve to be highly commended for publishing these techniques. A tremendous way to train outside of the gym ecosystem." —V. R., Bangalore, India

Very Informative

"*Convict Conditioning 2* is more subversive training information in the same style as its original. It's such a great complement to the original, but also solid enough on its own. The information in this book is fantastic-- a great buy! Follow this program, and you will get stronger."
—Chris B., Thunder Bay, Canada

Just as brilliant as its predecessor!

"Just as brilliant as its predecessor! The new exercises add to the Big 6 in a keep-it-simple kind of way. Anyone who will put in the time with both of these masterpieces will be as strong as humanly possible. I especially liked the parts on grip work. To me, that alone was worth the price of the entire book."
—Timothy Stovall / Evansville, Indiana

If you liked CC1, you'll love CC2

"CC2 picks up where CC1 left off with great information about the human flag (including a version called the clutch flag, that I can actually do now), neck and forearms. I couldn't be happier with this book."
—Justin B., Atlanta, Georgia

From the almost laughably-simple to realm-of-the-gods

"*Convict Conditioning 2* is a great companion piece to the original Convict Conditioning. It helps to further build up the athlete and does deliver on phenomenal improvement with minimal equipment and space.

The grip work is probably the superstar of the book. Second, maybe, is the attention devoted to the lateral muscles with the development of the clutch- and press-flag.

Convict Conditioning 2 is more of the same - more of the systematic and methodical improvement in exercises that travel smoothly from the almost laughably-simple to realm-of-the-gods. It is a solid addition to any fitness library."
—Robert Aldrich, Chapel Hill, GA

Brilliant

"Convict Conditioning books are all the books you need in life. As Bruce Lee used to say, it's not a daily increase but a daily decrease. Same with life. Too many things can lead you down many paths, but to have Simplicity is perfect."—Brandon Lynch, London, England

Convict Conditioning 2
Advanced Prison Training Tactics for Muscle Gain, Fat Loss and Bulletproof Joints
By Paul "Coach" Wade
#B59 $39.95
eBook $19.95
Paperback 8.5 x 11 354 pages
261 photos, charts and illustrations

Mid-Level   Advanced

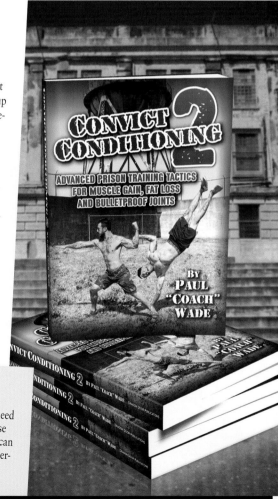

— TABLE OF CONTENTS —

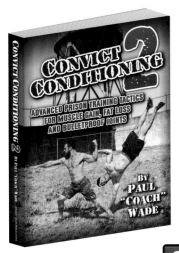

Convict Conditioning 2

Advanced Prison Training Tactics for Muscle Gain, Fat Loss and Bulletproof Joints

By Paul "Coach" Wade
#B59 $39.95
eBook $19.95

2 Mid-Level
3 Advanced

Paperback 8.5 x 11 354 pages
261 photos, charts and illustrations

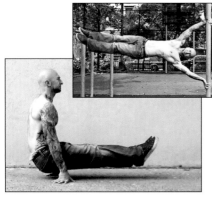

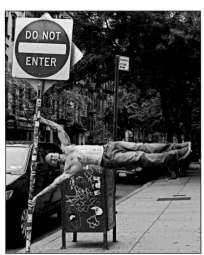

Foreword
The Many Roads to Strength by Brooks Kubik

Opening Salvo:
Chewing Bubblegum and Kicking Ass

1. Introduction: *Put Yourself Behind Bars*

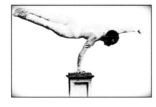

PART I: SHOTGUN MUSCLE

Hands and Forearms

2: Iron Hands and Forearms: *Ultimate Strength —with Just Two Techniques*

3: The Hang Progressions: *A Vice-Like Bodyweight Grip Course*

4: Advanced Grip Torture: *Explosive Power + Titanium Fingers*

5: Fingertip Pushups: *Keeping Hand Strength Balanced*

6: Forearms into Firearms: *Hand Strength: A Summary and a Challenge*

Lateral Chain

7: Lateral Chain Training: *Capturing the Flag*

8: The Clutch Flag: *In Eight Easy Steps*

9: The Press Flag: *In Eight Not-So-Easy Steps*

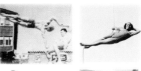

Neck and Calves

10. Bulldog Neck: *Bulletproof Your Weakest Link*

11. Calf Training: *Ultimate Lower Legs—No Machines Necessary*

PART II: BULLETPROOF JOINTS

12. Tension-Flexibility: *The Lost Art of Joint Training*

13. Stretching—the Prison Take: *Flexibility, Mobility, Control*

14. The Trifecta: *Your "Secret Weapon" for Mobilizing Stiff, Battle-Scarred Physiques—for Life*

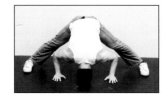

15: The Bridge Hold Progressions: *The Ultimate Prehab/Rehab Technique*

16: The L-Hold Progressions: *Cure Bad Hips and Low Back—Inside-Out*

17: Twist Progressions: *Unleash Your Functional Triad*

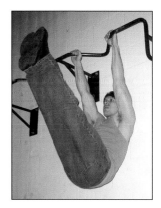

PART III: WISDOM FROM CELLBLOCK G

18. Doing Time Right: *Living the Straight Edge*

19. The Prison Diet: *Nutrition and Fat Loss Behind Bars*

20. Mendin' Up: *The 8 Laws of Healing*

21. The Mind: *Escaping the True Prison*

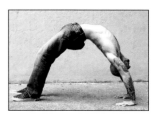

!BONUS CHAPTER!

Pumpin' Iron in Prison: *Myths, Muscle and Misconceptions*

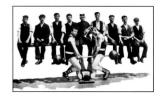

GET DYNAMIC, CHISELLED, POWER-JACK LEGS AND DEVELOP EXPLOSIVE LOWER-BODY STRENGTH— WITH PAUL "COACH" WADE'S ULTIMATE BODYWEIGHT SQUAT COURSE

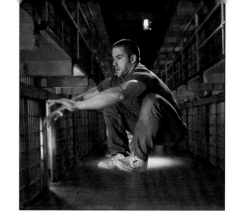

Paul Wade's *Convict Conditioning Ultimate Bodyweight Squat Course* explodes out of the cellblock to teach you in absolute detail how to progress from the ease of a simple shoulderstand squat—to the stunning "1-in-10,000" achievement of the prison-style one-leg squat. Ten progressive steps guide you to bodyweight squat mastery. Do it—and become a Bodyweight Squat Immortal.

This home-study course in ultimate survival strength comes replete with bonus material not available in Paul Wade's original *Convict Conditioning* book—and numerous key training tips that refine and expand on the original program.

A heavily and gorgeously-illustrated 80-plus-page manual gives you the entire film script to study at your leisure, with brilliant, precise photographs to remind you of the essential movements you absorbed in the DVD itself.

Paul Wade adds a bonus **Ten Commandments for Perfect Bodyweight Squats**—which is worth the price of admission alone. And there's the additional bonus of **5 major Variant drills** to add explosivity, fun and super-strength to your core practice.

Whatever you are looking for from your bodyweight squats— be it supreme functional strength, monstrous muscle growth or explosive leg power—it's yours for the progressive taking with *Convict Conditioning, Volume 2: The Ultimate Bodyweight Squat Course.*

WHY EVERY SELF-RESPECTING MAN WILL BE RELIGIOUS ABOUT HIS SQUATS...

Leg training is vital for every athlete. A well-trained, muscular upper body teetering around on skinny stick legs is a joke. Don't be that joke! The mighty squat is the answer to your prayers. Here's why:

- Squats train virtually every muscle in the lower body, from quads and glutes to hips, lower back and even hamstrings.

- Squat deep—as we'll teach you—and you will seriously increase your flexibility and ankle strength.

- All functional power is transmitted through the legs, so without strong, powerful legs you are *nothing*—that goes for running, jumping and combat sports as much as it does for lifting heavy stuff.

ARE YOU FAILING TO BUILD MONSTROUS LEGS FROM SQUATS—BECAUSE OF THESE MISTAKES?

Most trainees learn how to squat on two legs, and then make the exercise harder by slapping a barbell across their back. In prison, this way of adding strength wasn't always available, so cell trainees developed ways of progressing using only bodyweight versus gravity. The best way to do this is to learn how to squat all the way down to the ground and back up on just one leg.

Not everybody who explores prison training will have the dedication and drive to achieve strength feats like the one-arm pullup, but the legs are much stronger than the arms. If you put in the time and work hard, the one-leg squat will be within the reach of almost every athlete who pays their dues.

But the one-leg squat still requires very powerful muscles and tendons, so you don't want to jump into one-leg squatting right away. You need to build the joint strength and muscle to safely attempt this great exercise. Discover how to do that safely, using ten steps, ten progressively harder squat exercises.

IN THE STRENGTH GAME, FOOLS RUSH IN WHERE ANGELS FEAR TO TREAD

The wise old Chinese man shouted to his rickshaw driver: "Slow down, young man, I'm in a hurry!" If ever a warning needed to be shouted to our nation of compulsive strength-addicts, this would be it. You see them everywhere: the halt, the lame, the jacked-up, the torn, the pain-ridden—the former glory-seekers who have been reduced to sad husks of their former selves by rushing helter-skelter into heavy lifting without having first built a firm foundation.

Paul Wade reveals the ten key points of perfect squat form. The aspects of proper form apply to all your squats, and they'll not only unlock the muscle and power-building potential of each rep you do, but they'll also keep you as safe as you can be.

Bodyweight training is all about improving strength and health, not building up a list of injuries or aches and pains. They are so fundamental, we call them the Ten Commandments of good squat form.

Obey the Ten Commandments, follow the brilliantly laid out progressions religiously and you simply CANNOT fail to get stronger and stronger and stronger and stronger and stronger—surely, safely and for as long as you live…

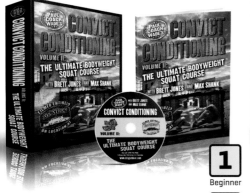

Convict Conditioning
Volume 2: The Ultimate Bodyweight Squat Course
By Paul "Coach" Wade featuring Brett Jones and Max Shank
#DVO84 $69.95
DVD 56 minutes with full color Companion Manual, 88 pages

1 Beginner
2 Mid-Level
3 Advanced

COMPLEX MADE SIMPLE

Having read both *Convict Conditioning* and *Convict Conditioning 2*, the complementary DVD series is an excellent translation of the big six movement progressions into a simple to follow DVD. The demonstration of movement progression through the 10 levels is well described and easy to follow.

As a Physical Therapist it is a very useful way to teach safe progressions to patients/clients and other professionals. I have already used Volume I (the push up progression) to teach high school strength coaches how to safely progress athletes with pressing activity and look forward to using volume 2 with these same coaches. I think anyone who studies movement realizes very few athletes can properly squat with two legs, let alone one.

You will not find an easier way to teach the squat. Well done again Paul. Look forward to the rest of the series."

—Andrew Marchesi PT/MPT, FAFS, Scottsdale, AZ

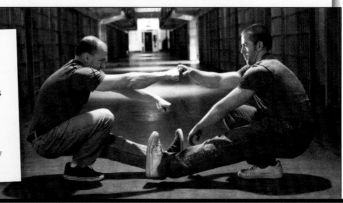

NAVY SEAL ON THE ROAD

"My whole team uses it. We can work out effectively anywhere and I mean any-where!"
—Tyler Archer, Navy

GET A ROCK-HARD, BRUTISHLY POWERFUL UPPER FRAME AND ACHIEVE ELITE-LEVEL STRENGTH— WITH PAUL "COACH" WADE'S PRISON-STYLE PUSHUP PROGRAM

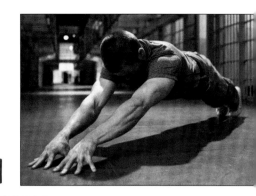

Paul Wade's *Convict Conditioning* system represents the ultimate distillation of hardcore prison bodyweight training's most powerful methods. What works was kept. What didn't, was slashed away. When your life is on the line, you're not going to mess with less than the absolute best. Many of these older, very potent solitary training systems have been on the verge of dying, as convicts begin to gain access to weights, and modern "bodybuilding thinking" floods into the prisons.

Thanks to Paul Wade, these ultimate strength survival secrets have been saved for posterity. And for you...

Filmed entirely—and so appropriately—on "The Rock", Wade's *Convict Conditioning Prison Pushup Series* explodes out of the cellblock to teach you in absolute detail how to progress from the ease of a simple wall pushup—to the stunning "1-in-10,000" achieve-ment of the prison-style one-arm pushup. Ten progressive steps guide you to pushup mastery. Do it—and become a Pushup God.

This home-study course in ultimate survival strength comes replete with bonus material not available in **Paul Wade's** original *Convict Conditioning* book—and numerous key training tips that refine and expand on the original program.

A heavily and gorgeously-illustrated 80-plus-page manual gives you the entire film script to study at your leisure, with brilliant, precise photographs to remind you of the essential movements you absorbed in the DVD itself.

Paul Wade adds a bonus **Ten Commandments for Perfect Pushups**—which is worth the price of admission alone. And there's the additional bonus of **5 major Variant drills** to add explosivity, fun and super-strength to your core practice.

Whatever you are looking for from your pushups—be it supreme functional strength, monstrous muscle growth or explosive upper-body power—it's yours for the progressive taking with *Convict Conditioning, Volume 1: The Prison Pushup Series.*

AWESOME RESOURCE FOR COACHES & STRENGTH DEVOTEES

"I am using this manual and DVD not just for my own training, but for the training of my athletes. It shocks and amazes me how varsity high school athletes can NOT perform a solid push up.... not even 1! Getting them to perform a perfect push up requires regressions, progressions, dialing in the little cues that teach them to generate tension and proper body alignment, ALL of which carry over to other exercises.

This manual is an awesome resource for Coaches. It can & should be used to educate those you train as well as shared with your staff. For those who have a love for strength, you will respect all the details given for each and every push up pro-gression and you will use them and apply them.

As a Strength devotee for over 2 decades, I've been through the grinder with free weights and injuries, push ups are something I **KNOW** I'll be doing for the rest of my life which is why I RESPECT this course so much!

The lay out of this manual and DVD are also BIG time impressive, the old school look and feel fires me up and makes me wanna attack these push ups!"
—Zach Even-Esh, Manasquan, NJ

I RECOMMEND IT

"I fully expected to be disappointed with **Paul Wade's** *Convict Conditioning, Volume I: The Prison Pushup Series*. John Du Cane will tell you: I am not a fan of some of the stuff in these books. It's been said by others that this might be one of the most striking DVDs ever made. It's on location in Alcatraz and the graphics are pretty amazing. So, yes, stunning. This DVD from Wade is stunning and very cool.

The manual that supports the DVD is very helpful as much of the material is done too well in the DVD. Many of us need to take some time looking at the DVD then flipping the manual back and forth to 'get it.'

Once again, there are parts of this DVD and the series that rub me the wrong way. Having said that, I am frankly amazed at the insights of the product here. As a coach, I am better than when I popped the box open. I have a whole set of tools, and the progressions, that I can use tomorrow with my group. That to me is the testimony that people should hear from me: I watched it and I applied it instantly! This one 'gets it.' You can apply what you learn instantly and know where you are going from there. I highly recommend it."
—Dan John, Master RKC, Burlingame, CA

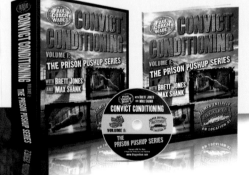

1 Beginner	
2 Mid-Level	
3 Advanced	

Convict Conditioning
Volume 1: The Prison Pushup Series
By Paul "Coach" Wade featuring Brett Jones and Max Shank
#DV083 $69.95
DVD 59 minutes with full color Companion Manual, 88 pages

DEMONIC ABS ARE A MAN'S BEST FRIEND—DISCOVER HOW TO SEIZE A SIX-PACK FROM HELL AND OWN THE WORLD... LEG RAISES

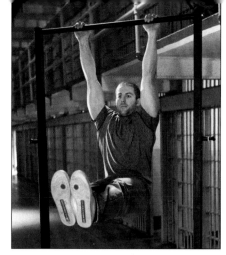

Paul Wade's *Convict Conditioning 3, Leg Raises: Six Pack from Hell* teaches you in absolute detail how to progress from the ease of a simple Knee Tuck—to the magnificent, "1-in-1,000" achievement of the Hanging Straight Leg Raise. Ten progressive steps guide you to inevitable mastery of this ultimate abs exercise. Do it, seize the knowledge—but beware—the Gods will be jealous!

This home-study course in ultimate survival strength comes replete with bonus material not available in **Paul Wade's** original *Convict Conditioning* book—and numerous key training tips that refine and expand on the original program.

Prowl through the heavily and gorgeously-illustrated 80-plus-page manual and devour the entire film script at your animal leisure. Digest the brilliant, precise photographs and reinforce the raw benefits you absorbed from the DVD.

Paul Wade adds a bonus **Ten Commandments for Perfect Bodyweight Squats**—which is worth the price of admission alone. And there's the additional bonus of **4 major Variant drills** to add explosivity, fun and super-strength to your core practice.

Whatever you are looking for when murdering your abs—be it a fist-breaking, rock-like shield of impenetrable muscle, an uglier-is-more-beautiful set of rippling abdominal ridges, or a monstrous injection of lifting power—it's yours for the progressive taking with *Convict Conditioning, Volume 3, Leg Raises: Six Pack from Hell*

PRISON-STYLE MID-SECTION TRAINING—FOR AN ALL SHOW AND ALL GO PHYSIQUE

When convicts train their waists, they want real, noticeable results—and by "results" we don't mean that they want cute, tight little defined abs. We mean that they want thick, strong, muscular midsections. They want *functionally* powerful abs and hips they can use for heavy lifting, kicking, and brawling. They want guts so strong from their training that it actually hurts an attacker to punch them in the belly. Prison abs aren't about all show, no go—a prison-built physique has to be all show and all go. Those guys don't just want six-packs—they want six-packs from Hell.

And, for the first time, we're going to show you how these guys get what they want. We're not going to be using sissy machines or easy isolation exercises—we're going straight for the old school secret weapon for gut training; progressive leg raises.

If you want a six-pack from Hell, the first thing you need to do is focus your efforts. If a weightlifter wanted a very thick, powerful chest in a hurry, he wouldn't spread his efforts out over a dozen exercises and perform them gently all day long. No—he'd pick just one exercise, probably the bench press, and just focus on getting stronger and stronger on that lift until he was monstrously strong. When he reached this level, and his pecs were thick slabs of meat, only then would he maybe begin sculpting them with minor exercises and higher reps.

It's no different if you want a mind-blowing midsection. Just pick one exercise that hits all the muscles in the midsection—the hip flexors, the abs, the intercostals, the obliques—then blast it.

And the one exercise we're going to discover is the best midsection exercise known to man, and the most popular amongst soldiers, warriors, martial artists and prison athletes since men started working out—the leg raise.

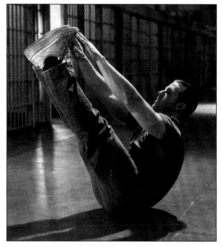

You'll discover ten different leg raise movements, each one a little harder than the last. You'll learn how to get the most out of each of these techniques, each of these ten steps, before moving up to the next step. By the time you get through all ten steps and you're working with the final Master Step of the leg raise series, you'll have a solid, athletic, stomach made of steel, as well as powerful hips and a ribcage armored with dense muscle. You'll have abs that would've made Bruce Lee take notice!

THE TEN COMMANDMENTS YOU MUST OBEY TO EARN A REAL MONSTER OF AN ATHLETIC CORE

Paul Wade gives you ten key points, the "Ten Commandments" of leg raises, that will take your prison-style core training from just "okay" to absolutely phenomenal. We want the results to be so effective that they'll literally shock you. This kind of accelerated progress can be achieved, but if you want to achieve it you better listen carefully to these ten key pointers you'll discover with the DVD.

Bodyweight mastery is a lot like high-level martial arts. It's more about *principles* than individual techniques. Really study and absorb these principles, and you'll be on your way to a six-pack from Hell in no time.

The hanging straight leg raise, performed strictly and for reps, is the Gold Standard of abdominal strength techniques. Once you're at the level where you can throw out sets of twenty to thirty rock solid reps of this exercise, your abs will be thick and strong, but more importantly, they'll be functional—not just a pretty six-pack, but a real monster of an athletic core, which is

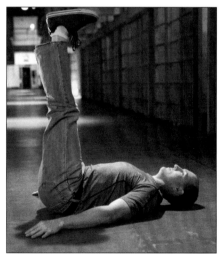

capable of developing high levels of force.

Hanging will work your serratus and intercostals, making these muscles stand out like fingers, and your obliques and flank muscles will be tight and strong from holding your hips in place. Your lumbar spine will achieve a gymnastic level of flexibility, like fluid steel, and your chances of back pain will be greatly reduced.

The bottom line: If you want to be stronger and more athletic than the next guy, you need the edge that straight leg raises can give you.

ERECT TWIN PYTHONS OF COILED BEEF UP YOUR SPINE AND DEVELOP EXTREME, EXPLOSIVE RESILIENCE—WITH THE DYNAMIC POWER AND FLEXIBLE STRENGTH OF ADVANCED BRIDGING

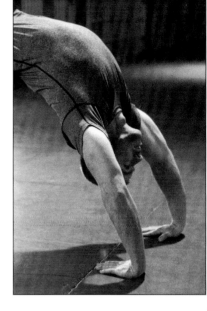

Paul Wade's *Convict Conditioning* system represents the ultimate distillation of hardcore prison bodyweight training's most powerful methods. What works was kept. What didn't, was slashed away. When your life is on the line, you're not going to mess with less than the absolute best. Many of these older, very potent solitary training systems have been on the verge of dying, as convicts begin to gain access to weights, and modern "bodybuilding thinking" floods into the prisons. Thanks to Paul Wade, these ultimate strength survival secrets have been saved for posterity. And for you…

Filmed entirely—and so appropriately— on "The Rock", Wade's *Convict Conditioning Volume 4, Advanced Bridging: Forging an Iron Spine* explodes out of the cellblock to teach you in absolute detail how to progress from the relative ease of a Short Bridge—to the stunning, "1-in-1,000" achievement of the Stand-to-Stand Bridge. Ten progressive steps guide you to inevitable mastery of this ultimate exercise for an unbreakable back.

This home-study course in ultimate survival strength comes replete with bonus material not available in **Paul Wade's** original *Convict Conditioning* book—and numerous key training tips that refine and expand on the original program.

Prowl through the heavily and gorgeously-illustrated 80-plus-page manual and devour the entire film script at your animal leisure. Digest the brilliant, precise photographs and reinforce the raw benefits you absorbed from the DVD.

Paul Wade adds a bonus **Ten Commandments for Perfect Bridges**— which is worth the price of admission alone. And there's the additional bonus of **4 major Variant drills** to add explosivity, fun and super-strength to your core practice.

Whatever you are looking for from your pushups—be it supreme functional strength, monstrous muscle growth or explosive upper-body power—it's yours for the progressive taking with *Convict Conditioning Volume 4: Advanced Bridging: Forging an Iron Spine.*

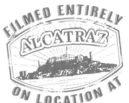

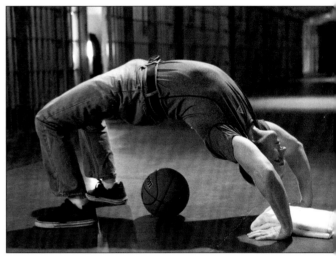

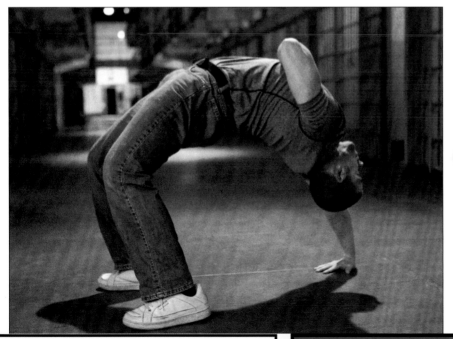

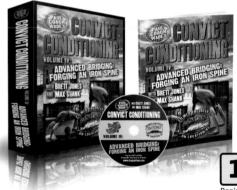

TAP INTO THE DORMANT ANCESTRAL POWER OF THE MIGHTY PULLUP—
TO DEVELOP A MASSIVE UPPER BACK, STEEL-TENDON ARMS, ETCHED ABS AND AGILE SURVIVAL STRENGTH

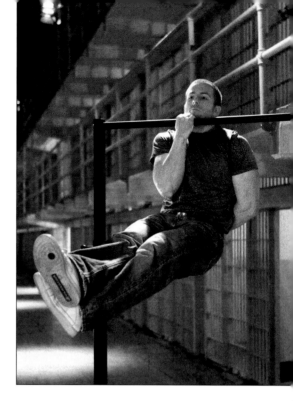

P aul Wade's *Convict Conditioning* system represents the ultimate distillation of hard-core prison bodyweight training's most powerful methods. What works was kept. What didn't, was slashed away. When your life is on the line, you're not going to mess with less than the absolute best. Many of these older, very potent solitary training systems have been on the verge of dying, as convicts begin to gain access to weights, and modern "bodybuilding thinking" floods into the prisons. Thanks to Paul Wade, these ultimate strength survival secrets have been saved for posterity. And for you…

Filmed entirely—and so appropriately— on "The Rock", Wade's *Convict Conditioning Volume 5, Maximum Strength: The One-Arm Pullup Series* explodes out of the cellblock to teach you in absolute detail how to progress from the relative ease of a Vertical Pull—to the stunning, "1-in-1,000" achievement of the One-Arm Pullup. Ten progressive steps guide you to inevitable mastery of this ultimate exercise for supreme upper body survival strength.

This home-study course in ultimate survival strength comes replete with bonus material not available in **Paul Wade's** original *Convict Conditioning* book—and numerous key training tips that refine and expand on the original program.

Prowl through the heavily and gorgeously-illustrated 80-plus-page manual and devour the entire film script at your animal leisure. Digest the brilliant, precise photographs and reinforce the raw benefits you absorbed from the DVD.

Paul Wade adds a bonus **Ten Commandments for Perfect Pullups**—which is worth the price of admission alone. And there's the additional bonus of **4 major Variant drills** to add explosivity, fun and super-strength to your core practice.

Whatever you are looking for from your pullups—be it agile survival strength, arms of steel, a massive upper back with flaring lats, Popeye Biceps or gape-inducing abs—it's yours for the progressive taking with *Convict Conditioning Volume 5, Maximum Strength: The One-Arm Pullup Series.*

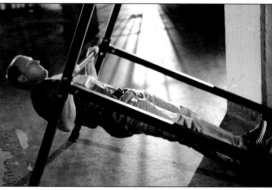

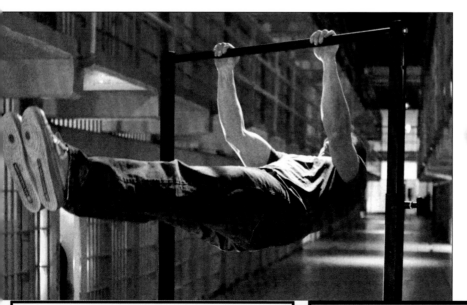

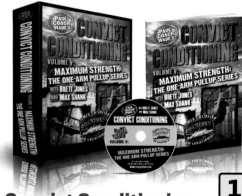

Convict Conditioning

Volume 5: Maximum Strength: The One-Arm Pullup Series
By Paul "Coach" Wade featuring Brett Jones and Max Shank
#DV088 $59.95

1 Beginner

2 Mid-Level

3 Advanced

Al Kavadlo's Progressive Plan for Primal Body Power

How to Build Explosive Strength and a Magnificent Physique—Using Bodyweight Exercise Only

What is more satisfying than owning a primally powerful, functionally forceful and brute-strong body? A body that packs a punch. A body that commands attention with its etched physique, coiled muscle and proud confidence…A body that can PERFORM at the highest levels of physical accomplishment…

Well, both **Al Kavadlo**—the author of *Pushing the Limits!*—and his brother **Danny**, are supreme testaments to the primal power of body culture done the old-school, ancient way—bare-handed, with your body only. The brothers Kavadlo walk the bodyweight talk—and then some. The proof is evident on every page of *Pushing the Limits!*

Your body is your temple. Protect and strengthen your temple by modeling the methods of the exercise masters. Al Kavadlo has modeled the masters and has the "temple" to show for it. Follow Al's progressive plan for primal body power within the pages of *Pushing the Limits!*—follow in the footsteps of the great bodyweight exercise masters—and you too can build the explosive strength and possess the magnificent physique you deserve.

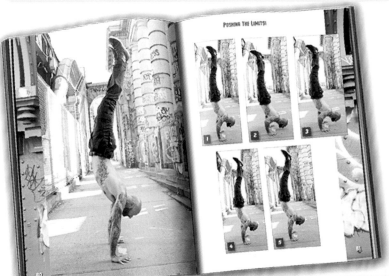

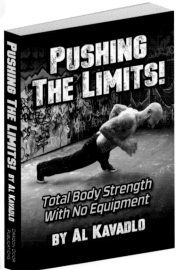

Pushing the Limits!
Total Body Strength With No Equipment
By Al Kavadlo
#B69 $39.95
eBook $19.95
Paperback 8.5 x 11   224 pages
240 photos

1 Beginner   **2** Mid-Level   **3** Advanced

Stretching and Flexibility Secrets To Help Unlock Your Body–Be More Mobile, More Athletic, More Resilient And Far Stronger...

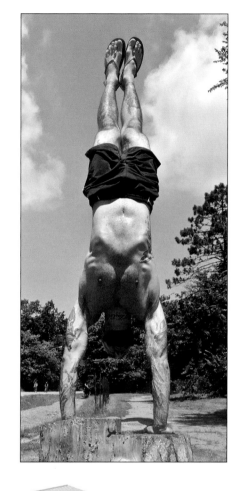

"The ultimate bodyweight mobility manual is here! Al Kavadlo's previous two Dragon Door books, *Raising the Bar* and *Pushing the Limits*, are the most valuable bodyweight strength training manuals in the world. But strength without mobility is meaningless. Al has used his many years of training and coaching to fuse bodyweight disciplines such as yoga, martial arts, rehabilitative therapy and bar athletics into the ultimate calisthenics stretching compendium. *Stretching your Boundaries* belongs on the shelf of any serious athlete—it's bodyweight mobility dynamite!"

—"COACH" PAUL WADE, author of *Convict Conditioning*

"In this book, Al invites you to take a deeper look at the often overlooked, and sometimes demonized, ancient practice of static stretching. He wrestles with many of the questions, dogmas and flat out lies about stretching that have plagued the fitness practitioner for at least the last decade. And finally he gives you a practical guide to static stretching that will improve your movement, performance, breathing and life. In *Stretching Your Boundaries,* you'll sense Al's deep understanding and love for the human body. Thank you Al, for helping to bring awareness to perhaps the most important aspect of physical education and fitness."

—ELLIOTT HULSE, creator of the **Grow Stronger** method

"An absolutely masterful follow up to *Raising The Bar* and *Pushing The Limits, Stretching Your Boundaries* really completes the picture. Both easy to understand and fully applicable, Al's integration of traditional flexibility techniques with his own unique spin makes this a must have. The explanation of how each stretch will benefit your calisthenics practice is brilliant. Not only stunning in its color and design, this book also gives you the true feeling of New York City, both gritty and euphoric, much like Al's personality."

—MIKE FITCH, creator of **Global Bodyweight Training**

"Stretching Your Boundaries is a terrific resource that will unlock your joints so you can build more muscle, strength and athleticism. Al's passion for human performance radiates in this beautifully constructed book. Whether you're stiff as a board, or an elite gymnast, this book outlines the progressions to take your body and performance to a new level."

—CHAD WATERBURY, M.S., author of *Huge in a Hurry*

"Al Kavadlo has done it again! He's created yet another incredible resource that I wish I had twenty years ago. Finding great material on flexibility training that actually enhances your strength is like trying to find a needle in a haystack. But look no further, because *Stretching Your Boundaries* is exactly what you need."

—JASON FERRUGGIA, Strength Coach

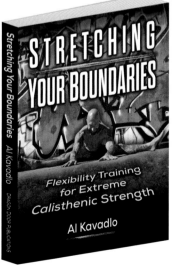

Stretching Your Boundaries
Flexibility Training for Extreme Calisthenic Strength
By Al Kavadlo
#B73 $39.95
eBook $19.95
Paperback 8.5 x 11 214 pages
235 photos

Beginner   Mid-Level   Advanced

Go Beyond Mere "Toughness"— When You Master The Art of Bar Athletics and Sculpt the Ultimate in Upper Body Physiques

> "*Raising the Bar* is very likely the most important book on strength and conditioning to be published in the last fifty years. If you only ever get your hands on one training manual in your life, make it this one. Buy it, read it, use it. This book has the power to transform you into the ultimate bar athlete." — Paul "Coach" Wade, author of *Convict Conditioning*

Raising the Bar
The Definitive Guide to Bar Calisthenics
By Al Kavadlo
#B63 $39.95   eBook $19.95
224 pages, 330 Photos

1 Beginner   **2** Mid-Level   **3** Advanced

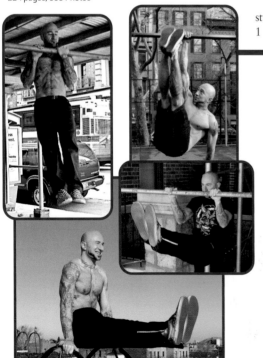

Raising the Bar breaks down every type of exercise you can do with a pull-up bar. From the basic two arm hang, to the mighty muscle-up, all the way to the elusive one arm pull-up, "bar master" Al Kavadlo takes you step by expert step through everything you need to do to build the chiseled frame you've always wanted.

Whether you're a die-hard calisthenics enthusiast or just looking to get in the best shape of your life, *Raising the Bar* will meet all your expectations—and then some!

The message is clear: you can earn yourself a stunning upper body with just 3 basic moves and 1 super-simple, yet amazingly versatile tool.

And what's even better, this 3 + 1 formula for upper body magnificence hides enough variety to keep you challenged and surging to new heights for a lifetime of cool moves and ever-tougher progressions!

Cast in the "concrete jungle" of urban scaffolding and graffiti-laden, blasted walls—and sourced from iconic bar-athlete destinations like Tompkins Square Park, NYC—*Raising the Bar* rears up to grab you by the throat and hurl you into an inspiring new vision of what the human body can achieve. Embrace Al Kavadlo's vision, pick up the challenge, share the Quest, follow directions—and the Holy Grail of supreme upper body fitness is yours for the taking.

"With *Raising the Bar*, Al Kavadlo has put forth the perfect primal pull-up program. Al's progressions and demonstrations make even the most challenging exercises attainable. Anyone who is serious about pull-ups should read this book." —Mark Sisson, author of *The Primal Blueprint*.

A Kick Ass Encyclopedia of Bodyweight Exercises

"Al Kavadlo has put together a kick ass encyclopedia of the most powerful and most commonly used bodyweight exercises amongst the various groups of bodyweight masters.

From the most simple form of each exercise progressing to the most challenging form of each exercise, Al covers it. As a Coach and bodyweight training addict I loved all the variations shown. This book is far beyond just pull ups and there are countless exercises for upper body and abs. Al covers what is probably EVERY exercise he knows of, uses and teaches others, breaking down proper techniques, regressions and progressions. This is HUGE for the trainers out there who do NOT know how to adapt bodyweight exercises to each individual's fitness level.

If you're a fan of bodyweight training, between this book and *Convict Conditioning* you can turn your body into a deadly weapon!!!" —Zach Even-Esh, Manasquan, NJ

"Al has put together the companion manual for all the crazy bar calisthenics videos that you find yourself watching over and over again—a much needed resource. Within this book is a huge volume of bar exercises that will keep your pullup workouts fresh for years, and give you some insane goals to shoot for."
—Max Shank, Senior RKC

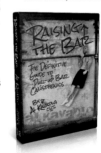

Raising the Bar
The Definitive Guide to Bar Calisthenics
DVD with Al Kavadlo
#DV090 $29.95
224 pages, 330 Photos

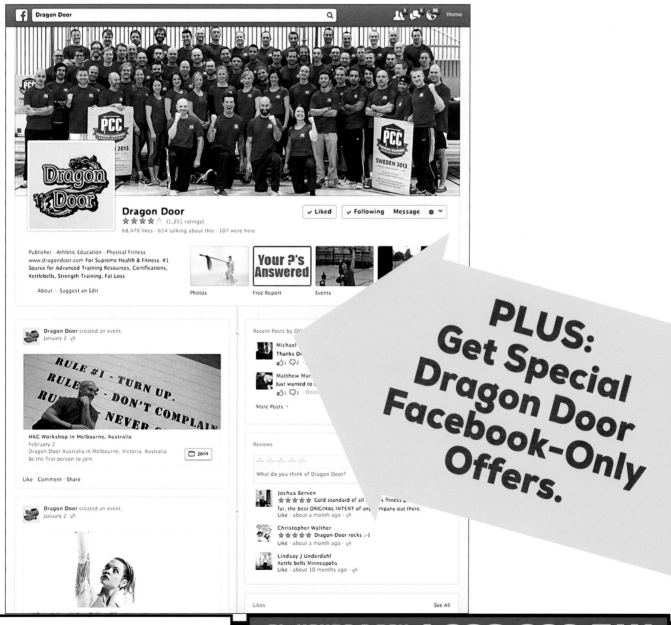

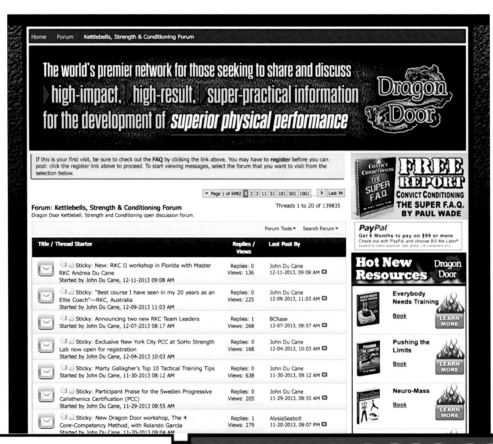

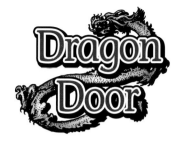

1·800·899·5111
24 HOURS A DAY • FAX YOUR ORDER (866) 280-7619
O R D E R I N G   I N F O R M A T I O N

Telephone Orders For faster service you may place your orders by calling Toll Free 24 hours a day, 7 days a week, 365 days per year. When you call, please have your credit card ready.

Customer Service Questions? Please call us between 9:00am– 11:00pm EST

Monday to Friday at 1-800-899-5111. Local and foreign customers call 513-346-4160 for orders and customer service

100% One-Year Risk-Free Guarantee. If you are not completely satisfied with any product—we'll be happy to give you a prompt exchange, credit, or refund,

as you wish. Simply return your purchase to us, and please let us know why you were dissatisfied—it will help us to provide better products and services in the future. *Shipping and handling fees are non-refundable.*

Complete and mail with full payment to: Dragon Door Publications, 5 County Road B East, Suite 3, Little Canada, MN 55117

Please print clearly
Sold To: **A**

Name_____

Street_____

City_____

State _____ Zip _____

Day phone*_____
Important for clarifying questions on orders

Please print clearly
SHIP TO: *(Street address for delivery)*   **B**

Name_____

Street_____

City_____

State _____ Zip _____

Email_____

Warning to foreign customers:
The Customs in your country may or may not tax or otherwise charge you an additional fee for goods you receive. Dragon Door Publications is charging you only for U.S. handling and international shipping. Dragon Door Publications is in no way responsible for any additional fees levied by Customs, the carrier or any other entity.

ITEM #	QTY.	ITEM DESCRIPTION	ITEM PRICE	A OR B	TOTAL

HANDLING AND SHIPPING CHARGES • NO COD'S
Total Amount of Order Add (Excludes kettlebells and kettlebell kits):

$00.00 to 29.99	**Add $6.00**	$100.00 to 129.99	**Add $14.00**
$30.00 to 49.99	**Add $7.00**	$130.00 to 169.99	**Add $16.00**
$50.00 to 69.99	**Add $8.00**	$170.00 to 199.99	**Add $18.00**
$70.00 to 99.99	**Add $11.00**	$200.00 to 299.99	**Add $20.00**
		$300.00 and up	**Add $24.00**

Canada and Mexico add $6.00 to US charges. All other countries, flat rate, double US Charges. See Kettlebell section for Kettlebell Shipping and handling charges.

Total of Goods	
Shipping Charges	
Rush Charges	
Kettlebell Shipping Charges	
OH residents add 6.5% sales tax	
MN residents add 6.5% sales tax	
TOTAL ENCLOSED	

METHOD OF PAYMENT ____CHECK ____M.O. ____MASTERCARD ____VISA ____DISCOVER ____AMEX

Account No. (Please indicate all the numbers on your credit card)   EXPIRATION DATE

☐☐☐☐ ☐☐☐☐ ☐☐☐☐ ☐☐☐☐   ☐☐/☐☐

Day Phone: ( )_____

Signature: _____ Date: _____

NOTE: *We ship best method available for your delivery address. Foreign orders are sent by air. Credit card or International M.O. only. For* **RUSH** *processing of your order, add an additional $10.00 per address. Available on money order & charge card orders only.*

Errors and omissions excepted. Prices subject to change without notice.

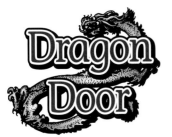

1·800·899·5111
24 HOURS A DAY • FAX YOUR ORDER (866) 280-7619
O R D E R I N G   I N F O R M A T I O N

Telephone Orders For faster service you may place your orders by calling Toll Free 24 hours a day, 7 days a week, 365 days per year. When you call, please have your credit card ready.

Customer Service Questions? Please call us between 9:00am– 11:00pm EST

Monday to Friday at 1-800-899-5111. Local and foreign customers call 513-346-4160 for orders and customer service

100% One-Year Risk-Free Guarantee. If you are not completely satisfied with any product—we'll be happy to give you a prompt exchange, credit, or refund,

as you wish. Simply return your purchase to us, and please let us know why you were dissatisfied—it will help us to provide better products and services in the future. *Shipping and handling fees are non-refundable.*

VISA   MasterCard   AMERICAN EXPRESS Cards   DISCOVER NOVUS

Complete and mail with full payment to: Dragon Door Publications, 5 County Road B East, Suite 3, Little Canada, MN 55117

Please print clearly

Sold To: A

Name_____

Street _____

City _____

State _____ Zip _____

Day phone*_____
* Important for clarifying questions on orders

Please print clearly

SHIP TO: *(Street address for delivery)*   B

Name_____

Street _____

City _____

State _____ Zip _____

Email _____

Warning to foreign customers:
The Customs in your country may or may not tax or otherwise charge you an additional fee for goods you receive. Dragon Door Publications is charging you only for U.S. handling and international shipping. Dragon Door Publications is in no way responsible for any additional fees levied by Customs, the carrier or any other entity.

ITEM #	QTY.	ITEM DESCRIPTION	ITEM PRICE	A OR B	TOTAL

HANDLING AND SHIPPING CHARGES • NO COD'S
Total Amount of Order Add (Excludes kettlebells and kettlebell kits):

$00.00 to 29.99	**Add $6.00**	$100.00 to 129.99	**Add $14.00**
$30.00 to 49.99	**Add $7.00**	$130.00 to 169.99	**Add $16.00**
$50.00 to 69.99	**Add $8.00**	$170.00 to 199.99	**Add $18.00**
$70.00 to 99.99	**Add $11.00**	$200.00 to 299.99	**Add $20.00**
		$300.00 and up	**Add $24.00**

Canada and Mexico add $6.00 to US charges. All other countries, flat rate, double US Charges. See Kettlebell section for Kettlebell Shipping and handling charges.

Total of Goods	
Shipping Charges	
Rush Charges	
Kettlebell Shipping Charges	
OH residents add 6.5% sales tax	
MN residents add 6.5% sales tax	
TOTAL ENCLOSED	

METHOD OF PAYMENT ____CHECK ____M.O. ____MASTERCARD ____VISA ____DISCOVER ____AMEX

Account No. (Please indicate all the numbers on your credit card)   EXPIRATION DATE

☐☐☐☐ ☐☐☐☐ ☐☐☐☐ ☐☐☐☐   ☐☐/☐☐

Day Phone: ( )_____

Signature: _____ Date: _____

NOTE: *We ship best method available for your delivery address. Foreign orders are sent by air. Credit card or International M.O. only. For* **RUSH** *processing of your order, add an additional $10.00 per address. Available on money order & charge card orders only.*

Errors and omissions excepted. Prices subject to change without notice.

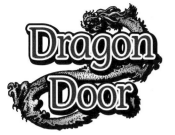

1·800·899·5111

24 HOURS A DAY • FAX YOUR ORDER (866) 280-7619

O R D E R I N G   I N F O R M A T I O N

   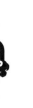

Telephone Orders For faster service you may place your orders by calling Ioll Free 24 hours a day, 7 days a week, 365 days per year. When you call, please have your credit card ready.

Customer Service Questions? Please call us between 9:00am– 11:00pm EST

Monday to Friday at 1-800-899-5111. Local and foreign customers call 513-346-4160 for orders and customer service

100% One-Year Risk-Free Guarantee. If you are not completely satisfied with any product—we'll be happy to give you a prompt exchange, credit, or refund,

as you wish. Simply return your purchase to us, and please let us know why you were dissatisfied—it will help us to provide better products and services in the future. *Shipping and handling fees are non-refundable.*

Complete and mail with full payment to: Dragon Door Publications, 5 County Road B East, Suite 3, Little Canada, MN 55117

Please print clearly

Sold To: A

Name_____

Street _____

City _____

State _____ Zip _____

Day phone*_____
* Important for clarifying questions on orders

Please print clearly

SHIP TO: *(Street address for delivery)*   B

Name_____

Street _____

City _____

State _____ Zip _____

Email _____

Warning to foreign customers:
The Customs in your country may or may not tax or otherwise charge you an additional fee for goods you receive. Dragon Door Publications is charging you only for U.S. handling and international shipping. Dragon Door Publications is in no way responsible for any additional fees levied by Customs, the carrier or any other entity.

Item #	Qty.	Item Description	Item Price	A or B	Total

HANDLING AND SHIPPING CHARGES • NO COD'S
Total Amount of Order Add (Excludes kettlebells and kettlebell kits):

$00.00 to 29.99	Add $6.00	$100.00 to 129.99	Add $14.00
$30.00 to 49.99	Add $7.00	$130.00 to 169.99	Add $16.00
$50.00 to 69.99	Add $8.00	$170.00 to 199.99	Add $18.00
$70.00 to 99.99	Add $11.00	$200.00 to 299.99	Add $20.00
		$300.00 and up	Add $24.00

Canada and Mexico add $6.00 to US charges. All other countries, flat rate, double US Charges. See Kettlebell section for Kettlebell Shipping and handling charges.

Total of Goods	
Shipping Charges	
Rush Charges	
Kettlebell Shipping Charges	
OH residents add 6.5% sales tax	
MN residents add 6.5% sales tax	
Total Enclosed	

METHOD OF PAYMENT ____Check ____M.O. ____Mastercard ____Visa ____Discover ____Amex

Account No. (Please indicate all the numbers on your credit card)   EXPIRATION DATE

☐☐☐☐ ☐☐☐☐ ☐☐☐☐ ☐☐☐☐   ☐☐/☐☐

Day Phone: (   )_____

Signature: _____ Date: _____

NOTE: *We ship best method available for your delivery address. Foreign orders are sent by air. Credit card or International M.O. only. For* **RUSH** *processing of your order, add an additional $10.00 per address. Available on money order & charge card orders only.*

Errors and omissions excepted. Prices subject to change without notice.